# Occupational Therapy Treatment Goals for the Physically and Cognitively Disabled

Claudia Kay Allen, MA, OTR, FAOTA

Catherine A. Earhart, OTR

Tina Blue, OTR

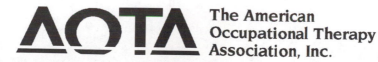

**AOTA** The American Occupational Therapy Association, Inc.

ISBN: 0-910317-72-0

PRINTED IN THE UNITED STATES OF AMERICA

# Table of Contents

*Dedicated to Mary Foto, OTR, FAOTA*

# Preface

Treatment goals are based on a prediction of how therapists can intervene to improve a patient's activity performance that has been impaired by a health problem. Improvement is determined by what the therapist knows and what the patient can and/or will learn to do. The hardest part of clinical practice is setting realistic treatment goals for patients who have learning difficulties. This book is designed to help therapists predict the rehabilitation potential for patients who have a cognitive disability. The book could also be used by fiscal intermediaries to make decisions about paying for rehabilitation services when a mental manifestation of a disease process is present. And finally the book can be used to do clinical research, with descriptive studies, comparison groups, and replications to examine treatment effectiveness.

The treatment goals suggested here are set in a paradigm that recognizes residual consequences of health problems. While the patient's medical condition is changing, goals are aimed at evaluating functional changes and explaining possible consequences. When the medical condition has stabilized, the therapist can work with patients and caregivers to reduce disabilities and handicaps. Reductions are made by teaching patients and caregivers how to circumvent residual impairments by safely using remaining abilities. Chapter 1 explains the value of rehabilitation services provided to people who have temporary and residual cognitive disabilities..

This text adds to a prior publication that addressed psychiatric diseases (Allen, 1985). With this publication, any diagnostic category that affects the mind (psychiatric or neurological) can be addressed by the cognitive levels. The 6 original cognitive levels have been expanded into 52 modes of performance in chapter 5. The longer scale is more sensitive to change within each cognitive level, and the transitions from one level to another can be described. The treatment goals suggested throughout the book address the 52 modes of performance. To avoid confusion, the original 6 cognitive levels have been retained, with a decimal system added to sequence the modes of performance.

When brain functioning is compromised, legal questions about patients' ability to manage their own affairs arise. The courts have the responsibility for deciding competency. Therapists are asked to describe observations of performance that become part of the database for legal decisions. Legal definitions represent socially agreed upon standards of performance. Chapter 2 contains definitions from American and English jurisprudence that are apt to have an impact on the social decisions made about providing assistance to the cognitively disabled. This chapter also raises questions about independence in doing functional activities and suggests further investigation of marginal ability to function independently. A brief description of the 6 cognitive levels that can be used to educate the general public about a cognitive disability is included in chapter 2.

Progress made in instrument development is reported in chapter 3. A new typology for the Routine Task Inventory (RTI) is described, and all of the activities are analyzed by the 6 original cognitive levels. Work that Theressa Burns has done in developing a standardized performance of activities from the RTI is presented. A larger version of the initial evaluation, the Allen Cognitive Level (ACL), test is presented by Kathy Kehrberg. Therapists will find all of the information needed to administer the tests in this chapter.

Rehabilitation potential is different during different phases of an illness. Acute, postacute, rehabilitation, and long-term care are defined. The expected outcomes and methods used to achieve those outcomes are suggested for these phases in chapter 4. Chapter 5 contains the model.

In chapter 6, processes required to complete many craft and work tasks are analyzed according to the 52 modes of performance. As of this writing it is not possible to do treatment effectiveness studies that can be substantiated by group replication. Group replication requires detailed descriptions of the treatment process. Chapter 6 aims at making it possible to examine the reliability and the validity of the treatment process, as prerequisites for examining treatment effectiveness.

Treatment goals that match the 52 modes of performance are presented in chapter 7. The RTI typology suggested in chapter 3 is used to categorize activities. Treatment goals for safe and effective performance are suggested, with goals that are aimed at the patient and the caregiver. Warnings for difficult-to-anticipate secondary effects are also included. Chapter 7 aims at mental impairments that have little or no localized effect on the motor system;

paralysis, paresis, and apraxia are not present to an appreciable degree. As of this writing the traditional split between neurology and psychiatry is still in place. The usual split is followed even though we expect to see overlap; this chapter simply reflects the realities of current practice.

A physical disability that is added to a cognitive disability is discussed by Tina Blue in chapter 8. An assumption is made that the reader has access to the physical disability literature commonly applied by therapists. It is further assumed that a new physical disability will require some new learning on the part of the patient and/or the caregiver. Guidelines for when and how to set treatment goals are offered. The chapter is organized according to personal care disabilities, body disposition disabilities, and dexterity and other physical disabilities.

When the physical disability stabilizes, the therapist directs treatment toward adaptive equipment. Tina Blue identifies the level of cognitive ability on the part of the patient required to learn the use of adaptive equipment safely and effectively. Equipment is analyzed according to the cognitive demand produced by these material objects and the type of cognitive compensation that the patient must make. The role of the caregiver is identified.

Case studies written by therapists working in a variety of treatment settings with various patient populations are presented in chapter 10. Case studies are used to illustrate the application of knowledge in a variety of age groups, diagnostic categories, socioeconomic conditions, and cultures.

Most of the book is devoted to helping therapists set treatment goals that maximize the patient's current ability to process information. The last chapter addresses the theoretical context that guides goal selection, treatment methods, and chapter formats. Some relationships with the social and health care sciences are identified along with needs for further research.

## Reference

Allen, C.K. (1985). *Occupational therapy for psychiatric diseases: Measurement and management of cognitive disabilities.* Boston: Little, Brown.

—*Claudia Kay Allen, MA, OTR, FAOTA*

# Chapter 1

# Professional Judgment

Claudia Kay Allen, MA, OTR, FAOTA

The knowledge presented in this book is different than the knowledge presented in many other occupational therapy and rehabilitation texts. The application of this knowledge is apt to place different demands on the therapist. This chapter identifies the differences, suggests guidelines to help apply the information, and recommends associated professional obligations.

The word *professional* refers to learned experts who are engaging in a vocation requiring knowledge. Judgment is based on that knowledge. The therapist forms opinions, estimates, or conclusions based on the circumstances presented by the patient as those circumstances relate to the therapist's knowledge. The quality of the therapist's knowledge is a major determinant of the responsibilities that the therapist is prepared to assume.

The worst case scenario occurs when therapists say "patients and others in the medical world don't understand what we do." The source of the difficulty can often be traced to ambiguities in the literature. "They don't understand" because the therapist cannot explain clearly. When a lot of therapists have trouble explaining, a deficiency in the literature can be identified.

Ambiguous knowledge uses language that is characterized by circumlocution and jargon and is usually hard to understand. Circumlocution is a roundabout or indirect way of saying something. Students are bewildered and confused by ambiguous knowledge. Faculty members explain that the author is using more words than necessary or words that are vague in meaning to explain an idea. Students may question the need to learn such information, and the real reason may be that this is all there

is to learn. Education, frames of reference, and theory building can, and have, acquired a bad reputation in these circumstances. The difficulty is in the ambiguity, not in the educational process or theory building as an academic exercise.

The knowledge presented in this text attempts to free therapists from ambiguity. Specific descriptions of behavior are given to make things as plain and obvious as possible. Ordinary language is used according to standard dictionary definitions to try to keep the ideas clear.

## Cautions and Warnings

An increase in the clarity of knowledge may be accompanied by an increase in the responsibilities that therapists are expected to assume. When general descriptions of dysfunction are used, a therapist can only imply that a problem exists. General descriptions are nonexclusive and widespread such as stress, poor self-concept, distorted body image, uncertainty, grief, deficiency of skills, role confusion, not accepted by peers. General descriptions tend to be either/or characteristics; the patient does or does not have deficiency. Many people have these problems and the need for and responsibility of the therapist are unclear. With general descriptions therapists can hint or suggest that something needs to be done, but they cannot be held accountable for such a statement.

Measures of improvement impose different degrees of accountability that seem to have a strong association with the length to the scale. The 6 cognitive levels, for example, allow therapists to caution people (Allen, 1985). Precautions advise people about possible harmful circumstances or conditions. Possibilities are likely to happen, other circumstances being equal. Precautions explain a need to be alert and prudent in hazardous situations. Therapists can use the 6 cognitive levels to identify hazardous situations and put people on their guard.

The 52 modes of performance presented in this text make it possible for therapists to warn people. Warnings speak plainly and usually in strong terms of possible harm or anything else unfavorable. A warning is more distinct and unmistakable than a caution. Warnings extend beyond harmful situations to include unfavorable or unwanted occurrences. The strength of the advice given by the therapist should be in proportion to the therapist's ability to predict. Predicting human behavior is more like forecasting the weather than foretelling what will happen in a science experiment. Therapists can use the modes of performance to say what is apt to happen, and to imply that there is a natural disposition for something to happen. Therapists should not use the modes of performance to imply precision in foretelling what will happen. There may be a natural disposition for the patient to forget to turn off the stove, but the therapist cannot say that an individual will forget to turn off the stove. The therapist has an obligation to warn people but cannot honestly say an unfavorable event will happen. Warnings place a greater responsibility on therapists and hold them accountable for giving authoritative and formal notice of easily understood events.

The modes of performance may also make therapists liable for fulfilling greater obligations to patients and their caregivers. All cautions and warnings must be documented in the patient's record. Because the list of warnings is lengthy, a special column was created for them in the chart in chapter 7. In practice, a checklist may be developed to ensure that these basic activities are covered. Advice should be given for those activities that are relevant to the individual and his or her circumstances. Documentation needs to include comments that apply to individuals in doing the basic activities and any other activities the person intends to do.

A greater involvement with families and other caregivers may emerge from the modes of performance. Several of the cases presented in chapter 10 contain innovative ways of reaching these people and may be examples of what could be done more often. Cautions and warnings give therapists the

unfavorable aspects of the disability, but the case studies point out the benefits of dealing with these difficulties in a candid manner. The modes of performance help people understand what it is exactly that they need to adjust to, making adjustment and planning clearer.

## Rehabilitation Potential

The patient's rehabilitation potential is a general prediction of possible benefits from services. The treatment goals in this book have been written as if there is a one-to-one correspondence between a mode of performance and treatment goal. That was done because it made reading and writing clearer, but this heuristic devise could be misleading in practice. The patient's rehabilitation potential is influenced by many factors: diagnosis, time since onset, compounding medical problems, finances, social support system. The mode of performance is expected to be a factor, and probably a heavily weighted factor, but not the only factor. Therapists are expected to be knowledgeable about other factors that need to be taken into consideration when setting long-term treatment goals. During the post-acute phase of an illness, the 6 cognitive levels may be about as precise as one can hope to be in predicting rehabilitation potential.

The modes of performance may be most helpful in identifying short-term treatment goals. The modes of performance identify what the patient can do now, with the condition as it is. By matching the complexity of the activity to the patient's current mode of performance, practicable short-term goals can be achieved.

The question is what should therapists do about possible changes in the patient's mode of performance. Therapists should look for a change on a regular basis. Therapists should probe for a higher mode by offering sensory cues from the next mode of performance. When the information is processed, change short-term goals to the next mode. When the information is rejected or causes frustration, continue with present short-term goals. When information from the present short-term goals causes frustration or confusion, rescue the patient by offering information from a lower mode. Change short-term goals to the lower mode. If no change in mode is detected, continue with practicable goals that match current mode.

If, for example, the current mode is 4.4, the

therapist would probe for 4.6 or higher. Short-term goals would be changed if success at a higher level is detected. Frustration or confusion with level 4.4 stimuli would suggest a lower mode. The therapist would rescue by offering 4.2 information. If that still caused difficulties the therapist would go to 4.0 information. The therapist should search for a higher mode and be alert to the possibility of going to a lower mode.

A mode of performance is assigned during a treatment session designed to evaluate the current mode. The frequency of evaluative sessions should be determined by the rate in which changes are expected and the importance of detecting small changes. The number given is the average performance observed during the session, usually lasting about an hour. Activities that have a lot of steps that differentiate between modes would be expected to provide the most valid evaluation. Assess improvement or deterioration from 1 day, week, month or year to the next by recording the average mode of performance in a specified time period.

The mode of performance can only be evaluated while the patient is doing an activity that is agreeable to the patient. The attempt to evaluate performance during any activity that the patient will agree to do is an ambitious undertaking for therapists. Considerable ingenuity in creating activities is frequently required. The analysis of processes in chapter 6 is provided to help therapists improve the reliability of their evaluations.

Motivation is not the only factor that can invalidate the therapist's evaluation. Training effects can be just as problematic. Any activity that the therapist has a patient do over and over again can produce a training effect. If people functioning at levels 3, 4, and 5 do an activity often enough their performance will improve. But improved performance in that activity will probably not predict performance in other activities or be an accurate measure of change. The most reliable evaluations need to eliminate training effects.

In some cases an exceptionally high or low step that is out of context with the rest of performance is observed. These exceptions are treated as artifacts and eliminated from the average score. There are numerous explanations for artifacts, and therapists should try to figure out which one applies to each artifact. The exceptions can have prognostic implications that are related to medication changes or the

natural course of the disease. A glimmer of a higher level with depression can, for example, suggest that this range of ability is still available to the patient. The medication may be accessing the ability. Conversely, a dip to a lower level may suggest that the patient is overmedicated or experiencing other biological changes. Artifacts can often be explained by the patient's education and work history. Closely related activities that have been done a lot in the past can improve performance in a step or an entire activity.

A screening tool, the Allen Cognitive Level (ACL) test, is available. The 1990 version is designed to correspond more closely with the modes of performance (S & S/Worldwide). A larger version is described in chapter 4. In practice, a therapist should administer the screening tool first and then observe performance in an activity. The activity should be set up to match the score on the ACL, with a potential to probe or rescue as needed.

Do an interview before trying to administer the ACL. Find out about the patient's education and work history, interests, spare-time activities, a recent typical day, and social support system. Therapists need this information, and rapport must be established before attempting a performance measure. Even then, some patients will refuse to try the ACL. Additional impairments can also make it impossible for some patients to do the ACL. When this happens, therapists have to make the best possible guess as to the patient's abilities and cognitive level. When patients cannot use their hands, as with spinal cord injuries or arthritis, the guess must be based on verbal performance. Computers, when available, may be helpful in making evaluations with patients who cannot use their hands.

When people can use their hands, the ACL can be used to screen out patients functioning at levels 1 and 2. If patients cannot grasp an object, then attempts to engage them in object manipulation can be avoided. No score on the ACL is given for levels 1 and 2.

When a score on the ACL is given, the score should be regarded as an initial evaluation that requires further evaluation. The ACL can be administered in a couple of minutes. Forecasting a mode of performance from such a short observation is bound to be inaccurate. The fact that it forecasts as well as it does for groups of people is amazing. Therapists should never base professional judgments about individual patients on the ACL alone.

## Professional Obligations for Change

Professional judgment about how hard to push a patient to function at a higher level of ability can be confusing. Guidelines for asking patients to process information from a mode of performance higher than the patient's current ability are as follows:

1. Do offer an opportunity to process information from the next mode for a brief period of time;

2. Do not force the patient to sustain functioning in any mode that causes confusion, frustration, or any other form of discomfort;

3. Do allow the patient to continue to struggle in a mode if that is his or her stated desire; do tell them that they are free to stop whenever they like; and

4. Do not allow your professional ego to get caught up in making the patient improve. Therapists are there to provide an opportunity for improvement to occur and to evaluate what happens. The "just right challenge" uses the patient's full capacity. Patient's have a natural tendency to use their full capacity when given the opportunity. Even when therapists give them things that are a little too easy, they have a tendency to make it a little more complicated on their own.

The motto "no pain, no gain" is not recommended for the cognitively disabled. Perseverance in asking patients to think above their current capacity can be so frustrating as to push people into a fight or flight response. While the patient may be blamed for being combative, the real cause of the behavior is the person who pushed the patient. This situation can be harmful and must be avoided.

Therapists can use their knowledge of the modes of performance to follow the patient's lead. The course of the disease may be improving, stabilizing, or deteriorating; it really does not alter the therapist's treatment methods. The therapist treats the cognitively disabled by recognizing current abilities and providing opportunities for those abilities to be used safely. The therapist's responsibilities do not end with treating the patient when residual disabilities exist. The therapist is obligated to teach others how to provide opportunities to use abilities and to warn the patient and others about harmful or unfavorable circumstances.

## Reference

Allen, C.K. (1985). *Occupational therapy for psychiatric diseases: Measurement and management of cognitive disabilities.* Boston: Little, Brown.

# Chapter 2

# Independence and Assistance in Doing Activities

## Claudia Kay Allen, MA, OTR, FAOTA

**D**efinitions of independence and a need for assistance are easily confounded by value judgments, cultural norms, historical conditions, and idiosyncrasies. Dealing with ordinary activities forces a consideration of different standards of performance; just how clean or dirty can the house be? Independence in doing functional activities occurs in a social context of what society will and will not permit that is operationally defined by the legal system.

In recent years the American legal system has taken a more active role in determining one's competency to manage one's own affairs. The change has affected therapists. Therapists are frequently asked to evaluate the need for a legal guardian or conservator when competency is in question. Other questions revolve around the need for power of attorney; child care versus foster care or removal of children from biological parents; living alone versus being sent to a nursing home or locked facility; referral to vocational services versus return to former employment or placement based on disability; or removal of a driver's license. Doing an evaluation that is fair to the patient and society is tough. This chapter seeks to clarify the current social expectations placed on ordinary American citizens judged to be independent in doing functional activities. To establish current social expectations as objectively as possible *Black's Law Dictionary* (1979) will be used. It is assumed that most readers will be providing services within the traditions of English and American jurisprudence. A different legal context would, of course, require a different set of social expectations. The need for assistance will be suggested by describing the behaviors associated with each of the cognitive levels.

A legal distinction is made between competency to manage one's own affairs and competency to stand trial. Competency to stand trial involves cooperating with one's attorney during a trial, a task that is not of concern here. Competency to stand trial has a long history of legal precedent but competency to manage one's own affairs is a relatively recent issue. A general recognition of different capacities to do these activities exists.

A free society allows for considerable freedom of choice in selecting an activity and determining the quality of performance. Individual differences are protected within a framework of social permission to be different. Society also puts some limits on the degree of individual differences that will be tolerated. The problem is: Where does one draw the line? Objective criteria are required, and legal decisions should be based on the best information available. For the following discussion jurisprudence is regarded as representing a summary of social science information. The information is applied to everyday life by a system of rules that govern the degree and type of individual difference that is permitted.

Cognitive level 6 represents a theoretical norm for independence in doing functional activities. The behavior pattern associated with this level is described and followed by a description of the sensorimotor information that is processed. The legal definitions are examined to see how the definition of level 6 corresponds with competency, reasonable conduct, negligence, eccentricity, health warnings, and mandates for social assistance. No presumption is made that the law represents a final definition of what is normal. The law is open to change as clearer understandings of reasonable expectations emerge. The advantage of jurisprudence is that the law can be oversimplified to give an overview of current social expectations to manage one's own affairs independently.

## Cognitive Level 6

Some specific behaviors that are often assumed to be a part of functional independence can be identified. Please note that the validity of these expectations has not been tested. There are, in fact, serious questions about the validity of these expectations for all citizens. The reason for outlining these expectations is a suspicion that many of us are practicing from a set of expectations that may be unfair to some patients because broader questions about educational bias and perhaps elitist biases can be directed to these legal standards. While far from perfect, the law represents the best attempts at current efforts to establish norms. The following description is offered in a spirit of supporting questioning and investigating of our assumptions about functional independence.

Functional mobility includes the capacity to read maps, follow signs and verbal directions, and remember routes previously traveled. Adjustments for physical limitations should be learned and precautions needed to prevent complications, such as falls or getting lost, should be comprehended. The effects that medications, abnormal anatomy, physiology, or endurance have on mobility should be anticipated and understood.

Functional communication abilities include the capacity to understand conversations and relate new information to planning and organizing future events. In an educated society the individual is expected to listen to speculations when verbally expressed and consider safety hazards. Communications go beyond one's own personal experience to consider the experiences/needs of others and to anticipate events that could have an impact on the lives of others. When reading, new information should be comprehended and applied to future actions. Writing can be done from an objective point of view, with an organized format, in a timely manner, and with consideration for the anticipated readership.

At home the individual can establish and follow a routine for maintaining food, clothing, shelter, and personal health. Plans for the future should be made including financial security, retirement, infrequent expenses, home maintenance, and seasonal changes. In the community the individual should adapt to such social changes as a push button telephone, answering machines, automatic tellers, credit cards, and the precautions printed on cleaning agents and grooming supplies.

At work or in social situations the individual should perform complex tasks by using speculations to plan activities, achieve precise results, avoid waste, and follow the most efficient and effective procedure. A schedule should be planned with adjustments in pace made as dictated by other perspectives, priorities, and time constraints. Verbal, written, and diagrammed instructions should be followed. Initiative in requesting clarifications, validation, or additional relevant information that may indirectly affect performance should be self-generated. Cooperation with other people through flexible fulfillment of roles to achieve overall function of the work, family, or social unit should be present. The individual should anticipate hazards, plan safety procedures, and understand the need to prioritize actions during an emergency.

The mental processes that are used to guide performance can be summarized as follows: Motor actions are premeditated by taking time to consider several possibilities and selecting the best course of action. The effects of planned motor actions are anticipated, and anticipation is used to prevent errors, accidents, injuries, or complications. Symbols, in the form of words, diagrams, and images are used to comprehend the meaning of the course of action in its entirety. Past experiences and prior knowledge are used to make judgments about the present situation, generalizing from prior experience. Current sensations and perceptions are selectively attended to. Attention is sustained for the time required to complete the intended course of action.

## Competence

Independence is a standard of performance that states that one can manage one's own affairs in a way that is self-sufficient or self-reliant. Within the legal context, competence is the right to manage one's own affairs. After the age of 18 years, adults are given the right to manage their own affairs unless a court of law determines that the mental capacity to exercise those rights is missing. The legal qualification for capacity is largely determined by cognitive ability. When reporting observations of behavior that might be used for legal purposes, therapists need to be aware of legal terminology and current legal standards.

Ability, capability, competence, and capacity are legal terms that are used interchangeably and applied to particular activities like making out a will, being a witness, voting, getting married, being responsible for a crime, or transacting ordinary business. The designated cognitive and physical abilities must match the requirements of the activity. Mental capacity or competence is defined in legal affairs by linking the activity to the cognitive demands of the activity. Mental capacity is the ability to understand the nature and effect of the act in which a person is engaged and the business he or she is transacting. Competence is a measure of intelligence, understanding, memory, and judgment relative to a particular transaction as will enable the person to understand the nature of his or her act.

Capacity is the ability to understand the nature and effects of one's acts. An incapacitated person is "anyone impaired by reason of mental illness, mental deficiency, physical illness or disability, advanced age, chronic use of drugs, chronic intoxication or other causes (except minority) to the extent that he/she lacks sufficient understanding or discretion to make or communicate responsible decisions concerning his/her person" (*Black's Law Dictionary*, 1979, pp. 684–685). Therapists should note that a physical disability, in and of itself, is not grounds for determining incapacity; understanding, discretion, or communication must be impaired. Ability, capability, competence, and capacity are legal terms used to connote the mental awareness of the ordinary citizen.

Most determinations of capacity focus on a mental understanding of the activity. Within the law of worker's compensation, earning capacity includes a rare consideration of physical ability. Earning capacity refers to "the capability of the worker to sell his/her labor or services in any market reasonably accessible, taking into consideration his/her general physical functional impairment resulting from accident, any previous disability, occupation, age at time of injury, nature of injury, and wages prior to and/or after injury" (*Black's Law Dictionary*, 1979, pp. 456–457). Earning capacity does not necessarily mean the actual earnings that one who suffers an injury was making at the time that the injuries were sustained. Earning capacity is based on training, experience, and possessed business acumen. Earning capacity incorporates physical ability into a cognitive framework. Testamentary and earning capacity place a priority on the cognitive understanding required to do the activity. Therapists should note the low priority placed on physical ability. The same low priority will be given to physical disability in the selection of treatment goals. The primary determinant of realistic treatment goals is the patient's cognitive ability.

The cognitive levels can be used as a part of the information used to determine a person's competency to manage his or her affairs. There is no set number for making the determination. Competency is linked to the activities that the individual intends to do. The social supports available to the individual may be taken into consideration.

## Reasonable Conduct

The law uses "ordinary" to identify baseline expectations for the average person. Care is a state of mind that expresses concern and attends to the needs of oneself or another. Ordinary care establishes the expectation that the average citizen has a duty to exercise concern in conduct toward others in circumstances in which injury may occur. Injury, in legal terminology, is broadly defined as any wrong or damage done to another, either to one's person, rights, reputation, or property. Injury is an invasion of any legally protected interest. This, of course, is a broader interpretation than the one used in medicine. I will use the broader definition throughout this chapter.

"Ordinary care is the degree of watchful attention that reasonably prudent persons exercise in the management of their own affairs to avoid injury to themselves or their property, or the persons or property of others" (*Black's Law Dictionary*, 1979, p. 193). Cognitive level 6 is meant to describe ordinary care.

A high degree of care is not the legal equivalent of ordinary care. A high degree of care is required in circumstances with a high risk of danger. A high degree of care is exercised by very cautious, careful, or prudent persons in risky situations. The assumption is made that the average person will be able to exercise a high degree of care when a potential for an accident or injury exists. Level 6 is also meant to describe a high degree of care; level 5 describes an inability to exercise either ordinary or a high degree of care.

A highest degree of care is not expected of ordinary citizens. The highest degree of care requires professional expertise. "The highest degree of care, or utmost care is the skill exacted by persons engaged in the same or similar business, when human safety is at stake" (*Black's Law Dictionary*, 1979, p. 193). Therapists are expected to exercise the highest degree of care exercised by all medical professionals. Health professionals share similar knowledge about preventing accidents, injuries, and medical complications that must be applied in practice in a very careful, skillful, and diligent manner. The highest degree of care is expected of medical professionals, but is not expected of the average citizen. Level 6 is not intended to include the highest degree of care.

Slight care is at the other end of the continuum and involves one's own affairs of slight importance. "Slight care may be exercised by persons of ordinary prudence or by persons of less than common prudence, who have a careless or inattentive disposition" (*Black's Law Dictionary*, 1979, p. 193). The law does make a distinction between circumstances that only merit slight care and circumstances that require ordinary care. If there is no risk of injury to self or others, slight care is acceptable. Levels 4 and 5 may be characterized by a slight degree of care, which worries therapists when warning patients about safety hazards.

Situations that require different degrees of care are taken into consideration in the activities analyzed for the cognitively disabled. The additions to the Routine Task Inventory (RTI) presented in chapter 3 divide reasonable conduct into out-of-the-ordinary events, following of safety precautions, and emergency conduct. Out-of-the-ordinary situations require slight care; safety precautions require ordinary care; and emergencies require a high degree of care. Therapists will certainly encounter situations that we have not thought of, and professional judgment will be required to warn patients and families about situations where reasonable conduct should not be assumed.

The amount of care demanded by the standard of reasonable conduct must be in proportion to the apparent risk. As the danger becomes greater, the actor is required to exercise greater caution commensurate with the risk. The amount of attention required is in proportion to the amount of danger in the present situation. This match between risk and care is similar to the match between ability and task demand proposed in the consequences model. What should be noted here is that the practice of rehabilitation proposed in this text corresponds to the legal view of risk and care.

## Negligence

The law of negligence describes actions that fail to conform with ordinary care. Negligence refers to the legal delinquency that results when a person fails to exhibit the care warranted by the circumstances, whether slight, ordinary, or high in degree. "Negligence is characterized by inadvertence, thoughtlessness, and inattention, or by the mistakes resulting from inexperience, excitement, or confusion" (*Black's Law Dictionary*, 1979, p. 931). The cognitively disabled do make mistakes because they do not process all of the information presented by the circumstances. Acts of negligence are predictable and protections from injury are required.

"Willful, wanton, reckless actions are intentionally done acts of an unreasonable character in disregard of a known risk that is highly probable" (*Black's Law Dictionary*, 1979, p. 932). Willful negligence usually implies a conscious indifference to the consequences with the implication that there is intent or a near willingness that the consequences occur. Willful actions are done without justifiable excuse. Here, the law makes a distinction between what the person will not do and what the person cannot do. Willful negligence assumes that the person knows what the consequences of his or her acts are; the cognitively disabled can only be held accountable for the effects that they understand. When the effects of these actions are not understood, the cognitively disabled should not be subject to the laws of negligence. Legal precedents need to be set to clarify this problem.

## Reasonable

The term *reasonable* provides a key to understanding another quality of thought that is expected of ordinary citizens. Reasonable is thinking, speaking, or acting according to the dictates of reason. In jurisprudence, reason is defined as "a faculty of the mind that distinguishes truth from falsehood, good from evil, and which enables the possessor to deduce inferences from facts or from propositions"

(*Black's Law Dictionary*, 1979, p. 1138). The expected quality of thought involves deductive reasoning and abstract thinking to interpret the nature of the action, the facts, and the circumstances surrounding the situation. Attention to the facts and circumstances surrounding a situation is a major feature in objectively evaluating the degrees of reasonable care that the person is able to exercise. Deductive reasoning and abstract thinking are not addressed by level 6, and are thought to be higher learning abilities.

Further clarification of what the law expects from the average person can be found in the cognitive demands for jury duty. A juror makes decisions based on reasonable doubt. Reasonable doubt that will justify acquittal is "doubt based on reason and arising from evidence or lack of evidence, and it is doubt that a reasonable person might entertain, and it is not fanciful doubt, is not imagined doubt, and is not doubt that a juror might conjure up to avoid performing an unpleasant task or duty" (*Black's Law Dictionary*, 1979, p. 1138). The reasonable inference rule states that the trier of facts may consider as evidence not only the testimony and real evidence presented at the trial but also "all inferences which may be reasonably drawn, though they are not necessary inferences" (*Black's Law Dictionary*, 1979, p. 1138). Juries are expected to make decisions after duly considering propositions, theories, hypotheses, probability, and/or the moral certainty of truth. Jury duty requires deductive reasoning about inferred circumstances described to the jury. Once again this quality of thought is regarded as beyond the limits of level 6.

Law enforcement officials are guided by the definition of ordinary/reasonable when making arrests, taking people into custody, or exercising force within the definitions of reasonable and probable cause, reasonable belief, reasonable force, reasonable suspicions, and reasonable grounds. Decisions based on facts, circumstances, and the credibility of informants must be made within a range of suspicion before a course of action can be taken. The law enforcement officials' decisions are reviewed to be sure that they are not immoderate or excessive. Decisions judged to be fair and suitable, then, are based on the officer's knowledge of the facts and given circumstances and the officer's interpretation of that information. Once again the social standard for ordinary thought involves an interpretation of the present situation. Some of this information is

covered by level 6, but assessing credibility within a range of suspicion would require processing additional information.

Two other legal terms can be used to clarify the expected cognitive ability of the average citizen: *prudent* and *diligent*. To be a prudent, a person must have or show acute mental discernment with a keen practical sense to determine a line of conduct. Functionally, the person is circumspect in adapting the means to achieve an end. The quality of thought associated with prudent actions is wise, judicious, careful, discreet, circumspect, and sensible. Diligence describes the duration and intensity of attention directed toward vigilant activity. Terms associated with attentive and persistent activity include steadily applied, active, sedulous, laborious, unremitting, and untiring. Prudent actions are planned and require deductive reasoning to select, from several options, the best course of action. Diligent actions are sustained for the period of time required to complete the planned course of action.

Reasonable, prudent, and diligent seem like very high expectations when looked at from the perspective of the cognitively disabled. A broad gap seems to exist between the minimum level of care that one needs to be able to exercise to live safely in the community and the legal view of reasonable. Some people live at home alone at level 4. A reliance on old models and new associations (level 4) produces inflexible behavior, making it difficult to exercise slight care in out-of-the-ordinary situations. A reliance on new associations and the formation of new models (level 5) neglects secondary effects, making it difficult to consider risks that are highly probable. Speculative sensorimotor models are added at level 6 and are a part of ordinary care. Many of the patterns of thought required to be reasonable and avoid negligence are beyond level 6. I wonder if these higher levels of ability are available to the average person.

## Eccentricity

English and American jurisprudence take great care to exclude eccentricity and personal idiosyncrasies from rulings on mental capacity. A free society, by definition, permits eccentric and idiosyncratic behavior. Of particular interest to rehabilitation therapists are some exclusions from the determinations of insanity. Uncleanliness, slovenliness, neglect of person and clothing, and offensive and disgusting habits do not, in and of themselves, constitute unsoundness of mind. One can still be judged to be capable of managing oneself and one's own affairs when these behaviors are present. Being dirty and disgusting is perfectly okay when questions about competency are raised. These behaviors are frequently indicators that a medical problem exists, but that is not always so. These behaviors, in and of themselves, cannot be used to determine competency.

A positive legal description of the competency to do two activities is fairly well-defined: to make out a will and to earn a living. Testamentary capacity to make out a will is "that measure of mental ability which is recognized in law as sufficient mind and memory to intelligently understand the nature of business in which one is engaged, to comprehend generally the nature and extent of the property which constitutes one's estate, and which one intends to dispose of, and to recollect the objects of one's bounty" (*Black's Law Dictionary*, 1979, p. 1322). A person is said to meet the necessary qualifications "when he/she understands: the nature and extent of one's property; one's relationship to the people named in the will and to any people disinherited; what a will is; and the transaction of simple business affairs" (*Black's Law Dictionary*, 1979, p. 1322). Insane delusions, eccentricity, personal idiosyncrasy, and mania that cannot reasonably be expected to affect disposition do not affect testamentary capacity. The implication of this ruling is that symptoms of a mental disorder do not incapacitate a person unless the symptoms interfere with the activity in question. Symptoms alone are also insufficient evidence for rulings on capacity.

Evaluating ability to do an activity is complicated in a free society. A failure to do an activity may be explained by a lack of ability, a lack of motivation, or idiosyncratic preferences. A free society honors all of these explanations. A failure to get dressed properly can, for example, be attributed to all three explanations. Motivation seems to be the explanation that comes to mind first. Maybe the individual does not want to dress properly. Ability cannot be evaluated when a person refuses to do a functional activity; all one can say is that the person refuses to accept the standards of functional performance. Carl, for example, refuses to dress properly by wearing a hospital nightgown that opens in the back while walking down a crowded corridor. Carl's ability to dress properly cannot be evaluated from this example of behavior. To evaluate ability to function one must have the necessary material objects and a stated desire to use them properly. Carl must have a bathrobe and agree to put it on in the customary manner. With cognitively disabled people this agreement is essential. Without agreement the assessment of disability is vulnerable to motivational questions. Efforts to be fair and objective in evaluating ability are frequently tangled up in disagreements about the patient's, as well as the families' motivation. Sometimes a lack of motivation is unjustly ascribed to a lack of ability, or vice versa.

The spirit of a free society allows for the expression of idiosyncratic and eccentric behavior. Deviation from the norm may be an expression of personal freedom. Carl may enjoy the stir he creates by exposing himself in the hospital corridor. Some deviations from the norm can be accepted as a part of functional independence. There are some values that health care professionals often share, but they are not always shared by patients. A free society can tolerate a wide range of out-of-the-ordinary behavior involving slight care. As long as no injury is done to self or others, unusual behavior is accepted and legally protected.

## Health Warnings

What one does to preserve one's health is also largely a matter of personal choice. Health care professionals give patients advice and issue warnings about health hazards. Our responsibility is to provide the information. What the patient does with the information is a matter of choice. Those rules seem simple enough until one considers a cognitive disability. What are the health care provider's obligations when a patient does not process information very well? As of this writing, many patients' rights advocates ignore the information-processing difficulties of psychiatric patients and argue for a full range of choice. The choices include consent to treatment, refusal of treatment, consent to participate in research, agreements to give up property, the right to be homeless, and the right to risk health complications and reduced life expectancy. The trouble is that their choices are seldom made with ordinary care. The cognitive levels attempt to operationally define the degree of care that the cognitively disabled person can exercise in a risky situation. I see this as a continuation of the traditional occupational therapy mission: To promote the use of as much ability, choice, and individual differences as possible, while protecting patients from harm.

From a cognitive standpoint it is interesting to note that the law of evidence does make a distinction between competency and credibility. Competency denotes the personal qualification of the witness and is determined by the court before evidence is given. Credibility is the veracity of the testimony and is determined by the jury after the testimony is given. Currently the distinction between competency and credibility is not made in the law of insanity. A clearer distinction would be beneficial to insanity decisions. Competency to understand the situation should be established before listening to the credibility of the patient's consent or refusal.

## Social Assistance with Activities

The determination of the amount of social assistance that a society is required to provide for a person who is unable to manage his or her own affairs is also addressed by the law. In seeking to define affairs, the law also provides lists of activities. The activities are listed under maintenance and supportive care. Maintenance is the minimum assistance that an individual is legally bound to provide for another person. Maintenance is frequently used when there is a legal relationship between people that states that one person is bound to financially support the other, such as father and child or husband and wife. Food, clothing, and shelter are the primary inclusions but such items as "reasonable and necessary transportation or automobile expenses, medical and drug expenses, utilities and household expenses" (*Black's Law Dictionary*, 1979, p. 859) are also included. Maintenance includes self-care and community living tasks, with a primary emphasis on self-care.

The term "support" contains a broader sense that would enable one to live in a degree of comfort suitable and becoming to a station in life. Support provides assistance for anything "requisite to housing, feeding, clothing, health, proper recreation, vacation, travel expenses or other proper cognate purposes; also proper care, nursing and medical attendance in sickness, and suitable burial at death" (*Black's Law Dictionary*, 1979, p. 1291). Supportive assistance considers the quality of life of the exceptional person with special advantages, usually wealth.

These definitions suggest that the social welfare system may be held responsible for providing assistance with maintenance activities, but not with supportive activities.

Supportive care activities extend beyond legal necessities to include concerns about the quality of life. Recreational activities, religious practices, cultural pleasures, and community events are included. The selection of supportive care activities is influenced by an individual's values and cultural background. The range of opportunities to engage in supportive care activities is largely determined by one's financial status. Therapists aim at maximizing supportive care activities when the opportunity and desire are available. The contents of this book will place an emphasis on self-care and maintenance activities, which are apt to be the priority for most patients.

Public health and social welfare policies are substitutes for family obligations for maintenance care. Private health insurance policies also tend to cover maintenance activities. As a rule the broader definition of activities pertains to those who are fortunate enough to have personal and/or familial resources. To translate those definitions into practice, treatment goals that aim at improving recreation, vacation, and travel activities will probably have to be paid for privately. Private pay patients may request assistance with a wide range of activities that are tailored to their unique circumstances. Health insurance policies are apt to regard maintenance activities as reasonable and necessary. In most cases therapists can honor requests for services that improve the following maintenance activities: bathing, grooming, dressing, toileting, eating, walking, exercising, taking medication/vitamins, housekeeping, doing laundry, obtaining and preparing food, traveling routinely, shopping, budgeting paying bills (rent, utilities, medical), and caring for others (children, parents, spouse).

Independence in doing functional activities requires the ability to manage one's own affairs. Maintenance activities identify the minimum tasks that one should be able to manage. Most of these activities are listed under self-awareness and situational awareness disabilities in chapter 4. The need for assistance with occupational role and social role disabilities are less clearly established within the law. Documentation of objective criteria for the need for assistance may be a contribution that needs to be made by rehabilitation therapists.

Jurisprudence lacks specificity about the quality of performance expected while doing maintenance activities. Caregivers charged with providing assistance to people with a cognitive disability need more specificity to protect individual differences while fulfilling social obligations.

The recent passage of the Americans with Disabilities Act (ADA, 1990) is apt to place different legal demands on therapists. ADA extends civil rights protections to the disabled in five areas: employment, public accommodations, transportation, state and local government services, and telecommunications. The list reflects awareness of physical disabilities, but cognitive disabilities can be included. A major difficulty in promoting the integration of the cognitively disabled is that the disability is invisible. The difficulty is frequently compounded at level 4 because these people rarely recognize their disability. People whose maximum ability is level 4 may be incorporated into the work force with the help of therapists. To achieve that goal therapists will probably need to do a lot of education to help other people understand what to expect. The six cognitive levels seem to provide an adequate understanding for many people.

## Assistance in Doing Functional Activities

Assistance is required when a person is incapacitated and cannot do ordinary activities safely. As of this writing the lay public and many health care professionals do not understand the assistance needed by the cognitively disabled. Educating other caregivers and the public becomes an important part of a therapist's job.

There are two descriptions of the cognitive levels in this book. The general description provided in this chapter gives a basic understanding of the levels that are often used for general education purposes. The levels are associated with the confinements of the medical condition, as limits on behavior. Limitations describe the negative consequences of medical conditions. Remaining abilities are described by the information that can be processed during activity performance. These descriptions correspond with prior publications (Allen, 1982; 1985; 1988; Allen & Allen, 1987).

## Level 1: Automatic Actions

People are often in a hospital bed with side rails up to keep them from falling (level 1). Unless agitated or in pain, they tend to lie still and stare into space. Moaning or crying in response to pain may be heard. A few responses to external stimuli can be elicited.

Withdrawal from a noxious stimuli is the first response seen when coming out of a coma. Turning the head to locate a stimulus follows. Head turning may be associated with chewing and swallowing and a soft diet can be tried. Pureed foods, and not liquids, come first to prevent the risk of choking. People may need to be fed, or people may eat soft food with their fingers or drink out of a cup when it is placed in their hand.

Any activity that is done sitting up is apt to be a problem because these patients do not hold their bodies up against gravity. They tend to slide down and out of whatever they are sitting in: bed, chair, wheelchair, or bathtub. Various positioning devices are available to hold them in place. Bathing, grooming, and dressing require a tremendous amount of nursing care. Some variability in the amount of cooperation that can be elicited can be detected. For a few seconds the person may hold still, hold an extremity up, roll over. Little cooperation with toileting should be expected. The patient may have no awareness of the need to void, but the caregiver may be able to schedule the time for a bowel movement.

Walking, which was included in the original description of level 1, has been moved to level 2 (Allen, 1985). Therapists working with traumatic brain injury have been helpful in refining the descriptions of levels 1 and 2.

Information processing is very slow and the therapist may need to wait several minutes to get a response from a cue. Each response to a cue will probably last for a moment or two. With continuous cuing some people can continue to cooperate for a few minutes, which can be long enough to greatly reduce the burden of care.

To establish patterns of movement the therapist observes movements of the head and torso that are adjusted in a simple stimulus and response manner. These movements are not timed. Speech is limited to nonverbal responses like screaming and crying. Pain is resisted.

Motor responses may be accompanied by changes in the autonomic nervous system. Some retrieval of stored sensorimotor models may occur and are most apt to relate to the instinctive need to eat and drink. Level 1 is a system that is barely open to external stimuli. Change in the level of arousal occurs when stimuli are related to an instinctive need for survival. The distinction between levels 1 and 2 is that motor responses are elicited by another person or pain at level 1. Motor actions are self-initiated at level 2.

## Level 2: Postural Actions

The first self-initiated motor action is to stay sitting in an upright position, which requires pushing the body up against gravity to keep from sliding down in one's seat. Be careful when these people sit down, because they are not apt to look to see if the chair is there. Grooming, dressing, and bathing still require a lot of nursing care and may be easier when the patient is sitting down. Even though they can stand, some people actively resist standing in a shower and sitting on a stool in the bathtub. A specially designed chair that fits over the bathtub may be more acceptable to them. Most of dressing must be done for the patient while sitting down.

Some support for sitting/standing balance while pulling pants up may be needed. The patient is aware of the caregiver's help, and spontaneous movements of the extremities while grooming, dressing, and bathing may occur, like pointing a hand toward the top of the sleeve. The rest, like inserting the hand, pulling the sleeve up over the arm, and moving the garment around the back, must be done by the caregiver.

If there is no damage to the motor cortex, people functioning at level 2 are apt to be up and walking around, very slowly. Some awareness of the external environment is noted when they walk through doorways and around large pieces of furniture, but they usually do not know where they are going. They may say they are going to the bathroom without knowing where the bathroom is. With guidance and enough time they may be able to walk there. Some awareness of the need to void and hold it can be expected, along with some accidents. A slow walk to other locations, like the dinner table or outside, may feel like a fine accomplishment to them.

Eating may be accomplished by sitting at the table and using a spoon or a cup. Eating is as slow as walking, and they may need frequent reminders to keep eating until they finish. Eating is also apt to be messy, and ways of controlling the damage are

needed. There are a few people who eat nonedible objects who are usually functioning at level 2. They are apt to swallow anything that they find in front of them.

The therapist observes patterns of movement in the torso that are spontaneous adjustments to overcome the effects of gravity. Movement patterns in the upper and lower extremities may be self-initiated and seem to be done because they feel good and are not timed. Speech may contain verbal and nonverbal yes/no responses as well as single words, such as own name, bed, or bathroom.

Instinctive sensory associations to the effects of gravity are formed. Stored sensorimotor models for walking and doing other gross motor actions are retrieved. The information processed is related to moving body parts or holding still. The system is open to information that restricts movement such as doors, stairs, furniture, and binding clothing. The patient may grab onto things for stability, but this is not reliable. The sociocultural context is not processed, and these people are apt to wander off and get lost, engage in bizarre gestures, or tug on clothing. The distinction between levels 2 and 3 is that grasp is limited to achieving postural stability at level 2.

## Level 3: Manual Actions

People use their hands to grasp and move objects at level 3. The stimulus is provided by placing an object in front of them and telling them what to do or demonstrating the required motion. Soap and wash cloth, toothbrush, hairbrush, food, and clothing can be placed in front of them, and they will do some of the necessary actions. The quality of performance is unreliable because they do not sequence themselves through the customary steps to complete the task.

When bathing they may get in and out of the bath or shower without assistance and use bathing articles. They may require assistance to adjust water temperature, to apply bathing articles to all body surfaces and rinse, to scrub hard enough to remove soil, to avoid too much pressure to delicate areas, and to dry all body surfaces. To make sure all of these are done, someone must be with them while they bathe.

A similar pattern is seen in dressing. They can put on basic garments, including shirt, pants, skirt, underwear, and shoes and socks. Someone will probably have to tell them to get dressed, select the clothes, and lay them out for them. The way they put their clothes on may reflect their not paying attention to the effect of what they are doing. They put things on inside out, backward, out of sequence with underwear on top, or shoes on the wrong feet. Whatever they are doing they may stop before they are done and require constant cueing to finish.

Eating, with all the lower levels, is usually the activity that is done best of all. At level 3 they often sit down at the table and eat their food without constant cueing (level 4). Eating seems to be hard wired into the brain and is the activity that is least apt to be equivalent to the pattern of performance seen in doing other activities. At level 3 they may request help with cutting their meat. According to the activity analysis criteria requests for help should occur at level 4. Clinical experience suggests that this is not true. The RTI2 has been changed to reflect clinical experience with eating.

Toileting is more consistent with the activity analysis criteria. They will go to the toilet, lower their garments, sit down and void, but they may get stuck there. Cueing to use toilet paper and get up off the toilet may be required. Reminders to wash hands, zip zippers, and tuck in shirttails are usually needed.

Walking can be the biggest problem, because they are apt to wander about aimlessly and get lost. In an unprotected environment they are apt to pick up and use anything they happen to find in their wanderings. What they will do with objects is unpredictable, and often amusing. Care needs to be taken to "disability proof" their living environment to remove hazards. Outside of the living environment an escort is needed.

Some participation in household activities can be elicited by placing the customary object in front of them and directing them to wipe a surface, peel a vegetable, fold the linen, or do some other repetitive motion. Household activities tend to be elective at level 3 because the quality of performance may be incomplete or done very slowly, making little real contribution to household chores. The real purpose may be to give the disabled person something to do. If so, other activities involving crafts, music, or walking may be preferred. A special effort has to be made to get people at level 3 to do anything. Without that effort they often sit and do nothing, stare at the television, or wander aimlessly.

The therapist observes movements of the hands to grasp and move objects located right in front of the person. The sensory association is for an external object that can be picked up and moved. The sensorimotor model retrieved is for a manual action, usually an action that is repeated over and over again. The effects that manual actions have on material objects may not be noticed or checked unless they grab something that hurts. Speech is usually confused, but a few objects and actions can be named.

Tool use, the use of an external object to do an action to one's self or to an external object, occurs at level 3. The instinctive use of the hands to pick up and apply objects that are found by chance is present. The information that is processed is for the action, not the sequence of actions. The sociocultural context may be supplied by the artifacts, like a toothbrush that is laid out by another person. These artifacts may be recognized and used but not preserved for later use. The object is put down without consideration of a need to clean it or put it away.

The distinction between levels 3 and 4 is that the completion of the goal is only recognized after the task is "done" at level 3. During the process of doing the task, someone else must sequence the person through the necessary steps. The sense of completion is internal and may not correspond with social standards for getting the job done.

## Level 4: Goal-Directed Actions

Having a goal in mind makes a big difference at level 4 because these people can sequence themselves through the steps of the activity to get the job done. Most of their self-care activities can be done independently with small errors of no real concern. They may look a little odd, but that can be tolerated. Taking medication can be a major self-awareness problem when they get confused about what the medicine does and does not do for them. Refusing to take medications or not recognizing and reporting adverse reactions are common concerns with people functioning at level 4.

The disability becomes more apparent in the performance of household activities. The house may get messy and dirty and the laundry may not be done very often. Their diet may be restricted to a few simple things that require little or no preparation. Spending money is apt to a vulnerable activity. A daily allowance for daily purchases is the safest way to manage their money. Cash and checks are apt to get lost or stolen. Bills are not paid with ease; they tend to neglect them or worry about them a lot. A budget may have little meaning to them.

Many people manage to get by living alone in the community at level 4. They generally follow a routine for doing household activities in a way that avoids ordinary hazards. When something different happens that does not match their usual way of doing things, the disability is a concern. They will notice changes that are clearly visible and request help. The person who is asked to help may be contacted with such frequency as to regard the disabled person as a burden or a nuisance. Their requests for help often involve trivial matters of no real threat to them or anyone else. The concern is that many real threats are unnoticed, and one worries about their blundering into an accident or injury. Frequent on-site checks to identify and remove hazardous materials and tools is a good safety precaution.

The poor quality of performance that one can get by with at home is not well-accepted in the community. People of working age are not able to hold jobs unless special circumstances are created for them. When special circumstances are created they may be dedicated to the job and compliant with job routines once the routines are learned. They may not get to spare time activities unless someone reminds them to go and organizes the activity for them.

Social roles are usually strained. The only meaning that may be communicated is a demand for help, often made by interrupting others. Directions on how to adjust to unusual situations have to be demonstrated, one step at a time. Verbal directions given over the telephone or left on a list of things to do usually confuse them or are ignored. Teaching them to learn to do anything new may take months of repetition before they learn it. If they have a physical disability, learning to use a piece of adaptive equipment can be tedious.

They may be given simple tasks to keep them participating in family activities, when the family organizes the task for them. They can do routine tasks for dependents but cannot solve problems for them. Other social contacts are often arranged for them. Conversations are apt to be limited to short answers to questions or telling the same story over and over. They are poorly informed about current events and have little to add to the conversation.

Therapists may need to initiate the movements required to get the necessary objects for patients to do a specific task. The effects of actions are noticed and adjusted to match a memory of the usual outcome of an activity or to match a sample of a project. Movements go through a self-directed sequence of steps to get the task done. These movements are timed, usually wanting to get the task done within an hour, or at least today. While these patients are quiet most of the time, they do request needed objects or ask for assistance to correct mistakes.

The sensory associations formed are for the striking features of material objects. Striking features include linear direction, color, shape, and number up to four. The sensorimotor models retrieved are memories of how to do routine activities or simple steps of activities. The effects that motor actions have on material objects are checked, and mistakes that fail to match a memory of how the objects should be are noticed. Mistakes that fail to match a physical sample of a craft project are also noted. Flexibility in departing from the memory or the sample may not be present, especially if motivation is high.

Habit patterns to do routine activities with very little thought are used, but at level 4 executing habit patterns takes a lot more effort. There is a tenacious reliance on stored sensorimotor models. The information that is processed is how to do an activity. An awareness of sociocultural standards of performance is present, and an effort is usually made to comply with those standards. Cultural understanding is concrete and usually related to the immediate choice or experience of an activity. Conceptualization, abstraction, and logical thinking are impaired, but can be misleading when people have a vocabulary that incorporates abstract terms.

The distinction between levels 4 and 5 is that learning is limited to rote learning at level 4. Rote learning is memorizing the steps to do a new activity without flexibility to understand, verify, or change the steps.

## Level 5: Exploratory Actions

Flexibility to change the steps is present at level 5. The first changes are continuous adjustments in neuromuscular effects, like variations in pressure and strength. Learning by doing occurs through the process of trial and error.

Self-care is intact at level 5 and most of these activities are done without difficulty: grooming, dressing, bathing, feeding, and toileting. Once again, taking medications can be a problem, but at level 5 it is because they do not understand medical concepts, like side-effects or temporary discomforts.

Household activities are done better than at level 4. Housekeeping is improved because they notice and remove less striking dirt like cobwebs, crumbs, hair, and fingerprints. They also adjust the amount of pressure used when they scrub so that stubborn stains are apt to be removed. The laundry is done more often because more of the dirt is seen. Clothes are separated by color for washing and for dry cleaning. Hot meals are prepared, and variation in the diet exists. Shopping, spending money, and talking on the telephone too long are the activities that are apt to cause problems. Over-extended credit, purchases of luxuries, or underspending that causes undue hardship may occur.

A failure to anticipate events produces many minor annoyances at level 5. They "forget" to do things ahead of time: get a prescription refilled, buy stamps, take clothes to the cleaners, buy birthday cards, make a grocery list and take it with them, preheat the oven, note the time when the parking meter will expire or the roast will be cooked.

Participation in major role activities in the community can be done with supervision. Watches, calendars, clocks, and appointment books may be used to follow a schedule. A self-centered focus on personal schedule and preferences is apt to guide major role and spare-time activities. Supervision is required to plan a schedule of activities, consider secondary effects that one's activities might have on others, and make sure that obligations are met on time. Spare-time activities that follow a regular schedule, or are done on the spur of the moment, are apt to be more successful than those that require planning ahead.

The phrase "an accident waiting to happen" may have been invented to describe people functioning at level 5. They can learn a safety procedure but following it consistently is a problem. They may act impulsively without considering the consequences. Learning is focused on immediate effects of actions, and secondary effects are not anticipated. These people should be warned to avoid activities of high risk for serious accidents or injury. Short cuts may be taken without considering the repercussions. When an emergency does arise, they are apt to have difficulties with selecting priorities, considering secondary effects, and coordinating their efforts with others. A failure to coordinate their efforts with others is the crux of their social role disability. The meaning they communicate is personal, without

considering the point of view of others. They may not place the interests of family members above their own or engage in give and take gracefully. Other people are often alienated by a failure to cooperate, collaborate, or consider the rights of others. If they supervise others, they are often bossy bosses. As citizens, they are apt to have a personal view of current events.

Therapists observe changes in the neuromuscular effects that the individual makes on material objects. Neuromuscular changes produce a different effect on the tangible properties of objects that can be detected by one of the five senses. Trial and error occurs as changes in actions, tools, and sequences are explored. Personal preferences guide the selection of the desired effect. Talking and working at the same time may be observed.

Sensory associations are formed for the subtle cues of material objects. Subtle cues include the surface and spatial properties of an object. The effects of motor actions are noted and changed to discover new sensorimotor models. New sensorimotor models are stored and can be retrieved for later use, which is learning by doing.

Fine-motor coordination and dexterity require concentrated effort at level 5. An instinctive interest in variability, exploration, discovery, and play opens the system up to inventing new courses of action. All of the physical features of the external environment can be explored. Personal values and choices may be regarded as more important than social or cultural standards of performance. A hedonistic quality of living for the personal pleasures of the moment may be evident. The difference between levels five and six is that planning a future course of action and understanding secondary effects must occur in the presence of objects at level 5.

## Level 6: Planned Actions

Anticipating secondary effects and planning in the absence of material objects occurs at level 6. Therapists observe for pauses to stop and think before acting at level 6. Persistence in solving the problems that do occur is expected, but many mistakes are predicted and therefore avoided. Mistakes are corrected within the context of the social situation as it relates to the specific activity being done. Individual priorities in accepting or correcting mistakes are expressed.

Speech includes a discussion of several courses

of action and a projection of what might happen. Images, words, and other symbols can be used in place of sensory associations. Several sensorimotor models for courses of action can be retrieved and used to form a new course of action. Sensorimotor models, new and old, can be compared and judged to select the best course of action.

Fine-motor coordination and dexterity are executed with ease while talking, listening, or thinking about something else. At level 6 the system is open to all of the social, cultural, and historical information available to the person, to be processed as the individual pleases.

## References

Allen, C.K. (1988). Cognitive disabilities. In S. Robinson (Ed.), *Focus*. Rockville, MD: American Occupational Therapy Association.

Allen, C.K. (1985). *Occupational therapy for psychiatric diseases: Measurement and management of cognitive disabilities.* Boston: Little, Brown.

Allen, C.K. (1982). Independence through activity: The practice of occupational therapy (psychiatry). *American Journal of Occupational Therapy, 36,* 731–739.

Allen, C.K., & Allen, R.E. (1987). Cognitive disabilities: Measuring the social consequences of mental disorders. *Journal of Clinical Psychiatry, 48,* 185–191.

*Americans with Disabilities Act of 1990,* Public Law 101-336, July 26, 1990.

*Black's Law Dictionary* (5th ed.) (1979). St. Paul, MN: Western Publishing.

# Chapter 3

# Reporting Occupational Therapy Services

## Claudia Kay Allen, MA, OTR, FAOTA

The 1990s contain an opportunity for occupational therapy to get back on the track of being concerned with functional outcomes that make a real difference in the way people live. While we have always claimed that improved function was the essence of our services, the 1970s and 1980s forced practice into measurable treatment objectives. Function is hard to measure. Occupational therapists had to resort to measuring symptoms and impairments. Finally we have figured out a way to measure function when the ability to function is restricted by brain pathology. Now we can stop depending on measures of symptoms and impairments and by primarily concerned with the way people live.

The shift to functional outcomes is apt to have a big affect on the way therapists report the services they provide. A legitimate concern for the affect this is apt to have on the people who pay for occupational therapy services needs to be addressed. This chapter discusses function from the perspective of the insurance industry that pays for most services in the United States. As of this writing, the insurance industry is very supportive of a shift toward functional outcomes.

As defined by Blue Cross of California, a functional outcome must be:

- Meaningful;
- Utilitarian; and
- Sustainable over time.

A "meaningful" outcome is an ability to do an activity that is valued by the patient and/or the caregiver so that the patient is able to function safely at home (or wherever the patient resides) or in major and spare-time roles. A "utilitarian" outcome is the most economical, effective, and efficient means of doing the activity within the safety constraints of the individual's living situation and social roles. A "sustainable" outcome is one that can be maintained by the patient outside of the clinical environment over a period of time.

A functional outcome must be established for individuals. There is no predetermined list of activities that can be applied to all patients. You will need to find out what activities are relevant to the individual and his or her social support system. You will also need to think about the patient's medical condition and predict the affects that the course of the disease are apt to have on the functional outcome. And you will need to predict how long it is going to take and how much it will cost to produce that outcome. The clinical reasoning required to select and predict functional outcomes for the cognitively disabled can get very complicated.

*Medical necessity* and *skilled services* are insurance industry terms for defining who needs care and the quality of care required. Definitions of these terms are used to establish referral and discharge criteria that establish the range of services covered by insurance.

Medical necessity occurs when there is a reasonable expectation that significant improvement in the patient's overall safety or functional ability will occur. In general, medical necessity reduces the consequences of illness or injury. Prevention of highly likely complications is also included. As of this writing the medical necessity for maintaining the remaining abilities of the disabled is not usually covered by insurance policies or Medicare.

The need for skilled services establishes the difference between therapists, trained aides, and the average person. If activities can be done safely and effectively with the assistance of a nonskilled caregiver, therapy services are not needed. Skill is the knowledge that the therapist has to prevent complications, maximize remaining functional abilities, protect the patient's safety, and engage in activities. An understanding of disease processes must be combined with an ability to analyze activities to fulfill these goals.

Establishing medical necessity and the need for skilled services are the common ways of justifying the value of services. The quality of a therapist's justification often determines payment for services rendered. Therefore, the purpose of this chapter is to define the medical necessity and subsequent need for skilled services within the continuum of care for mental disorders.

Four phases of illness are addressed by therapists. The *acute phase* occurs when the patient is not medically cleared to engage in any activities. The *postacute phase* occurs when the patient is medically cleared to engage in some activities. The *rehabilitation phase* occurs when the patient is cleared to engage in all activities that the individual is still able to do. The *long-term care phase* occurs when residual disabilities place the person at a social disadvantage. The phases of the healing process are major factors in determining what the therapist is expected to do.

## Acute Phase

From a consequences perspective, the acute phase occurs when the patient has not been medically cleared to engage in any activities. Therapists are evaluating and treating symptoms of the disease and/or reducing impairments. The medical model is used to select treatment goals and report treatment effectiveness. Examples include preventing deformities with splints or positioning devices, reducing edema, maintaining range of motion, and evaluating change in the cognitive level when patients are a danger to self or others. During the acute phase the medical condition is changing, and a return to some degree of functional ability is expected. Treatment may occur in an inpatient or outpatient setting, depending on the patient's medical condition. When the knowledge of a therapist is needed during the acute phase, a degree of residual disability is usually expected and complications are

expected, and/or prevented. Treatment effectiveness can be measured by a reduction in disability and/or prevention of complications.

## Postacute Phase

The postacute phase occurs when the patient has been medically cleared to engage in selected activities. The medical condition is still improving, and small degrees of change can be measured by using the decimal system provided in chapter 5. Evaluation is the service provided during most of the therapist's contacts with the patient. Preventing complications also occurs during the postacute phase. When the cognitive level stabilizes, therapists make discharge recommendations about the amount of assistance needed. Treatment effectiveness can be measured by the prevention of complications, accuracy of evaluations, and accuracy of discharge recommendations.

### Expectations for Therapists

The expected outcome is a recommendation of the least restrictive environment that the patient can function in safely at the time of discharge. The outcome is achieved by:

1. Establishing a baseline for the cognitive level at the time of referral with an estimate of the cognitive level at discharge; the discharge estimate can be used as a long-term goal; the short-term goals can be to provide activities that match the current level of ability and to probe for the next level;

2. Reporting symptoms of other diagnostic categories that might help with differential diagnosis;

3. Measuring change in symptoms, impairments, and disabilities;

4. Identifying the point in time when functional stability is reached;

5. Interpreting the meaning of any residual symptoms, impairments, or disabilities to the treatment team by describing the quality of performance and need for assistance to be expected after discharge.

### Referral Criteria

The patient meets the DSM R criteria and/or the ICD9 criteria for a medical diagnosis that is associated with a cognitive disability.

• *Medical necessity* is defined as a need for an evaluation of change in the cognitive level and a need for functional assessment to assist with discharge planning.

- *Skilled services* are defined as services that are trained to have adequate knowledge of the cognitive levels to accurately detect small changes in cognitive ability; sufficient medical knowledge to associate changes in the cognitive level with changes attributed to medical treatments and the natural course of the disease; sufficient knowledge of activity analysis to evaluate the cognitive complexity of any activity that the patient expresses an interest in doing after discharge; knowledge of community resources and judgment to predict compliance with recommendations.

Top priority is given to patients who have an expected change in life style after discharge. The change may be caused by a new physical and/or cognitive disability. Questions about changes in their social situation, like continuing to live with the family or living alone, are referral criteria. Questions about legal status, such as power of attorney or a legal guardian, are also given a high priority. These situations suggest that a major change in the person's life has occurred or is being considered. Major adjustments often suggest a need to refer the person to rehabilitation services.

When changes in psychotropic drugs are being made, the cognitive levels can be used to monitor medication effectiveness. Depressed people make this a challenge because they are not particularly interested in doing any activity. Furthermore they are apt to argue that doing a craft project will have no effect on their symptoms of depression, which is probably true. Convincing these people to do an activity to the best of their ability is a therapeutic challenge. Be candid about the reason for the evaluation; negotiate activities and a schedule that can be tolerated; and help the patients identify behaviors that they can associate with medication effectiveness.

The presence of mental retardation is apt to have an effect on the formation of new sensorimotor models as well as the number of stored sensorimotor models available for use. Treatment and discharge expectations may need to be adjusted down to allow for this additional difficulty. Interviews of family members and observations of performance may be required. If concerns about the person's safety remain, a referral to rehabilitation services is indicated.

The presence of Alzheimer's disease predicts a long-term decline in functional abilities, with variations in the rate of decline. Plan treatment goals and discharge recommendations for current abilities and adjust to decline after it occurs.

The presence of a stroke or brain injury predicts an improvement in functional abilities, most of which occur during the 1st year after injury. Make discharge recommendations based on current abilities and adjust these recommendations as improvement occurs. Consider the restriction that a cognitive disability will have on achieving physical goals such as ambulation and dexterity. Try to be realistic about the improvement in cognitive ability you predict for the next month and year. Keep track of patterns of improvement to improve your predictive validity. These patterns are used in the insurance industry to predict rehabilitation potential.

Each treatment plan should indicate the diagnosis (DSM III-R; Axis I, II, and III, or ICD9) and related health factors. The difficulty is that there is an enormous list of impairments in ICIDH. In the postacute phase it is easy to get sidetracked into doing extensive evaluations of little practical importance to the individual or the expected discharge situation. Lengthy evaluations are expensive and often unnecessary. Select impairments that are most apt to influence your discharge recommendations for this individual, and justify your selections.

During the postacute phase use the decimal system to evaluate the cognitive level weekly, when possible. A more frequent evaluation is apt to be subject to some normal fluctuations in ability. A change in the decimal number is an indication for a change in short-term goals and a check on the accuracy of the long-term goal.

If the cognitive level does not change from one week to the next, as predicted by the pattern of improvement associated with the diagnosis, time of onset, and medical interventions, further evaluation may not be reasonable or necessary. The exception would be further questions about discharge recommendations, but waiting on discharge placement does not constitute a reasonable and necessary need for services. Therapists can discharge patients from services that are no longer reasonable and necessary even though the patient remains in a hospital setting.

Many patients seen during the postacute phase are functioning at cognitive levels 3 and 4, with treatment goals aimed at teaching the caregiver. When the disability is new, family members have a lot of adjusting to do. Grieving over the loss of ability to do activities and the loss of major features of the patient's personality may not be possible during the postacute phase. Try to help families understand the burden of care required to protect the patient's safety. Document denial of disability and keep a written record of warnings issued (see safety checks in chapter 7). Provide the family with a written explanation of the disability, making the explanation as individualized as is possible. If the person is going to another health care agency, send a profile of the cognitive level to the agency. Be as resourceful as you can in finding ways to get information about the cognitive disability to long-term caregivers.

### Documentation

The patient's record should include the evaluation, progress notes, and discharge summary.

*Patient evaluation:* The purpose of the evaluation is to determine both the medical necessity and appropriate type of skilled service needed, including the following:

- The symptoms of diagnosis expressed during activity performance during the initial evaluation; include prior to admission for psychiatric patients;

- The symptoms of any other medical diagnosis expressed during activity performance that might assist with differential diagnosis;

- The cognitive level at the time of referral; you can report the ACL score if you think it is correct; if not, report your clinical impression;

- An estimate of the cognitive level predicted at discharge based on past responses to treatment, the usual pattern of the postacute treatment process, and the way the individual with a medical history has been functioning during the past year;

- An estimate of the least restrictive environment that the patient can function in safely at the time of discharge.

*Progress notes:* Improvements in the patient's cognitive level and reductions in symptoms and impairments are included. Interpret the meaning of these changes by noting associated medical treatments, correspondence with your predicted cognitive level at discharge, and your predicted discharge recommendations. If no change has occurred, say

so and explain what you think that means. Include warnings about safety hazards and efforts made to teach caregivers.

*Discharge notes summary:* A restatement of the original estimates of the need for cognitive assistance and discharge recommendations should be included with a review of the individual patient's course of treatment with an explanation for changes in the original estimates. Include information given to long-term caregivers.

## Rehabilitation

The rehabilitation phase occurs when patients are medically cleared for engaging in all functional activities that they are still able to do. The medical condition has stabilized, and there is little noticeable improvement in signs and symptoms, impairments, physical disability, or cognitive level. Therapists may improve the quality of performance by providing adaptive equipment, arranging for protective environments, and teaching caregivers how to provide assistance to compensate for the disability. The expected outcome is an improvement in doing activities safely. Treatment effectiveness can be measured by an increase in activities that the individual does, that are sustainable over time, with the assistance that is needed, and with reduced accidents or injuries.

The rehabilitation phase is an area of occupational therapy practice that needs to be strengthened. The myth is that this phase of the illness will not be paid for by third party payers. Within Medicare terminology, rehabilitation would be called "setting up a maintenance program," which is paid for by Medicare. Medicare tends to set the standard for what other insurance companies cover. Safety in doing meaningful activities is the issue of concern.

To strengthen this area of practice, occupational therapists need to think about improvement in a different way. During the acute and postacute phases, change occurs on a vertical axis; an increase in cognitive or physical ability can be expected. When no further increase in ability can be expected, therapists need to think about change on a horizontal axis. The horizontal axis is where therapists really maximize the patient's remaining abilities. To maximize remaining abilities, therapists need to consider what the person can and cannot do. Demands that are beyond remaining abilities must be avoided, while demands within the range of ability are provided. A numerical sequence of demands tells the therapist what the patient can and cannot do. A patient functioning at level 4.4 can be expected to do everything at 4.4 and below, but nothing at 4.5 and above. Change is made by getting the patient to do everything that he or she would like to do within his or her range of ability. Safety is protected by warning the patient and other caregivers about demands that are beyond the patient's ability.

Much of the motivation for writing this book has been derived from a desire to improve rehabilitation and long-term care. What happens to people who must live with the consequences of a health problem is our major concern. A lot of contemporary practice focuses on measuring improvements in impairments that occur during the acute and postacute phases of the illness. In recent years very little has been written or done about improving the activity performance of people who live with functional limitations. Part of the neglect can be traced to difficulties in measuring small changes in functional limitations, which chapter 5 addresses. Another part of the neglect can be attributed to not knowing how to improve activity performance. To improve the performance of activities, occupational therapists need to know how to analyze activities. The activities most commonly used in practice have been analyzed by Earhart and Blue in chapters 6 and 9. Therapists will still need to learn how to do an activity analysis so that other activities that are meaningful to individuals can be improved. Chapter 5 contains a suggestion for verifying your ability to do an accurate analysis. The origins of our profession are in rehabilitation and long-term care, but occupational therapists need to increase their knowledge of these phases of illness and activity performance.

## Expectations for the Therapist

The expectation is that the therapist will use the patients' remaining abilities to help patients fit into normal community activities in spite of the presence of intractable impairments and disabilities. Practice includes providing the patients/caregivers with an objective understanding of realistic needs for assistance and by preventing secondary complications that could produce further disability. The outcome is achieved by:

- Obtaining the patient's functional history in doing activities prior to the onset of the disability from the patient/significant others;

- Identifying expected changes in life style and

selecting priorities for change with the patient and the significant others;

- Analyzing selected activities to identify steps that the patient probably can and cannot do;

- Clarifying the necessary adjustment to the loss of abilities while the patient is doing activities, including on-site testing in the community;

- Advocating the legal rights of the cognitively disabled person;

- Teaching the use of environmental compensations to the patient and significant others; and

- Discussing use of environmental compensations on follow-up, making any indicated changes.

### Referral Criteria

The patient meets the DSM III-R criteria and/or the ICD9 criteria for a diagnosis that is associated with a long-term cognitive disability.

- *Medical necessity* is defined as a need for assistive devices, environmental modifications, or the protection of others to do activities safely and effectively.

- *Skilled services* are defined as services that are trained to have sufficient medical knowledge to recommend realistic precautions while patients are doing activities, sufficient knowledge of activity analysis to determine the cognitive complexity of activities that the patient is interested in doing and to suggest other possible activities; sufficient knowledge of how to make environmental substitutions to compensate for disabilities; and sufficient knowledge of how to teach caregivers to provide the assistance necessary to protect the patient's safety while doing activities.

Many rehabilitation programs are designed for the physically disabled who are functioning at cognitive level 6. Treatment programs aimed at compensating for a cognitive level 5 are available (Dougherty & Radomski, 1987). On-site training is required at cognitive levels 3 and 4; skilled services are justifiable to locate community placements and set up training procedures. People who stabilize at cognitive levels 3 through 6 qualify for rehabilitation services when there is a disability of recent onset, a recent change in the severity of the disability, or a recent recognition of the need for assistance.

Questions about where the disabled person is going to live are usually answered by the time the patient gets to this phase of the illness. Now the questions are about safety and assistance in that living environment as well as the disabled person's occupation of time. The treatment setting is a major determinant of referral criteria for the cognitively disabled. Outpatient clinics can be effective with patients and caregivers functioning at cognitive level 6, and effectiveness will probably decline when they are functioning at level 5. Therapists may be able to overcome the difficulties of working with people at level 5 in a clinic by doing home visits, job-site visits, as well as explorations of the neighborhood. People functioning at cognitive levels 3 and 4 need to have training procedures set up where they are going to be doing the activity with the people who will be providing long-term assistance. If the patient moves, or changes place of supportive employment, a new training procedure will probably be necessary.

During the rehabilitation phase a clear distinction needs to be made between what the patient does spontaneously and what the patient does when cued by the therapist. Therapists modify the way an activity is set up and the way directions are given to get an improvement in performance. The improvement is produced by the therapist's interventions. These interventions are taught to long-term caregivers to sustain the improvement.

Skilled services are required to teach lay people how to maximize the abilities of the cognitively disabled. The difference between will not and cannot must be explained within the context of the activities that the individual does. Without objective clarification conflicts and avoidance of the disabled person are apt to occur. Even with explanation, conflicts are hard to diminish unless this problem is addressed over a period of time.

When improvement in a physical or cognitive disability can be attributed to medication, medication compliance must be evaluated. This is a major factor with the cognitively disabled, who often deny the presence of a disability and refuse to take psychotropic drugs. The strength of the social support system in getting the necessary patient cooperation needs to be evaluated and warned about the problems of noncompliance.

The selection of the activity matters a great deal to the patients and their caregivers. Meaningless activities usually equal meaningless services. To make services meaningful, therapists must be prepared to analyze any activity that is important to the individuals. The activities analyzed on the Routine Task Inventory (RTI) provide a starting place. Interviews and frequent discussions of what the disabled person is doing or would like to do are necessary to discover other activities.

Patients and caregivers can disagree about which activities are important. The cognitively disabled often refuse to do things without understanding the consequences of their refusal. Or, they do the reverse and insist on doing things without understanding the consequences. Verbal warnings given by therapists may not be computed. Sometimes the only hope of preventing serious injury is to allow the patient to experience minor pain to recognize the danger. Even then, the patient may not be reliable in following safety precautions, and caretakers need to be warned.

Perhaps the most difficult situation occurs when a cognitively disabled person has a cognitively disabled caregiver. Some other form of social support is required by both people. If there is no family or significant other available, contact the appropriate social welfare agency, such as the public guardian's office.

As the patient and caregiver adjust to the realities of living with a disability, a change in priorities is apt to occur. The change may be as great as selecting a different activity or as small as change in activity procedure. When the patient can do the activity safely with the prompting of another caregiver, then skilled care is no longer required.

Rehabilitation programs can be physically and mentally exhausting. If the patient complains about being tired or falls asleep during treatment sessions, the frequency and duration of the sessions should be reduced to a level tolerated by the patient.

If it becomes apparent after a reasonable period of time that the patient, family, or caregiver will not or is not able to learn or be taught, then further teaching would cease to be reasonable and necessary.

## Documentation

*Patient evaluation:* The purpose of the evaluation is to determine both the medical necessity and the appropriate type of skilled service, and should delineate the following:

- The functional history of the patient prior to onset of the disability;
- The expected changes in life style and the patient/ caregiver awareness of those changes;
- The nature of the social support system currently available to the patient;

- The symptoms of diagnosis expressed during performance at the present time;

- The degree of cognitive assistance required at the present time, with an estimate of any expected change;

- Identification of activities that are important to the patient/caregiver;

- Long-term treatment goals that identify the activities selected, the estimated assistance needed at discharge, and an estimate of the frequency and duration required to achieve the goal;

- Short-term treatment goals that identify the methods used and the sequence in which the activities will be addressed, including safety hazards expected.

*Progress notes:* Improvements in the patient's activity performance per the estimated long-range goal are reported. The need for continuation of skilled services should be noted, with the necessary modifications in the treatment plan.

*Discharge summary:* A restatement of the original estimate of need for assistance in doing the selected activities is included with a review of the patient's course of treatment. An explanation for changes made in the treatment goals is also included.

## Long-Term Care

From a rehabilitation perspective, long-term care occurs when disabled people have residual abilities that cannot be used in customary activities. Long-term care is the provision of a community-based activity program designed for people who are functioning at cognitive levels 3 and 4. The activity program reduces the handicap of no occupation, maintains the individual's maximum level of function, and prevents secondary complications.

## Expectations for Therapists

The expected outcome is to maintain current functional abilities within a supportive social context and to avoid secondary complications that produce

**Table 3.1 Physical and cognitive assistance codes from Medicare Intermediary Manual Part III, 1990; code physical and cognitive assistance separately***

"*Total Assistance* is the need for 100 percent assistance by one or more persons to perform all physical activities and/or cognitive assistance to elicit a functional response to an external stimulation. A cognitively impaired patient requires total assistance when your documentation shows external stimuli are required to elicit automatic actions such as swallowing or responding to auditory stimuli.

"*Maximum Assistance* is the need for 75 percent assistance by one person to physically perform any part of a functional activity and/or demonstrated cognitive assistance to perform gross motor actions in response to direction. Due to lack of awareness of other people or objects in the environment, proprioceptive stimulation and/or one-to-one demonstration is required to move the patient.

"*Moderate Assistance* is the need for 50 percent assistance by one person to perform physical activities or constant cognitive assistance to sustain/complete simple repetitive activities safely. The patient requires intermittent one-to-one cueing (physical or verbal) to sequence through and complete an activity. Constant supervision is required to halt perseverative actions or prevent unsafe, erratic, or unpredictable actions.

"*Minimum Assistance* is the need for 25 percent physical assistance by one person for physical activities and/or visually cued cognitive assistance to perform functional activities safely. A cognitively impaired patient requires minimal assistance if your documentation indicates help is needed in performing known activities to correct repeated mistakes, to check for compliance with established safety procedures, or to solve problems with unexpected hazards.

"*Standby Assistance* is the need for supervision by one person for the patient to perform new activity procedures which were adapted by the therapist for safe and effective performance. A patient requires standby assistance when errors and the need for safety precautions are not always anticipated by the patient.

"*Independent Status* means that no physical or cognitive assistance is required to perform functional activities. Patients at this level are able to implement the selected courses of action, consider potential errors and anticipate safety hazards in familiar and new situations. These patients would not be candidates for services unless another medical reason explained the need, like suicidal thoughts."

*\*Medicare Intermediary Manual Part III, 1990.*

increased health and social welfare needs. This outcome is achieved by the following methods:

• Obtaining a functional history that identifies activities done in the past that the individual may still be able to do;

• Providing activities that are acceptable to the individual and avoiding activities that are apt to be rejected;

• Recognizing residual limitations that will require modifications in the usual activity procedure and tactfully making the necessary modifications;

• Replicating a sense of the individual's usual place in the culture of the community as closely as possible;

• Replacing deviant behavior with behavior that is more socially acceptable;

• Arranging for participation in normal community events whenever economically feasible and socially acceptable;

• Working with available social support systems to maintain the highest level of function by explaining the difference between cannot and will not;

• Arranging for access to the social welfare system and health care resources when needed;

• Assisting other caregivers in making environmental compensations that reduce the burden of care or improve functional abilities; and

• Facilitating departure from the long-term-care system whenever changes in the disability or the social welfare system (such as money for supportive employment) permit.

### Referral Criteria

The patient meets the DSM III-R criteria and/or the ICD9 criteria for a diagnosis that is associated with a cognitive disability:

• *Medical necessity* is defined by meeting the following criteria:

- Patients who have been or are expected to be disabled longer than 6 months with no expected change in the degree of assistance required for a physical and/or a cognitive disability as defined by Medicare, Part B (1990), and

- Patients who are handicapped to the extent that they are unable to participate in an occupational use of time within the usual community schedule (minimum or moderate cognitive assistance), and

### Table 3.2  Occupational handicaps (ICIDH, 1980)

"Customarily occupied includes routine tasks, school, work, play/leisure, and social activities according to ordinary community standards for the quality of performance and the time scheduled for doing these activities.

"Intermittently unoccupied is a temporary interference with customary activities caused by short-term signs and symptoms of a disease. The time away from customary activities can be brief, like a few hours with a headache. The limited activity may also remove a class of hazardous activities, as with epilepsy and driving.

"Curtailed occupation is a overall decrease in the quality of performance of all desirable activities, although able to manage a restricted participation in these activities.

"Adjusted occupation is a reliance on environmental adaptations for full participation in desirable activities. Environmental adaptations are broadly defined to include people and objects. Objects include adaptive equipment, prosthetics, orthotics, special purchases or changes in home and work space necessary for safe and effective participation. People include the reliance on caregivers for special assistance. When modifications are in place, the individual is able to engage in full-time occupation within the normal range of community events.

"Reduced occupation is a decrease in the amount of time that the individual is able to do customary activities. The quality of participation is not restricted.

"Restricted occupation is participation in activities that are modified to enhance the remaining abilities of disabled people. Special circumstances are created for safe and effective participation and are sustained for customary periods of time.

"Confined occupation is a decrease in the amount of time and the quality of the activity. Special circumstances are created for a reduced period of time.

"No occupation is no participation in safe and effective activities because no special circumstances exist, unable to participate in special circumstances, or unwilling to participate in special circumstances" (pp. 195–198).

- Patients who are not so disabled as to be bed ridden or unable to do any activity (total or maximum cognitive assistance), and patients who will accept other disabled people as their peers, and

- Patients who refrain from drug and alcohol abuse, and

- Patients whose behavior does not represent a danger to self or others.

• *Skilled services* are defined as services trained to have sufficient medical knowledge to take precautions to avoid the secondary complications of long-term disabilities; sufficient knowledge of activity analysis to match task demands to the person's remaining abilities; sufficient skill to do parts of the activity that the individual is unable to do; and sufficient skill to do a wide range of activities that interest different individuals.

The occupational handicap scale in ICIDH can be used to put the overall benefit of long-term care in perspective. Both the quality of the activity and the time spent in doing the activity are included (Table 3.1). Time is easier to measure but is often misleading without a qualitative measure. Documentation of participation should include attendance and the individual's involvement in doing activities.

Participation in a community-based activity program is voluntary, requiring the cooperation and motivation of the disabled person. Skilled services match activities provided to the individual's interests, sense of accomplishment, and remaining abilities. The certified occupational therapy assistant (COTA) has the knowledge required to analyze activities and match task demands to the remaining abilities of the individual. The occupational therapist has the knowledge required to recognize and prevent medical complications, make referrals to other health and social welfare agencies, and help other caregivers understand the difference between cannot and will not.

When activities are provided for groups of disabled people, some activities are apt to have more appeal than others. Program planning and documentation must demonstrate a consideration of the individual's interests and desires. When activities are rejected, an effort should be made to offer alternatives.

The frequency and duration of the activity program must be adjusted to the level tolerated by the patient. Documentation must show an awareness of how long performance can be sustained before a deterioration in ability to function occurs.

An individual may become bored with the available activities or too disabled to continue to participate in doing the available activities. For services to be considered reasonable and necessary, the individual must participate in doing the activities. Continuation of skilled treatment is based on continued participation. The following discharge criteria indicate when services are no longer reasonable and necessary:

• Patients who are so disabled as to be bedridden or unable to do any activity, or

• Patients who are so improved as to be able to engage in regular occupations within the community, or

• Patients who will not accept other disabled people as their peers, or

• Patients who cannot refrain from drug and alcohol abuse, or

• Patients whose behavior presents a danger to self or others.

## Documentation

*Patient evaluation:* The purpose of the occupational evaluation is to determine both the medical necessity of and the appropriate type of skilled service, and should contain the same information found in the rehabilitation evaluation.

*Progress notes:* Since stabilization of the occupational handicap is the expected outcome, progress notes should document any departures from this expectation. Report any improvements or deterioration of impairments, disabilities, or handicaps, with possible explanations for the change. Changes should also be reported to the physician and family.

Documentation must also contain the individual's response to the activities provided, with an ongoing record of preferences and dislikes. Any progress made in expanding the desirable activities available to the individual should be noted.

*Discharge summary:* The reason for discharge must be clearly stated with the patient's and long-term caregiver's response to discharge. Include any referrals made to other parts of the health and social welfare system.

## Codes

Rehabilitation services are delivered in the context of a health care system that uses codes to identify problems and to report treatment outcomes. During the acute phase, the *International Classification of Diseases,* 9th edition, codes are used, with associated signs and symptoms. During the post-acute phase, attention should shift to the *International Classification of Impairments, Disabilities and Handicaps.* Patients begin to do activities during the post-acute phase and experience the consequences of a health problem. Impairments restrict activity performance. Impairment codes, like perceptual difficulties, can be used to identify problems that are thought to limit performance of activities. By the time the patient reaches the end of the postacute phase, the therapist must be thinking about needs for assistance to make discharge recommendations. The Medicare assistance codes listed on Table 3.1 can be used to record general expectations (Medicare Intermediary Manual Part III, 1990). These codes combine physical and cognitive disabilities, which can be very confusing in clinical practice. You may choose to rate the need for physical assistance and cognitive assistance separately. The Western Physical Performance Analysis (WPPA) provides a reliable measure of the need for physical assistance.

Rehabilitation focuses on disabilities. The disability codes identify most of the activities that the person will be doing and the amount of assistance needed. Revisions in the behavior disabilities codes are suggested in this text. Long-term care focuses on reducing occupational handicaps (Table 3.2). A cognitive disability can be expected to produce a handicap in all of the survival roles, but long-term care reduces the occupational handicap.

## Conclusion

The acute and postacute phases measure improvement on a vertical axis; an increase in the cognitive level is a vertical axis improvement. The modes of performance described in chapter 5 are sensitive to change within the cognitive level and can also be used to measure change on the vertical axis. Natural healing and medical interventions can cause the improvement. With the exception of naturally occurring complications, like contractures, improvement does not depend on the patient's motivation, learning ability, or social support system. Verification of improved ability to function does require the patient's cooperation, but a lack of cooperation does not necessarily mean that no improvement has occurred. Resourceful therapists can usually find an

activity that the patient will agree to do and base an assessment of improvement on that activity. On the vertical axis, treatment goals and measures of treatment effectiveness can be stated and achieved with very little reliance on psychological or social factors. The intent is not to say that this is the best way to do it, but to merely state that it can be done with good results. The results that do occur depend on psychological and social factors that prevent complications and discharge planning.

All good results do depend on psychological and social factors during the rehabilitation and long-term-care phases, referred to as the horizontal axis. An improvement in the safe performance of activities that are meaningful, utilitarian, and sustainable is expected. The clinical reasoning required to select treatment goals, recognize a need and negotiate a change or modification of treatment goals, and measure improvement, must account for individual differences. An evaluation of the individual and social support systems is essential to successful treatment.

The functional history should identify the highest level of function that the patient has ever achieved, including education and work histories as well as a prior life style. The patient's understanding and acceptance of his or her condition, prior and expected improvements, goals, and temperament need to be evaluated. The family and any other expected long-term caregivers should be evaluated according to the same factors. The living situation and any other environments in which activities will be done, need to be evaluated to protect the patient and community. Community resources such as friends, volunteers, self-help groups, advocates, other health care providers, legal advisors, and social welfare agencies need to be evaluated for each individual case. To make a real difference in the way people live with a disability, a systematic evaluation of a large number of psychological and social influences must be done. The expected discharge date and placement needs to be evaluated according to the patient's and family's attitudes toward the plan.

## References

Dougherty, P.M., & Radomski, M.V. (1987). *The cognitive rehabilitation workbook.* Rockville, MD: Aspen Publishers.

*Medicare Intermediary Manual Part III.* (September 1990). Claims Processing, Transmittal #1487,

Section 3906. Baltimore: Health Care Financing Administration.

*Western Physical Performance Analysis.* Western Neurocare, PO Box 170, Tustin, CA 92681-0170.

World Health Organization. (1980). *International Classification of Impairments, Disabilities, and Handicaps (ICIDH).* Geneva: Author.

# Chapter 4

# Evaluation Instruments

Claudia Kay Allen, MA, OTR, FAOTA
Kathy Kehrberg, OTR, MSW
Theressa Burns, OTR

**P**rior to administering any of these standard evaluation tools, the therapist should establish a method for getting to know the patient and finding out what requests for services the patient and other caregivers have. The most common format is a functional interview. The purpose of the interview is to learn as much as possible about the individual's functional history and how the consequences of an illness are changing the individual's ordinary activities. The specific questions asked during the interview are influenced by the phase of the illness described in chapter 4. What should be noted here is that all of these assessment tools assume that a functional history has been taken and that the tools are being used to clarify the consequences of a health problem.

A therapist frequently needs to evaluate a patient's cognitive ability during the performance of any activity that the patient will agree to do. Refusals to try to do standardized tests are common, as are plausible excuses for poor performance. A fair and objective evaluation of cognitive ability is based on the assumption that the patient wants to do the activity. Therapists need to be very flexible in offering activities that are appealing to individuals. To be that flexible therapists must be prepared to analyze any activity. This chapter, in conjunction with chapters 5, 6, and 7, describes the process of learning how to do an activity analysis with confidence.

Two of the standardized evaluation instruments that have been developed to measure the cognitive levels are discussed in this chapter. The Allen Cognitive Level (ACL) test gives a quick estimate of the person's current ability to learn. The individual is asked to do three leather lacing stitches. The most recent version of the ACL is presented in Appendix A. Kehrberg has developed a larger version that is discussed in Part II of this chapter.

The Routine Task Inventory (RTI) describes behaviors that may be observed while a person is doing selected activities. Common tasks that are apt to be difficult for the cognitively disabled are identified. Behavior that may occur while doing these activities is described according to the 6 cognitive levels in Appendix B. Questions that can be asked while obtaining a self-report are also suggested. The same format can be easily converted to obtain a caregiver report.

The RTI aims at describing a broad range of activities that an individual might do in the community. Evaluations done in the hospital or outpatient settings cannot replicate natural settings. A standardized observation of performance in doing several activities seems to be the most practical and objective way of measuring performance abilities in these settings. In part III of this chapter Burns presents a standardized performance measure that can be administered in about 45 minutes (Appendix C).

The chapter aims at sharing new information about instruments that are being developed to encourage a wider investigation into instrument development and to further such development. The chapter also aims at opening evaluation up so that any activity that is meaningful to the patient or the caregiver can be directly evaluated.

## Part I: Allen Cognitive Levels (ACL) and the Routine Task Inventory (RTI)

*Claudia Kay Allen*

The ACL is an initial performance measure that can

be administered to patients functioning at levels 3 through 5. Greater cooperation is usually achieved by talking to patients before asking them to try the leather lacing. The initial interview contains questions that help the therapist understand what kind of services are indicated and what the individual's functional history is like. A chart review is often done before the interview, thus providing a medical history. Education, work, other major roles, and use of spare time histories provide a functional understanding of the individual. The patient is also asked how he or she expects to benefit from the services offered (Allen, 1985).

The information exchanged during the initial interview is heavily influenced by the patient's cognitive level. At level 3 very little information is exchanged. The patient may be able to answer a few questions about education and work history, but making sense out of what he or she says is often difficult. The patient may not know that anything is the matter with him or her, and has no idea of how he or she might benefit. At level 4 the patient can usually give a coherent functional history. Some of the facts may be distorted or delusional, but the story is easy to repeat. When asked how he or she expects to benefit from services, the patient may deny that there is anything the matter with him or her. When a physical problem is present, the patient is apt to identify that as the only problem. Unrealistic goals for the future are common. More realistic treatment goals are stated at level 5. An awareness of a new cognitive deficit is usually present, and adjusting to it is difficult.

An interview can also be a formal meeting between the therapist and another caregiver. When the cognitive level has stabilized, the caregiver's request for services may be as important, or more important, than the patient's. Therapists working in outpatient clinics may find that scheduling an interview with the caregiver is especially helpful in establishing treatment goals.

## Allen Cognitive Level

The ACL test provides a quick estimate of the patient's current capacity to learn. This performance test is usually administered at the end of the initial interview. Therapists use the score as a guideline for the treatment goals that are achievable at the present time. The test has been in clinical use since 1973. Three versions have been subjected to reliabil-

ity and validity investigation as previously published: Allen Cognitive Level-Original (ACL-O); Allen Cognitive Level-Expanded (ACL-E); and Allen Cognitive Level-Problem Solving (ACL-PS).

The first version (ACL-O) has a simple 5-point scale, measuring levels 2-6. Interrater reliability was established using a Person-product correlation as $r = .99$ (range of levels 2-6, $N = 32$) (Allen, 1985). The validity of using the ACL to place patients in an occupational therapy group that matched their cognitive level was established as $r = .76$ ($N = 23$). The Brief Psychiatric Rating Scale was used to investigate concurrent validity as $r = -.53$ at admission to the hospital and $r = .43$ at discharge (Allen, 1985). The Block Design of the Wechscler Adult Intelligence Scale (WAIS) was also used for concurrent validity as $r = .46$ at admission ($N = 32$) and $r = .40$ at discharge ($N = 32$) (Allen, 1985). An investigation of 50 nondisabled subjects found a significant correlation between education ($r = .50$), occupation ($r = .53$), and social position ($r = .51$). The Hollingshead Two-Factor Index of Social Position was used to establish education, occupation, and social position (Allen, 1985). Similar mean ACL-O scores and differentiations between populations were found in Israel in schizophrenic, depressed, and control populations (Katz & Heimann, 1990). In the adult populations under the age of 65, age and sex did not seem to affect the test scores. The predictive validity of the ACL-O was investigated to identify placement in work following a 3-week prevocational evaluation. A significant association was found, Chi square = 33,54, $p < .001$., $N = 32$. None of the subjects scoring a 3 was recommended for work. Level 4 subjects were recommended for supported or sheltered work. The higher levels were divided between open employment/education and supported employment (Katz & Heimann). The lack of sensitivity as well as other flaws have led to replacing the ACL-O with two other versions.

Interest in investigating populations where little change in the cognitive level was expected led to lengthening the score sheet (ACL-E). While revising, we also added a twist in the leather lacing for every patient, rather than leaving the twist to chance. Newman (1987) established the interrater reliability as 95% ($N = 21$). Test-retest reliability was established as $rs = .75$ ($N = 22$) using Spearman's rank correlation (Newman, 1987). A revised edition of the WAIS, (WAIS-R) investigated the relationship with learning potential (N = 40, range of scores of 3.0 to 6.6). Significant correlations were found with the following subtests using Spearman's Correlation Coefficients: Block design r = .62, Object assembly r = .55, Picture arrangement r = .59, Digit symbols r = .59, Digit span r = .54, Performance scale IQ r = .55, Verbal scale IQ r = .41, and Full-scale IQ r = .47. Correlations with the other subtests were not significant: Picture completion r = .28, Vocabulary r = .23, and Arithmetic r = .39. The results of this study demonstrate a relationship between the ACL-E and "the factors considered to be essential for organizing and processing information, that is learning" (Mayer, 1988, p. 183). The reliability and validity derived from a more sensitive measure is encouraging and enlightening.

Josman & Katz (1991) developed the ACL-PS, which asks the subject to first try to do each stitch by looking at the stitch; if the subject is not able to do it by looking, then by following verbal instructions, and finally by following a demonstration. The ceiling effect of the ACL-O was removed by the ACL-PS in the control group of normal adolescents. The different types of information used to learn to do the single cordovan stitch provided a range of scores. Somewhat more confusing was that the psychiatric inpatient adolescents also used a range of different types of information to do the whip and running stitches (Josman & Katz, 1991; Katz & Heimann, 1990). The ACL-PS was used in a study of 10 patients who had suffered cerebrovascular accidents (CVAs) and 10 patients with traumatic brain injuries (TBIs) at 3 months postinjury and after 2 months of therapy. The average score was the whip stitch, performed independently. No significant change between pre- and posttest was found, which was consistent with the anecdotal report of the therapists who reported little change. Some clues about the relationships between impairments and disabilities are available in this study. The Lowenstein Occupational Therapy Cognitive Assessment (LOTCA) Battery was used, which measures a number of impairments. Significant correlations between the ACL-PS and the LOTCA, with the highest being between the ACL-PS and visuomotor organization, r = .69 (Katz & Heimann, 1990).

While working on the development of chapter 5, we decided that more refinements in the ACL were needed (see Appendix A). Since we seem to keep changing this instrument, this version is called

the ACL-90, for the revisions made in 1990. The range of scores is 3.0 to 5.8, which seems to be more logically related to what leather lacing can measure. The ACL-E ranged from 1.0 to 6.6, but that length does not correspond with the refinements made in this text. Three stitches were added instead of 2 because some patients seem to get lucky, but they have not really learned how to do the stitch. The ACL-PS method of giving directions has been added to the single cordovan stitch, and the score sheet. The score sheet allows "prompts" in place of "verbal directions," a factor that comes out of our clinical experience of testing people who speak so many different languages. Prompts can include pointing to an error. The ACL-PS directions were not added for the whip or running stitches, because I am uncertain about how much they add or where they would fit on the score sheet. The ACL-90 was reviewed by N. Katz (personal communication, 1991) and will be used in future studies by each of us. A time lag is to be expected as studies using previous versions have not been published as of this writing. A test manual and kit for the ACL-90 is commercially available (Allen, 1990).

The biggest clinical irritant in using the ACL is visual impairments. If people cannot see the leather lacing, they cannot correct or learn from their mistakes. The larger version is a welcome solution to some of these problems. Patients who experience left-handedness, one-handedness, and hand tremors also raise questions about the test's validity, but not as great as those questions raised by vision problems. Being deaf or unable to understand the verbal directions poses the least difficulty as demonstrations and gestures can be substituted. When these difficulties occur, therapists often administer the test but have less confidence in the test score. Therapists who encounter these or other difficulties often are encouraged to revise the test. The CVA/TBI study tried another modification of placing the ACL in a vise for subjects who could not hold it themselves. The concern about this modification, expressed by the authors, is that the complexity may have been downgraded by fixing the directionality of the instrument (Katz & Heimann, 1990). Another possibility is to place the leather in an adapted embroidery hoop that swivels (T. Blue, personal communication, August 1991).

For patients who cannot use their hands, a verbal test may be required. The work being done by

Katz on Class Inclusion (CI) may solve this problem. Class inclusion focuses on the relationship between and within classes. The input is both visual and auditory, and the output is verbal. Katz has been examining the relationship between CI, ACL, and the Risk Object Classification (ROC) tests, and a pattern across the life span in patient and control populations is emerging. The relationships between classification and the activities of daily living are still ambiguous (Katz & Heimann, 1990). The more detailed analysis of the cognitive levels presented in chapter 5 suggests that the content of the information classified is an important consideration. Williams' discovery that psychiatric patients could not classify flowers but could classify by color and shape makes sense within that context (Allen, 1985).

The ACL is a visuomotor task that provides an estimate of a person's ability to learn to do other visuomotor tasks. The strength of the associations with other tasks seems to be related to the requirements for processing visuomotor information. It is obvious that the sensorimotor system processes additional kinds of information. I would expect a weaker association with other kinds of information. An initial test with validity for the blind would be helpful.

## Routine Task Inventory

Most psychological tests focus on a part of brain functions, like visuomotor or classification. Measures of impairments are abundant and many deficits can be detected. Fewer instruments exist to measure disability and most of the literature focuses on physical disabilities (Feinstein, 1987; McDowell & Newell, 1987; Reed, 1991). The trouble with this situation is that practice is impairment driven. An improvement in an impairment can be measured, but one wonders if it really makes a difference to the individual. The meaning to the individual becomes apparent while the person is doing an activity. The evaluation of activity performance is, therefore, regarded as more important than the evaluation of impairments.

Instruments that are specific enough to achieve interrater reliability and sensitive enough to detect the changes that therapists make, did not exist in 1984. The original RTI was undertaken to overcome a serious deficiency in the basic science literature. Discussions of ordinary activities in psychology, sociology, and anthropology tend to be too broad and general. The situation is scary because a failure to evaluate specifics means that we cannot investigate treatment effectiveness. In 1984 Earhart, Heyings, Heimann, and I decided to rely on our experiences with patients to describe behavior. The original list of activities was taken from Lawton & Brody (1969). Earhart and I have continued to rely on clinical experience to describe behavior. Our goal is to get occupational therapy ready to develop a lot of instruments for evaluating activity performance.

The notion that this goal was achievable was given a big boost by the work done by Heyings, Heimann, and Wilson (Heyings in Allen, 1985; Heimann, Allen, & Yerxa, 1989; Wilson, Allen, McCormack, & Burton, 1989). Heyings did pioneer work in recording responses to an Alzheimer's functional evaluation by focusing of the cognitive difficulties that were largely ignored (Allen, 1985). Heimann did the initial reliability and validity study on the RTI. Significant interrater ($r = .98$) and test-retest ($r = .91$) reliabilities were established. The most encouraging finding was the internal consistency with an alpha coefficient of .94 ($N = 41$). Further examination of the Pearson correlations between the activities enhanced confidence in the criteria for evaluating the cognitive complexity of activities.

Internal consistency examined task equivalence among all the activities on the RTI. The Pearson correlations were between two activities. If therapists are going to be able to analyze any activity that the patient wants to do, internally consistent criteria must be established, which seems to be possible. The alternative would be to develop a detailed description of behavior for a seemingly endless list of activities. The Spearman's rank correlation between the ACL-O and the RTI was $r = .54$ (range 3-6, $x = 4.39$, $SD = .86$) for concurrent validity (Heimann, Allen, & Yerxa, 1989).

The correlation between the ACL-O and the RTI was $r = .56$ in the second study, indicating that validity could be replicated in a different population ($N = 20$). Test-retest reliability was also replicated at $r = .99$. The Mini-Mental State (MMS) examination (Folstein, et al.) was also administered to this population, which suffered from senile dementia. The Spearman's correlation between the MMS and the RTI was $r = .61$, supporting the notion that mental impairments are associated with a decline in functional activities (Wilson, Allen, McCormack, & Burton, 1989).

There are three ways of evaluating the performance of activities: self-report, caregiver report, and observations of performance. All of these studies used caregiver report as a means of collecting data. The reliability of the patient is questionable at levels 1 through 4. The reliability of the caregiver can be influenced by privacy concerns, amount of contact with the patient, personal goals, and style of care giving. Observations of performance that objectively describe behavior usually have the greatest credibility. All three approaches are used in practice for a variety of reasons. The aim here is to make it possible for therapists to develop evaluations with all three approaches.

Observing the performance of a single activity is problematic. Poor performance can be excused by a problem with that activity, rather than a disability. If the activity has no meaning to the patient, poor performance can be explained by a lack of motivation or interest in the activity. A lack of face validity can raise reasonable doubts. The patient may not understand a connection between doing a craft activity and a discharge plan, even though it has been explained. The cognitively disabled rely on face validity. Observing the performance of several activities, some of which have face validity, has greater credibility when a pattern of disability is described.

The credibility of observations of performance is apt to be the greatest in the natural setting (at home or on the job). When access to the natural setting is not possible (in a hospital or an outpatient clinic) efforts need to be made to make the setting as close to natural as possible. The cost, in time and transportation, of obtaining observations of performance in a natural setting can be prohibitive. Observations made in a hospital or outpatient clinic are necessary for practical reasons. Burn's work (in this chapter) is a means of overcoming many of these difficulties by using standardized tasks that have face validity and can be done in a reasonable period of time.

Many caregivers are very reliable sources of information. The fastest way to evaluate the pattern of activity performance is to interview the caregiver. Conduct the interview in a way that the patient will not hear what the caregiver is saying. Therapists working in outpatient clinics may find this a particularly valuable way of establishing treatment goals.

A self-report may be helpful around level 4 when patients are unaware of their disability. Score the self-report according to what the patient says he or she can do. Score the observations according to what he or she does, and then compare the scores. This approach has been used when legal decisions must be made and seems to be fair to the patient.

Conducting the interview is, at least at the present time, part of the art of practice. While the performance of activities seems straightforward, ordinary activities have a way of getting very complicated. The following definitions of activities are provided to help therapist consider the most relevant factors during the interview or in setting up observations.

## Activity and Behavior Disability

The ICIDH format allows for the description of eight activities within each definition of a disability. An effort has been made to include those activities that are apt to be most important to most people. Table 4.1 outlines the activities selected. Tasks that are apt to be affected by a cognitive disability are identified.

### 1. Behavior Disability

A behavior disability is a cognitive disability, an incapacity to process the information required to do ordinary human activities safely. The activities are divided into the following categories: self-awareness, situational awareness, occupational role, and social role.

### 10. Self-Awareness Disability

A self-awareness disability is a disturbance in the ability to do self-care activities, including meeting the natural demands of one's body as well as the consequences of health problems that no longer require professional assistance. Self-awareness includes the activities one does to keep one's body clean, safe, healthy, comfortable, and attractive. The material objects one uses are fairly standard and cross-cultural. The universal nature of these activities makes it possible to list the steps required to complete each task with a good amount of specificity that is apt to be cross-cultural.

*10.0 Grooming* includes combing, brushing, setting, straightening, braiding, and curling hair; washing, shaving, using tweezers, and applying make-up to the face; cleaning, cutting, shaping, and polishing nails; brushing and flossing teeth; removing, cleaning, and reinserting dentures; washing,

**Table 4.1  Activities analyzed on RTI-2 as behavior disabilities**

| 10. | Self-awareness disability | 12. | Occupational role disability |
|---|---|---|---|
| .0 | Grooming | .0 | Planning/doing major role activities |
| .1 | Dressing | .1 | Planning/doing spare-time activities |
| .2 | Bathing | .2 | Pacing and timing actions |
| .3 | Walking/exercising | .3 | Exerting effort |
| .4 | Feeding | .4 | Judging results |
| .5 | Toileting | .5 | Speaking |
| .6 | Taking medications | .6 | Following safety precautions |
| .7 | Using adaptive equipment | .7 | Responding to emergencies |
| .8 | Other | .8 | Other |
| .9 | Unspecified | .9 | Unspecified |
| | | | |
| 11. | Situational awareness disability | 13. | Social role disability |
| .0 | Housekeeping | .0 | Communicating meaning |
| .1 | Preparing/obtaining food | .1 | Following instructions |
| .2 | Spending money | .2 | Contributing to family activities |
| .3 | Shopping | .3 | Caring for dependents |
| .4 | Doing laundry | .4 | Cooperating with others |
| .5 | Traveling | .5 | Supervising independent people |
| .6 | Telephoning | .6 | Keeping informed |
| .7 | Adjusting to change | .7 | Engaging in good citizenship |
| .8 | Other | .8 | Other |
| .9 | Unspecified | .9 | Unspecified |

drying, and putting lotion on hands. Washing and drying hair and other parts of the body are excluded. Care of the skin on the face and hands may be included, but application to the rest of the body should be included in bathing.

*10.1 Dressing* includes selecting and putting clothes on with a consideration of time of day, temperature, season, comfort, and how various garments go together. Dressing includes obtaining clothing from storage areas, dressing and undressing in a sequential manner, fastening and adjusting clothing and shoes, donning and doffing assistive or adaptive equipment, prostheses, or orthoses.

*10.2 Bathing* includes using soap, water, towel, and toiletries to clean, rinse, dry, moisturize, and deodorize body and hair. Bathing may be done anywhere: in bed, bathroom, tub, or shower. This category excludes grooming.

*10.3 Walking and exercising* includes awareness of how to move a normal body to different locations in space or through different movement patterns.

*10.4 Eating* includes sitting at the table, putting food in the mouth, cutting food into bite-sized pieces, chewing and swallowing without letting food escape, removing food that soils from face, hands, clothes, or eating area, adjusting pace and sequence according to food temperature, adjusting seasonings, and opening unusual packages.

*10.5 Toileting* includes recognizing the need to void, going to the bathroom, closing door, adjusting garments, sitting down, voiding, wiping body clean, readjusting garments, flushing, washing and drying hands, and leaving bathroom.

*10.6 Taking medication* includes recognizing the reason for taking medication, knowing when and how much to take, remembering to take, opening and closing containers, obtaining the correct amount, swallowing, and reporting adverse effects to the physician.

*10.7 Using adaptive equipment* includes recognizing a physical disability, recognizing an object as a substitute for normal ability, accepting the equipment, and learning to use the equipment.

*10.8 Other*

*10.9 Unspecified*

## 11. Situational Awareness Disability

A situational awareness disability is a disturbance in the ability to register and understand relations between objects in situations of daily living. Situational awareness includes the activities that one does at home and in the community that are basic to living in a social group. Once again the activities analyzed are common and probably cross-cultural.

*11.0 Housekeeping* includes recognizing the accumulation of dust, dirt, and clutter; getting cleaning supplies, sweeping, mopping, or vacuuming floors; washing, dusting and polishing furniture, windows, mirrors, utilities, and bric-a-brac; cleaning toilet, bath tub, shower, sinks in bathroom and kitchen, and counters; keeping drawers, closets, and cupboards tidy; picking things up and putting them away; deciding when things need to be repaired, replaced, or discarded; and emptying trash. This category excludes preparing food and sharing in family activities.

*11.1 Preparing/obtaining food* includes taking an inventory of food stuffs on hand, planning a balanced diet, preparing a grocery list, obtaining food, storing food, following a recipe, timing dishes, setting the table, serving food, cleaning the food preparation area and utensils, washing the dishes and the table, and discarding spoiled or uneaten food. This category excludes eating, and sharing in family activities.

*11.2 Spending money* includes understanding the value of local currency, recognizing situations that require payment for goods and services; being aware of current prices, calculations of cost, change, and remaining money; accounting for money spent; adjusting to price changes as well as changes in personal income; anticipating future purchases; paying bills; using credit; balancing a checkbook; and planning for financial security. This category excludes shopping.

*11.3 Shopping* includes deciding on items needed, visiting stores and malls to examine goods; checking mail order catalogues and advertised sales or specials; remembering intent to purchase; locating goods within a store; comparing goods and prices; recognizing budget and adjusting purchases according to what one can afford; deciding on method of payment; and protecting currency, checks, and credit cards from theft. Excludes spending money.

*11.4 Doing laundry* includes recognizing when clothes are dirty; placing them in a hamper; sorting according to method of cleaning and color; loading the washing machine or sink and washing; sorting for drying; loading the dryer; hanging or lying flat to dry; ironing by need and setting for fabric; hanging things up or folding; simple mending to replace buttons or holes in seams; and putting; clothing and linens away. Hand laundry, machine laundry, and dry cleaning are included.

*11.5 Traveling* includes using a vehicle as a means of conveyance for the self or objects inside buildings and around the community. Vehicles include carts, wagons, wheelchairs, bicycles, cars, buses, trains, and airplanes. Traveling may consist of selecting a destination; deciding on means of transportation and route and time to go and return; collecting objects needed for the trip; and finding one's way there and back. This category excludes walking and major role disability.

*11.6 Telephoning* includes understanding how to use the telephone; deciding to make a call; obtaining and dialing numbers; leaving messages; answering the telephone; relaying messages; accounting for time zone changes; recognizing an emergency and using emergency numbers and paying the telephone bill. The category excludes talking.

*11.7 Adapting to change in routine* includes recognizing out-of-the-ordinary situations presented by material objects; differentiating change from a hazard or an emergency; identifying different ways of adjusting; adjusting one's usual pattern of motor actions; and evaluating and refining one's course of action. Safety protocols already known by the individual are excluded as are responses to emergency situations.

*11.8 Other*

*11.9 Unspecified*

## 12. Occupational Role Disability

An occupational role disability is a "disturbance in the ability to organize and participate in routine activities connected with the occupation of time, not only confined to the performance of work" (ICIDH, 1980, p. 152). Occupational roles identify the activities that the individual does during the day, which may be done in isolation but are still constrained by social standards of performance. The list of activities that people do as a part of their occupational role is enormous. Cognitive abilities that are essential factors in doing a variety of activities are identified and analyzed.

*12.0 Planning/doing major role activities* is the organization of one's time to fulfill primary obligations such as going to work or school and being a homemaker. A major role includes following a schedule, informing, negotiating, and collaborating with others about changes in schedule, and considering secondary effects that changes in scheduled activities might have on others.

*12.1 Planning/doing spare-time activities* is the organization of one's time to do elective activities that may or may not require adherence to a schedule. Activities done with others have the same cognitive demands as major role activities. Activities done alone include scheduling one's own time and timing actions to avoid interfering with others.

*12.2 Pacing and timing actions* is the regulation of speed and energy within a given period of time. Pacing includes conserving, expending, or exhausting available energy within the constraints of available time. Timing includes regulating, calculating, adjusting, or setting a time period for frequency of repeated actions, sequence of steps, and duration to complete several steps.

*12.3 Exerting effort* is the physical and mental energy put forth to get something done. Moving includes the mental regulation of strength, range of motion, coordination, posture, and position in space while trying to get something done. Trying includes the mental regulation of concentration, persistence, and bringing back related memories while getting something done.

*12.4 Judging results* is the act of the mind in comparing the effect of one's actions on material objects and other people according to a social standard. The effects of placing objects can be judged according to location in a designated area, arrangement into groups that are alike, or by direction in following a real or imagined line. The effects of determining amount can be judged according to liquid measure, linear measure, equivalence, or completeness.

*12.5 Speaking* includes the volume, rate, and clarity of pronunciation with precise vocabulary and intelligible sentences. The content of speech includes an awareness of self, situation, and material objects. Speaking conforms with the social rules for language; it excludes communicating meaning.

*12.6 Following safety precautions* includes being aware of and complying with protocols for known hazards to prevent accidents and injuries and revising protocols to increase safety, efficiency, or comfort. Under ordinary circumstances hazards are noxious stimuli that produce temporary discomfort. The category excludes adjusting to change, responding to emergencies, and caring for dependents.

*12.7 Responding to emergencies* includes a response to a sudden, unexpected occurrence of urgency, requiring immediate action. Emergencies require recognizing sudden change, evaluating the change's potential severity as a serious threat to health or property damage, taking action to seek needed help, acting to reduce further accidents or injuries, and acting to provide aid. This category excludes adjusting to change, following safety precautions, and caring for dependents.

*12.8 Other*

*12.9 Unspecified*

### 13. Social Role Disability

A social role disability is a disturbance in a person's ability to meet social expectations when interacting with other people. Social roles identify the activities that are done with other people; the meaning of these activities is defined by the social context.

*13.0 Communicating meaning* is the act of perceiving, identifying, acknowledging, and accepting the impact that one's words have on other people. Meaning includes recognizing the intent and effect that is conveyed, denoted, signified, or understood by communicating with utterances, gestures, signs, and language. This category excludes speaking.

*13.1 Following instructions* is the act of perceiving, identifying, acknowledging, and accepting the directions given to one's self by other people. Instructions can be communicated with utterances, gestures, signs, or language. Instruction includes a systematic method of teaching, drilling, or training. Indoctrination and enlightenment are beyond the realm of rehabilitation and are excluded.

*13.2 Contributing to family activities* is giving

one's time and effort to tasks that are desirable to the family unit. The family unit includes the members of the household where the individual lives. If a patient lives alone and has no family, use the closest viable social group. Included is a consideration for the time and effort given versus demands made. This category excludes housekeeping, doing laundry, eating, obtaining and preparing food, shopping, and spending money.

*13.3 Caring for dependents* is watchful, conscientious effort to protect others from harm, accident, or injury. Dependents include children, adults who are sick or disabled, and animals. Caring includes recognizing hazards, preventing access to dangerous situations, warning others, and instructing in safety procedures. This category excludes adjusting to change, following safety procedures, and responding to emergencies.

*13.4 Cooperating with others* includes working or acting with another person(s) in an agreeable manner for a mutual benefit. This category excludes caring for dependents and supervising independent people.

*13.5 Supervising independent people* includes planning activities and influencing employees, subordinates, and peers. This includes making a differentiation between dependent and independent people and acting accordingly.

*13.6 Keeping informed* includes acquiring new information about local and world events to relate one's own activities to a social framework of conventions and expectations. This excludes engaging in good citizenship and spare-time activities.

*13.7 Engaging in good citizenship* is fulfilling one's duties and obligations as expected by society. Citizenship includes protecting the public from injury with ordinary and reasonable care. This excludes adjusting to change, following emergency procedures, responding to emergencies, and caring for dependents.

*13.8 Other*

*13.9 Unspecified*

## Activity Analysis

The rehabilitation literature contains descriptions of the above activities as they are affected by physical disabilities, which are usually much shorter. The longer descriptions are required because the impact of a cognitive disability is more pervasive. Thera-

pists may find these descriptions useful when discussing treatment goals with patients and caregivers. Common problems may be identified and individual priorities can be established. Therapists should expect to encounter additional problems not covered by these descriptions. When that occurs, therapists need to know how to analyze the cognitive complexity of those activities that are important to the individual.

To reduce the amount of analysis that therapists have to do, two forms of analysis are provided in this text: A general analysis by the 6 cognitive levels and a more detailed analysis by the modes of performance. The RTI-2 (Appendix B) contains the general analysis, and chapter 7 has a detailed analysis of self-awareness and situational activities. Different purposes may be achieved with these two types of descriptions. Longitudinal studies that describe the consequences of a disability for health care planning purposes may be chosen to use the RTI-2. Measures of treatment effectiveness may be detected by the modes of performance.

The reader should note that the rest of the book will not focus on occupational and social role disabilities. The most detailed description of role disabilities is located on the RTI-2. No attempt is made to analyze role activities because the tasks are so varied and heavily influenced by cultural differences. Therapists should use the modes of performance described in chapter 5 to analyze role performance activities. The processes described in chapter 6 and the activities described in chapter 7 can be used as examples of how to do an activity analysis according to the modes of performance. The most efficient way to do activity analysis is to specify what the activity consists of, as done in this chapter. Then apply the modes of performance of the activity to detect the cognitive demands of each step of the activity.

An alternative approach is to try to remember all of the steps and behaviors described, like remembering everything described in chapters 6 and 7. The human brain does not seem to be able to retain all of that information. When students have tried to remember lists of behaviors observed while doing activities, they usually lose the concept of a mode as a whole system. Accurate assessments of performance require an understanding of the modes as a unit of behavior. When students have tried to remember the steps of the activity and the modes, they usually understand the whole system as an integrated unit. And their evaluations and treatment goals improve.

To learn how to do an activity analysis, start with the easy material. Learn the descriptions of the self-awareness and situational awareness activities, most of which you already know. Select a mode of performance, like 4.4 and think about how that mode differs from the adjacent modes, like 4.2 and 4.6. Write down what you would expect to see in the self-awareness activities and then compare it to the descriptions in chapter 7. Remember that you can expect eating to be one cognitive level higher, like 5.4. Take the same mode and select an action from the beginning of chapter 6. Write down what you would expect to see and then compare it to the description. You can repeat that learning process with all of the modes, activities, and actions. This book is designed to give you feedback about the accuracy of your activity analysis so that you confidently can analyze any activity that is important to your patient.

## References

Allen, C.K. (1990). *Allen cognitive level test manual (with kit included)*. Colchester, CT: S & S/ Worldwide.

Allen, C.K. (1985). *Occupational therapy for psychiatric diseases: Measurement and management of cognitive disabilities*. Boston: Little, Brown.

Allen, C.K. (1982). Independence through activity: The practice of occupational therapy (psychiatry). *American Journal of Occupational Therapy, 36,* 731-739.

Earhart, C.A., & Allen, C.K. (1988). *Cognitive disabilities: Expanded activity analysis*. Colchester, CT: S & S/Worldwide.

Heimann, N. E., Allen, C. K., & Yerxa, E. J. (1989). The routine task inventory: a tool for describing the functional behavior of the cognitively disabled. *Occupational Therapy Practice, 1,* 67-74.

Josman, N., & Katz, N. (1991). Problem solving version of the Allen Cognitive Level (ACL) test. *American Journal of Occupational Therapy, 45,* 331-338.

Feinstein, A.R. (1987) . *Clinimetrics*. New Haven, CT: Yale University Press.

Katz, N., & Heimann, N. (1990). Review of research conducted in Israel on cognitive disability instrumentation. *Occupational Therapy in Mental Health, 10,* 1-15 .

Mayer, M.A. (1988). Analysis of information processing and cognitive disability theory. *American Journal of Occupational Therapy, 42,* 176-183 .

McDowell, I., & Newell, C. (1987). *Measuring health: A guide to rating scales and questionnaires*. New York; Oxford University Press.

Newman, M. (1987). Cognitive disability and functional performance in individuals with chronic schizophrenic disorders. Unpublished master's thesis, University of Southern California.

Reed, K.L. (1991). *Quick index of occupational therapy*. Gaithersburg, MD; Aspen Publishers.

Wilson, D.S., Allen, C.K. McCormack, G., & Burton, G. (1989). Cognitive disability and routine task behaviors in a community based population with senile dementia. *Occupational Therapy Practice, 1,* 58-66.

World Health Organization. (1980). *International classification of impairments, disabilities, and handicaps* . Geneva, Switzerland: Author.

## Part II: The Large ACL

*Kathy Kehrberg*

The ACL has been a useful screening tool for cognitive deficits in geriatric patients. It is used at the Minneapolis Department of Veterans Affairs Medical Center in the Geriatric Research and Clinical Center (GRECC) during initial evaluations of patients' functional abilities and deficits. It has also been used as a quick assessment tool to anticipate an inpatient's potential performance in individual self-care activities of daily living (ADLs) or in group activity sessions. The use of the ACL does not rely on the patient's verbal abilities. Persons with aphasia and word-finding problems can demonstrate their cognitive functioning level. Conversely, well-preserved verbal skills cannot obscure functional deficits that can be detected with the ACL.

The occupational therapists in this facility use both the ACL screening test and the Cognitive Performance Test (CPT) (also presented in this chapter) to provide complete evaluations and to monitor cognitive changes in persons who have been identified as having dementia and who return for follow-up appointments every 6 months. For both the initial visit and follow-up appointments, the patients typically see a neurologist, social worker, nurse clinician, psychometrist, and occupational therapist. Medical and psychological tests are ordered as needed to answer diagnostic questions. Patients and family members are then given information and ongoing support to deal with the cognitive changes that are being experienced by the patient and affect both patient and family. Often the question of driving cars and using farm equipment or other hazardous tools and machinery comes into question.

Once the Allen level of functioning is determined, therapists can alert family members to the amount and type of assistance the patient will require to complete daily activities. They can also recommend therapeutic approaches and specify safety concerns to the GRECC clinic team, patient, and family members.

One of the problems that the therapists have encountered in using the ACL is that older patients may experience difficulties in visual acuity due to failing eyesight, cataracts, and/or difficulty with fine-motor tasks due to arthritis or sensory impairment. Persons may be unable to distinguish the two sides of the brown flat lace on the ACL or be unable to untwist the lace as they attempt to do the whip and cordovan stitches. The running stitch presents fewer problems to older persons, but the holes may be hard to see and the sharp needle can be a hazard for more severely impaired patients who have put it in their mouth or poked it in the finger placed behind the empty hole.

It was these problems that led to the development of the large ACL, or LACL, for use in geriatrics. The LACL uses a brown shoelace for the running stitch, a wider lace painted white on the wrong side for the whip and single cordovan stitches, and a larger leather base with bigger holes, as demonstrated in Figure 10.1. The original base has been enlarged 1.41 times, and the holes follow the pattern shown in Figure 10.2. The score sheet and directions are from the ACL-E.

The validity of the larger tool was investigated through a controlled research study using 49 subjects matched for age and gender (Kehrberg, Mortimer, Kuskowski, & Shoberg, in preparation). All subjects were given both the ACL-E and LACL

tests in a split format to control for any practice effects. Concurrent validity was established with the Mini-Mental State Exam (MMSE) and the Routine Task Inventory (RTI). Scores on the LACL and the ACL-E correlated significantly ($p < .001$) with MMSE scores and with the scores on the physical and community subscales of the RTI. No significant difference was found between the scores on the ACL-E and LACL when controlled for practice effect and gender. The scores on the ACL-E and LACL were significantly correlated in both AD ($r = 0.95$, $p < .001$) and control subject groups ($r = 0.58$, $p < .001$). AD subjects were significantly impaired, compared to control subjects, on both lacing tests even when the effects of age (<75 years, >75 years), gender, and test order were controlled (LACL, $F(1, 71) = 73.96$, $p < .001$; ACL-E, $F(1,71) = 76.79$, $p < .001$).

In the AD group, the mean scores on the ACL-E were not statistically different across age groups (for ACL-E, $t(47) = 1.04$, n.s.; for LACL, $t(47) = 0.29$, n.s.). In the control group, age *was* significantly correlated in both the ACL-E ($r = -0.52$, $p < .01$) and LACL ($r = -0.51$, $p < .01$). When subjects above and below the age of 75 were compared, the mean score on both the ACL-E and LACL were significantly different. The older subjects did not perform as well as the younger subjects on both the ACL-E ($t(33) = 2.11$, $p < .05$) and the LACL ($t(33) = 2.45$, $p < .02$).

The original ACL-O research was carried out on adults up to the age of 60. While the control subjects in this study were selected because there was no known evidence of dementia or diminished capacities, these elderly controls did not have consistently top scores on the ACL-E or LACL. The mean ACL-E and LACL scores of control subjects <75 were also lower than the mean scores of those >75. One might surmise that "normal" elderly persons may, as a group, perform less well on this task without there being substantial impairment in independent functioning. For example, elderly persons may still be preparing food for themselves, but may no longer attempt to make the large, elaborate meals they prepared in the past. Minor impairments in older persons may include such factors as reduced speed or efficiency of performance.

The ACL-E allows for only two demonstrations to learn the single cordovan, the most complex stitch. Studies related to speed of learning and response rates in the elderly indicate there is a decline in those factors as persons age (Hale, Myerson, &

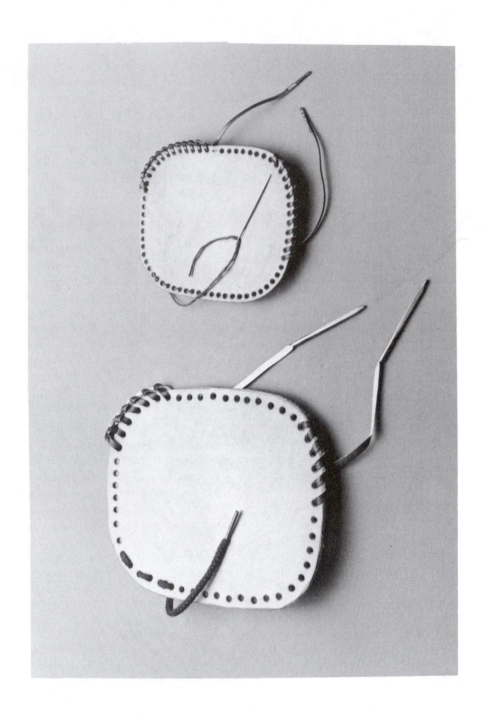

Figure 10.1   Brown shoelace used for running stitch in LACL

Figure 10.2 The enlarged ACL

## Materials

- 6–8 oz. cowhide (1/8" thick) for the base
- Very thin natural calf works well for the back pocket
- Two 36" pieces of dark brown florentine lace; Tandy # 5006*
- Two "life eye" latigo needles; Tandy #1213
- One 27" dark brown round braid shoe lace
- Small jar of white Cova Dye; Tandy #2041
- 11/64" drive punch—size 5 tube, Tandy #1768: handle #1767

(*Tandy Leather Company, PO Box 2934, Forth Worth, Texas 76113.)

## Assembly

Cover back side of wide lace with two coats of white dye; a small stencil brush or Q-tip works well. The front of the cowhide and the brown side of the lace can be covered with protective clear finish, such as Neat Shene from Tandy.

Attach the back leather pocket using Barge or rubber cement, along the entire lower edge of the pocket. When almost dry, press the pocket into the back as down in the drawing, but do not allow the top part of the pocket to fit flush to the kit; pull it out so the tabs of the pocket line up with the tabs from the front piece, matching the holes.

Attach the brown shoelace off to the side at the bottom of the pocket. Attach the lace for the other two stitches where each of the pocket's tabs are joined. Place a small piece of self-stick velcro inside the top of the pocket to help hold the pocket shut.

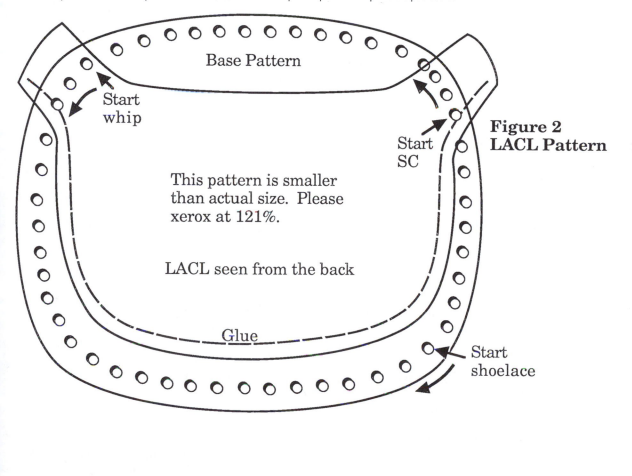

Base Pattern

Start whip

Start SC

Figure 2
LACL Pattern

This pattern is smaller than actual size. Please xerox at 121%.

LACL seen from the back

Glue

Start shoelace

Wagstaff, 1987; Rabbitt, 1980). In an article reviewing cognitive screening tools for use in geriatrics, Ritchie (1988) points out that there are very few elderly over 80 who do not experience the interactive effects of aging and several disease processes.

## Case Example

The following case example illustrates the value of the larger screening tool with this population.

Mr. K. initially came to the GRECC clinic in January of 1991 to be evaluated for possible dementia. He had been referred through one of the other medical clinics at the VA Medical Center. The patient is an 80-year-old widower, who has lived alone in his own home since his wife's death 11 years ago from amyotrophic lateral sclerosis (ALS). Mr. K. lives in a small town and has a married son nearby who checks in on him daily and helps manage his father's financial affairs. The son began to notice his father's memory problems approximately 1 year prior to the GRECC clinic visit. His father began to repeat comments and questions, misplace items, and was forgetting the names of familiar persons. Word-finding problems were noticed along with increased temporal confusion. Mr. K., however, did not feel that he was having any particular difficulties. There was no history or current symptoms of depression, hallucinations, or unusual behavior. Mr. K. reported sleeping well and had no appetite problems; his weight had been stable.

Past medical history included hypertension and adult-onset diabetes myelitis, treated in the past, but not at present. There was no known history of psychiatric or neurological problems. The patient suffered shrapnel wounds in World War Two, leaving him with residual right hand numbness from an ulnar nerve injury. Past surgeries included cholecystectomy in 1980, bilateral carpal tunnel repairs in 1980, bilateral knee arthroplasties in 1984, and left iridectomy in 1990. The patient has had arthritis for a number of years. He currently uses safety rails in the bathroom and depends on the use of a button hook to button his shirts,

Family history was significant for dementia in the patient's father, who was institutionalized for severe dementia prior to his death at age 75. Mr. K's four brothers died from strokes, heart attacks, or cancer. His two sisters are still living and in reasonably good health.

A physical examination revealed a mild to moderate dyspnea and a slightly elevated blood pressure that led to the consideration of medication possibilities. Mr. K. was not presently on any prescription medication. The resulting tentative diagnosis was primary degenerative dementia with superimposed orthopedic problems. A full dementia work-up was ordered, which included the ACL-E the Cognitive Performance Test.

Neuropsychological testing indicated the possibility of multifocal dysfunction as opposed to a progressive generalized dementia, and retesting was recommended again in 1 year,

## Occupational Therapy Evaluation

When Mr. K. was given the ACL-E, he was able to distinguish the right from the wrong side of the brown lace. He had managed to complete his whip stitches without significant twisting. When shown the whip stitch twist, he could recognize the error, but not manipulate the lace successfully to correct the error.

The patient was then given the LACL, which was much easier for him to handle with his arthritic hands. He was able to correct the twist mistake and continue with the single cordovan stitch, scoring 4.5. Mr. K's score on the LACL was more accurate as it did allow him to complete the task to the best of his cognitive abilities and he was not penalized because he lacked the physical ability to manipulate the smaller lace.

The score of 4.5 for this patient was fairly consistent with his overall performance on the complete CPT battery, where his total performance score was slightly better than level 4. Interviewing his son with the RTI showed 4.5 behaviors on the physical subscale and 4.3 on the community subscale.

Another situation where the LACL proves useful is when patients do not have corrective eye wear or have forgotten their glasses at home. In that situation, they may attempt the ACL-E, but not get an accurate score. They often are unable to adequately distinguish the two sides of the flat lace when doing the whip twist and cordovan stitches well enough to eliminate errors. Mr. K. had forgotten his glasses for his clinic appointment. He was able to identify the right and wrong sides of the flat lace prior to the task. When asked to correct the twist during the test, the two sides appeared more blurred to him when the stitches were close together and he could not proceed. When given the LACL, Mr. K. achieved a score of 4.7, which more accurately represented his cognitive abilities.

## Interpretation of Scoring

### Case Example of Mr. K.

At a family meeting with GRECC staff, the patient and his family were given the results from all the diagnostic tests and appropriate recommendations. The recommendations from occupational therapy specifically related to daily activities.

Mr. K. had a strong desire to remain as independent as possible in his own home. His son was willing to check on him daily and, as yet, had not encountered serious problems in the home. The son did most of the shopping, had power of attorney, and gave his Dad only small amounts of cash for incidentals. A housekeeper provided assistance with cleaning and so far, the patient had managed to do his own laundry. The son had noticed occasional dressing errors, and attention to personal hygiene had been diminishing. Mr. K. had been preparing his own breakfast and a light evening meal. He still insisted on driving to the Senior Center for his noon meal and often drove the car in the country to visit friends. He had had two car accidents prior to his cataract surgery and now felt that his driving was safe due to his improved vision.

Both family and GRECC staff encouraged the patient to discontinue driving. The Senior Center could be reached by walking or using the city bus, and Mr. K. was familiar with both of these options. His overall level of cognitive impairment also indicated that a more supervised living situation would be desirable. The fact that Mr. K.'s functional abilities were consistently at level 4+ or approximately level 4.5 was a cause for concern with his present living situation. The patient's lack of awareness of his deficits and his prognosis of continued decline led the staff to make recommendations for a safer environment. Other options and possibilities available in the patient's community were explored with the GRECC social worker.

### Other Situations

When discrepancies exist between the full functional battery (CPT) and the ACL screening tool, the therapist will look for explanations. Sometimes persons who have worked for years in jobs demanding good manipulative skills will perform slightly better on the ACL than the CPT. In those instances, their overall performance scores will be seen as more accurate and used to make specific recommendations. Patients with higher ACL scores often have the interest and desire to continue to do construction, carpentry, auto mechanics, or home maintenance tasks that they have done all of their life. They may begin to experience less success and more frustration in the process or be overconfident of their skills, and family members should be alerted to safety issues.

Conversely, significant difficulties with visuospatial relationships and new learning have been reflected by poorer ACL scores and somewhat better CPT scores as persons may continue to perform familiar daily tasks with slightly more success than they can achieve on the ACL screening test. In these cases, the lower ACL score will tend to more accurately predict the person's true abilities to handle new learning and problem-solving situations.

In summary, an adapted screening tool such as the LACL may not be needed with many patients, but it can be extremely useful in selected cases. Some elderly patients, who can see and manipulate both the ACL and LACL prefer the LACL because it is more comfortable to handle, and the larger size is easier for them to see. Since the LACL has not produced inflated scores and the research has found the results of the two versions comparable, the therapists at GRECC have used the LACL with patients who seemed less confident or apprehensive when initially given the ACL. For elderly patients who have significant visual and manipulative deficits, the LACL can provide accurate Allen level screening of cognitive performance abilities.

## References

Hale, S., Myerson, J., & Wagstaff, D. (1987). General slowing of nonverbal information processing: Evidence for a power law. *Journal of Gerontology, 42,* 131–136.

Kehrberg, K.L., Kuskowski, M.A., Mortimer, J.A., & Shoberg, T.D. (in preparation). *Validating the use of an enlarged, easier-to-see Allen cognitive level test in geriatrics.* Minneapolis: Geriatric Research Education and Clinical Center, Veterans Affairs Medical Center.

Rabbitt, P.M. (1980). A fresh look at changes in reaction time in old age. In E.G. Stein (Ed.), *The psychobiology of aging: Problems and perspectives* (pp. 425-445). New York: Elsevier.

Ritchie, K. (1988). The screening of cognitive impairment in the elderly; a critical review of current methods. *British Journal of Epidemiology, 41*(7), 635-643.

## Part III: The Cognitive Performance Test: An Approach to Cognitive Level Assessment in Alzheimer's Disease

*Theressa Burns*

### Introduction

Alzheimer's disease (AD), the most common form of a dementing illness, results in a progressive decline of cognitive and functional abilities. Medical services are geared to supporting the special needs of persons with AD, including assistance and supervision with activities of daily living (ADLs), and the prevention or remediation of excess disability. Services also support the care given by families and health care workers, for example, through education and training in caregiving techniques.

Comprehensive assessment of the patient and caregiver(s) provides information for making decisions such as those concerning a feasible living situation, supportive services (i.e., adult daycare, home health care, meals on wheels, etc.), and guardianship. Assessment is an ongoing process that identifies interventions appropriate to the changing status of the patient and available caregiving resources.

Assessment of the decline associated with AD has focused on changes in cognitive ability, the Mini-Mental State Examination (MMSE) being the most commonly used measure to assess progression (Folstein, Folstein, & McHugh, 1975). Although studies have shown that the MMSE score decreases over time in patients with AD, usually it reaches a floor in the later stages of the disease, and it may lack sensitivity in very mild patients (Naugle & Kawczak, 1989). Furthermore, the MMSE does not directly measure the clinical impact of the disease.

The assessment of functional abilities in Alzheimer patients has taken a variety of approaches, including caregiver report and direct observation of patient abilities. Several instruments have been developed specifically to stage function in demented individuals, including the Global Deterioration Scale (Reisberg, Ferris, Deleon, & Crook, 1982); Functional Assessment Stages (Reisberg, et al., 1984); and the Clinical Dementia Rating Scale (Hughes, Berg, Danziger, Coben, & Martin, 1982). All of these instruments rely on caregiver-derived information, which is essential for a comprehensive view of the patient. However, assessment by an informant in-

troduces the possibility of rater basis (Rubenstein, Schairer, Wieland, & Kane, 1984). Furthermore, it is not uncommon to see patients who have no caregiver, as in those who are living alone.

ADL performance tests for use with demented subjects have been developed to provide a more objective measure of function than caregiver report. Some rate the successful completion of selected ADL tasks or their components, while assessment of the cognitive complexity of the tasks is not a primary focus (Lowenstein, et al., 1989; Mahurin, DeBettignies, & Pirozzoio, 1991). Other observational ADL scales (Kapust & Weintraub, 1988; Sandman, Norberg, Adolfsson, & Hedley, 1986) assess specific cognitive impairments in demented patients. A third approach has been to evaluate the types of assistance required to complete specified tasks (Beck, 1988; Skurla, Rogers, & Sunderland, 1988). While these instruments are valuable in pointing out impairments and assistance needs in specific tasks or particular types of cognitive deficits that affect ADL performance, there is no easy way to generalize the findings to identify a global stage of functional deficit. The delineation of stages of function facilitates the measurement of change and provides boundaries and guidelines for stage-specific activity and care recommendations.

### Cognitive Performance Test

The Cognitive Performance Test (CPT) was developed to provide a standardized, ADL-based instrument for the assessment of functional level in AD. It differs from other ADL assessments in that its basis is Allen's information-processing system delineated by the cognitive levels. The focus in this instrument is placed on the degree to which particular deficits in information processing compromise common functional activities. The specific tasks that are selected, while having face validity, are less important than the manner in which patients respond to demands of varying complexity. Because performance is interpreted within the Allen model, the deficits observed on CPT tasks have implications for the performance of a wide variety of ADLs.

The CPT was initially conceived as a research instrument, to be used in longitudinal study of functional change over time, or for serial assessment to detect change in response to a pharmacological or environmental intervention. It has also proved very useful in clinical assessment of patients to predict their capabilities to function in various contexts. Previous studies suggest the applicability of cognitive level assessment to demented patients and support the predictive function of the model (Heyings, 1985; Kehrberg & Schoberg, in press; Wilson, Allen, McCormack, & Burton, 1989).

The CPT is composed of common ADL tasks for which the information-processing requirements can be systematically varied to assess the Allen cognitive level. Routine activities were selected since in dementia, performance anxiety tends to increase in unfamiliar or abstract activities. Furthermore, colleagues and families may understand to a greater degree ADL recommendations based on direct assessment in ADL. Administration of the entire battery takes approximately 45 minutes.

The test includes six tasks, entitled *Dress, Shop, Toast, Telephone, Wash,* and *Travel.* Each task requires standardized equipment, set-up, and methods of administration that involve the sequential elimination or inclusion of sensory cues as difficulty with performance is observed. For example, if difficulty is observed with locating a telephone number, the telephone book, which requires use of symbolic cues, is removed and the printed number is given. If dialing is not initiated, the number, requiring use of visual cues, is removed and nonspecific dialing is demonstrated (inclusion of manual cues) for imitation.

For each task, a specific set of verbal instructions is initially given to the subject. The tester then performs the standardized interactions that correspond to specific patient behaviors. In essence, the tester changes the task demands in response to deficit behaviors by controlling or simplifying the information-processing requirements of the task. Complete task protocols and administration procedures are given in Appendix C.

CPT tasks *Shop, Telephone,* and *Travel* score to level 6. *Dress, Toast,* and *Wash* score to level 5, since performance of these less complex tasks does not require level 6 ability and persons functioning at either level 5 or 6 would perform similarly on these tasks. A level score of 3.5 was added to each task since it appeared that some subjects continued to use visual cues and remain goal focused, hallmarks of level 4 performance, but they required additional verbal cues and support to complete, or nearly complete, each task. Clinically, the identification of behavior consistent with level 3.5 has been useful in determining the need for 24-hour supervision. The

total test score, with a range of 6 to 33, is obtained by summing individual task scores. Multiplying each Allen level by 6, or by the number of CPT tasks, gives the projected total CPT score for each of the cognitive levels. CPT scores that fall between the levels are used to indicate high or low functioning within a level.

Subjects should score at or close to the same level for all 6 tasks. However, since individual task scores may differ, the total CPT score is used as the average representation of performance. The fact that subjects may not score at the same level across tasks points to either deficiencies in the test itself, or that task behavior has a range that will normally fluctuate, a concept in concert with Allen's redefinition of the model as an open system (chapter 1). Statistical analyses of exact score agreement between tasks suggests that the validity of the CPT decreases as tasks are eliminated. However, administration of all 6 tasks appears to offer a valid representation of global task ability. (Spearman correlations between each individual task score and the CPT total score [item–scale correlations] were highly significant.)

Development of the CPT began in 1985, with Allen's first book. Therefore, CPT scoring reflects the descriptions of the cognitive levels at that time. The recent distinctions between a nonambulatory status at cognitive level 1, an ambulatory status at cognitive level 2, and the range from grasping to the manipulation of objects at cognitive level 3, do not hold true for the CPT. Persons can score at level 1 whether or not they are ambulatory, and persons need to grasp CPT objects in order to score at level 2. In testing, the difference between levels 1 and 2 is essentially the ability to attend to and grasp moving objects. The difference between levels 2 and 3 is the ability to manipulate objects in some meaningful manner. Thralow and associates (in press) have used the CPT extensively with persons functioning at the lower levels. Their studies demonstrate strong correlations between the CPT total score and scores from their nursing observation scales for the identification of Allen cognitive levels in four self-care tasks.

The CPT does not tap the full range of abilities associated with level 6 functioning. For example, persons who have reported difficulty with high-level ADLs such as managing finances, may perform the CPT without error. Further development of the CPT could include the addition of level 6 components to level 5 tasks; the redefinition and expansion of scores to more accurately reflect the current model or to increase sensitivity within each cognitive level; and the formal study and adaptation of the CPT to other diagnostic groups.

## Reliability and Validity Studies

Studies of the CPT were carried out at the Minneapolis VA Medical Center's Geriatric Research, Education, and Clinical Center (GRECC). A complete description of methodology and results is available in the literature (Burns, Mortimer, & Warmbler, 1991). Seventy-seven patients with mild to moderate Alzheimer's disease and 15 normal elderly controls were administered the CPT. The Alzheimer subjects were participants in a longitudinal study sponsored by the National Institute of Aging (Burns, Mortimer, & Warmbler), in which subjects were recruited in the early stages of AD and followed over time. Control subjects were recruited from a pool of normal volunteers, and had no history of cognitive impairment nor reported problems with ADL.

For the 77-AD patient sample, CPT was significantly correlated with MMSE (r = 0.67) and two measures of caregiver-rated ADL (Instrumental Activities of Daily Living: r = 0.64; Physical Self-Maintenance Scale: r = 0.49) (funding support was provided by the National Institute on Aging [1 PO1 AG06309] and the Veterans Administration). Cronbach's alpha and item-scale correlations were uniformly high, implying that similar constructs are measured by the 6 different ADL tasks.

Subsets of the AD patients were assessed again at 4 weeks, and at 1, 2, and 3 years following the initial evaluation. Interrater reliability at 4 weeks was 0.91 (N = 18); test–retest reliability at 4 weeks was 0.89 (N = 36). Changes in CPT scores over 1 year were studied in 64 patients, over 2 years in 45 patients, and over 3 years in 26 patients. Attrition was due to either institutionalization or death. A significant decline in mean CPT scores from entry to year 1 was observed. Mean scores continued to significantly decline from year 1 to year 2, and from year 2 to year 3. These data from the 4-year follow-up period demonstrate that scores on the CPT decline with progression of the disease. Scores of normal controls showed little overlap with the initial scores of patients.

Predictive validity of the CPT was studied in relation to risk of institutionalization over the total period of follow-up. Patients were divided into those with high (>25.2) versus low (<25.2) scores on the CPT at the time of entry into the study. For the group with low CPT scores, the time at which 50% of the patients were institutionalized was 624 days versus 1,294 days for those with high CPT scores. The difference in survivorship of these two groups was highly significant. These findings were compared with those for MMSE scores at entry in the same patient sample. No significant difference in survivorship was found when patients were divided into groups with MMSE scores greater than or less than 17.5. In addition to providing an index of function at a single point in time, and an index of change in function over time, the initial CPT score is predictive of the long-term risk of institutionalization.

## Case Study Example

Mr. Jones is a 68-year-old white male who was initially seen in the GRECC memory loss clinic on January 17, 1990. He was accompanied by his wife of 45 years. They live in their own home and have two adult children who are both married with families of their own. Mr. Jones completed a 10th grade education at 16 years of age. He then worked as a laborer, and for the past 20 years, owned his own brick-laying business. After an altercation with his son, who worked in the business with him, he retired in 1989. Mrs. Jones characterized this as a semivoluntary retirement.

Mr. Jones' memory loss and behavioral changes were first noted in 1986 at this worksite, where he had difficulty naming, locating, and using tools that he had used all of his working life. The memory loss progressed to the point where he was unable to remember names of people or places well-known to him. His wife noted that word-finding difficulties had increased in recent years. Additionally, he has developed problems with attention and concentration, and is unable to read or watch television. He continues to drive on occasion.

Mrs. Jones reported that her husband sleeps 12 to 14 hours a day. He avoids social events and will not go out without her. She has tried unsuccessfully to engage him in a variety of activities. She is able to leave him home alone for several hours at a time without concern for safety. She handles the finances, shopping, meal preparation, and management of the household.

Mr. Jones' symptoms are described as slow onset with a steady deterioration and no marked fluctuation in either memory or behavioral symptoms. His history and clinical presentation are consistent with Alzheimer's-type dementia. On the initial visit to the GRECC, MMSE was 22/30 ($\leq$23 is indicative of dementing illness), CPT score was 30/33 or Allen level 5; ACL was 4.7. Affect appeared blunted. Verbalizations were appropriate but limited, as was his general fund of knowledge.

Soon after his initial visit to GRECC, Mr. Jones was entered into the GRECC Adapted Work Program (AWP), a 3-morning-a-week sheltered workshop for veterans in the early to middle stages of AD. The AWP is based on Allen's model in that tasks are selected and adapted to the cognitive level of the worker. A high degree of routine and repetition with the same tasks are other aspects of the program. Based on his performance of the CPT, Mr. Jones was taught level 5 jobs including surgical towel inspection, measuring rag strips, sorting bandages and a variety of slings, and pick-up/delivery of tasks from hospital departments. He worked at a normal to fast pace, anticipating the daily schedule, and achieved good quality in his work. Socializing with coworkers was minimal and limited to interactions with one worker in particular. RTI scores from the work scale were as follows:

- Maintaining pace/schedule—level 6
- Following instructions—level 5
- Performing simple versus complex tasks—level 5
- Getting along with coworkers—level 5

Mr. Jones was reevaluated on July 18, 1991. The MMSE score declined from 22 to 20; ACL declined from 4.7 to 4.4; CPT total score declined from 30 to 27. Performance on the follow-up CPT was as follows:

- Dress—patient selected and donned an inappropriate coat and hat in response to the initial task directions (score level 4);
- Shop—patient was able to follow the multistep directions for item selection and payment. He determined the amount of money given for purchasing, but required cuing to obtain all of the money from the wallet. He checked price tags, and made an appropriate selection based on size and price. Payment was accurate for the dollar amount and inaccurate for the coin amount (score level 5);
- Toast—patient began this task with buttering. After redirection to the toaster, task follow through was accurate and complete (score level 4);

- Telephone—patient required specific directions for whom to call for the price of paint. Use of the telephone book was slow but functional. Dialing was accurate. His ability to obtain and immediately relay the information was good (score level 5).
- Wash—patient required concrete directions for the initiation of this task. Follow through was complete and accurate (score level 4).
- Travel—patient was not able to follow the test map. Following concrete, printed directions to locate the structure was accurate (score level 5).

### Impression

Mr. Jones' performance of the CPT indicates an Allen cognitive level of 4.5. Persons functioning at this level demonstrate mild to moderate deficits in task planning, reasoning, and problem-solving abilities. These deficits prevent efficient and error-free performance of high-level ADLs (managing finances, meals, medications, home maintenance, etc.), which need to be assisted, or done by others. The performance of self-care ADLs may require some minimal assistance in the areas of planning and judgment (i.e., obtaining appropriate supplies, following a schedule). Due to impaired judgment, independent living poses a significant risk at this functional level; however, this is not an issue for this patient. Mr. Jones demonstrated impulsive behavior during testing, including difficulty with contemplating task instructions. Impulsive behavior coupled with deficits in interpreting complex information pose concerns for safety in hazardous activities. Supervision of such activities and discontinuance of driving in the near future are recommended. Since last evaluated on January 17, 1990, Mr. Jones demonstrates functional decline from level 5 to level 4.5

Task performance in the AWP has not changed and RTI work-scale scores from the above categories remain the same. This phenomenon of functional maintenance in the AWP with concurrent decline noted in other areas is observed in a number of AWP participants and requires further investigation. Social interactions for Mr. Jones have increased dramatically since he entered the program. For example, he routinely brings treats to share and passes these out individually to each worker. Additionally, he initiates his own work based on the jobs available for the day. Although he continues to sleep excessively and remains passive at home, Mrs. Jones reports that her husband's mood has improved and that he looks forward to the AWP. Since beginning the program, Mr. Jones has maintained near-perfect attendance.

## Conclusion

With the aging of society and increase in the incidence of Alzheimer's disease, more health care and research dollars have been allocated to study not only the causes of AD, but also treatments such as pharmacological, behavioral, and environmental interventions. Consequently, the direct assessment of functional status and change in function is gaining in importance and in application to the development of activity interventions.

## Acknowledgment

Appreciation is extended to Dianne Timmer, OTR, MBA, Joan Thralow, OTR, Peggy Merchak, OTR, and James Mortimer, PhD for assistance with the development and study of the CPT.

## References

Beck, C. (1988). Measurement of dressing performance in persons with dementia. *American Journal of Alzheimer's Care and Related Disorders Research, 3,* 21–25.

Burns, T., Mortimer, J., & Warmbler, P. (in press). *The cognitive performance test: A new approach to functional assessment in Alzheimer's disease.*

Folstein, M.F., Folstein, S., & McHugh, P.R. (1975). Minimental state: A practical method for grading the cognitive state of the patient for the clinician. *Journal of Psychiatric Research, 12,* 189–198.

Heyings, L. (1985). Research with subjects having senile dementia. In Allen, C.K. (Ed.), *Occupational therapy for psychiatric disease: Measurement and management of cognitive disabilities* (pp. 339–365). Boston: Little, Brown.

Hughes, C., Berg, L., Danziger, W., Coben, L., & Martin, R. (1982). A new clinical scale for the staging of dementia. *British Journal of Psychiatry, 140,* 566–572.

Kapust, L.R., & Weintraub, S. (1988). The home visit: Field assessment of mental status impairment in the elderly. *Gerontologist, 28,* 112–115.

Kehrberg, K., & Schoberg, T. (in press). Manuscript in preparation. Minneapolis, MN: VA Medical Center, GRECC.

Lawton, M.P., & Brody, E. (1969). Assessment of older people. Self-maintaining and instrumental activities of daily living. *Gerontologist, 9,* 179–196.

Lowenstein, D., Amigo, E., & Dura, R., et al. (1991). A new scale for the assessment of functional status in Alzheimer's disease and related disorders. *Journal of Gerontology, 46,* 58–66.

Naugle, R.J., & Kawczak, K. (1989). Limitations of the mini-mental state examination. *Cleveland Clinical Journal of Medicine, 56,* 277–281.

Reisberg, B., Ferris, S., Deleon, M., & Crook, T. (1982). The global deterioration scale for assessment of primary degenerative dementia. *American Journal of Psychiatry, 139,* 1136–1139.

Reisberg, D., Ferris S.H., & Armand, R., et al. (1984). Functional staging of dementia of the Alzheimer's type. *Annals of the New York Academy of Science, 435,* 481–483.

Rubenstein, L., Schairer, C., Wieland, D., & Kane, R. (1984). Systematic biases in functional status assessment of elderly adults: Effects of different data sources. *Journal of Gerontology, 39,* 686–691.

Sandman, P.O., Norberg, A., Adolfsson, R., Axelsson, K., & Hedley, V. (1986). Morning care of patients with Alzheimer type dementia. A theoretical model based on direct observations. *Journal of Advanced Nursing, 11,* 369–378.

Skurla, E., Rogers, J., & Sunderland, T. (1988). Direct assessment of activities of daily living in Alzheimer's disease. *Journal of the American Geriatric Society, 36,* 97–103.

Thralow, J. (in preparation). St. Cloud, MN: VA Medical Center, Rehabilitation Medicine Service.

Wilson, D.S., Allen, C.K., McCormack, G., & Burton, G. Cognitive disability and routine task behaviors in a community-based population with senile dementia. (1989). *Occupational Therapy Practice, 1,* 58-66.

# Appendix A—Allen Cognitive Level Test, 1990

## Preparation for Testing*

The leather lacing and linen thread need to be attached to the piece of leather prior to testing as follows:

1. One third of the holes on the perimeter will be used for each of the 3 stitches.

2. Cut 15 inches of the linen thread and tie a big knot at one end and thread the needle on the other end. Working from left to right, or in a clockwise direction complete at least 3 sewing stitches.

3. Cut 2 pieces of leather lacing 30 inches long and securely attach the leather lacing needles. Do at least 3 single cordovan stitches with the other piece. Continue to work in a clockwise motion.

4. Check to make sure that your needles go through the holes easily and make any necessary modifications.

5. Optional. You can put a finish on your leather if you want to protect it from getting dirty. You can wrap the lacing around the leather when not in use, or you can make a pocket out of another piece of leather or an index card, adhered to the back, to tuck the lacing into while testing.

To prepare yourself to administer the test you should do the following:

1. Practice holding the leather so the patient can see what you are doing. You should be able to do this with all three stitches while standing or sitting on the patient's left or right.

2. Memorize the verbal directions and then put the demonstration and verbal directions together.

3. Think about the setting where you might be giving the test and pick a location that offers the best light and the fewest distractions.

4. Construct a brief interview that you can administer to get to know the patient before you administer the test. If you can establish rapport with the patient, you are less likely to get a refusal to try the test. Note this: busy therapists are often

---

*Allen, C.K. (1990). Distributed by S&S/Worldwide, Colchester, CT 06415. Item number HC-98.

tempted to skip the sewing stitch when the patient is coherent during the interview. The time saved is rarely worth what is lost. If the patient does the running stitches easily he/she gains confidence to try the harder stitches. If the patient complains of visual impairments later in the test, you may be able to rule that out based on how the running stitch was done.

5. Stop the test when an error is made and not corrected. Score the highest level achieved.

**Maintenance.** In time the leather lacing will get worn out by twisting a lot and getting dirty, and the linen thread will fray. Replace the lacing/thread when that happens.

## Directions

Show the patient the leather lacing stitches.

**Have you ever done anything like this before?**

If yes, find out how much and how long ago. On occasion, you will find a person who has done a lot of lacing and you are not testing new problem-solving abilities.

### Running Stitch:

**"I am interested in seeing how you follow directions and concentrate. I will show you how to do a stitch now, so carefully watch what I do."**

The therapist holds the leather project so that it is facing both the therapist and the patient. Hold the leather at eye level so that the top and bottom can be seen.

**"Take the needle and push it down through the next hole and pull the thread through the hole. Push the needle up through the next hole. Pull the needle through the hole and tighten it. Don't skip any holes. Now you do it."**

Hand the leather and the needle to the patient. These verbal directions and demonstrations can be repeated once if the patient cannot complete the stitch on the first attempt.

### Whip Stitch:

If the patient is able to complete the running stitch, the therapist goes on to the whip stitch. The whip stitch verbal directions and demonstrations can be repeated once if the patient cannot complete the stitch on the first attempt.

**"See how the leather lace has one rough side and one smooth, dark, shiny side. Always keep the smooth, dark side up as you do each stitch, being**

careful not to twist the lace. Now I will show you another stitch. Watch me carefully. Take the lace and bring it around to the front, over the edge of the leather. Push the needle through the hole and tighten it. Make sure the lace isn't twisted. Don't skip any holes. Now you do 3 stitches."

### Whip Stitch Cross and Twist:

If the cross and/or twist occur spontaneously, you do not need to repeat this/ these problems.

"I'm going to make a mistake to see if you can correct it."

The therapist takes the lacing and holds the lacing below the hole in the back and proceeds to push the needle through from front to back. The needle goes through the loop and forms a cross in back. Hand the leather back to the patient.

"Can you show me my mistake?" "Can you fix it?"

If the patient can point out and correct the cross error, demonstrate the twist. The therapist takes the whip stitch lacing and twists 2 stitches. Make both twists clearly visible. Hand the leather back to the patient.

"I have made another mistake." "Can you show me my mistake?" "Can you fix it?"

A whip stitch cross and twist cannot be scored if visual impairments or language comprehension are alternative explanations for being unable to do this part of the test. Scores of 4.0 to 4.4 can be confounded by these factors. When in doubt, continue the test by going on to the single cordovan stitch.

### Single Cordovan Stitch:

Hand the leather to the patient and point to this stitch.

"Can you figure out how to do this stitch by yourself?" "Please tell me what you are thinking as you try to solve this problem."

The therapist's response to the patient's comments should be as nondirective as possible. If the patient asks if he/ she is doing it right, say "what do you think? or "you decide" or "keep trying." If the patient says "that's not right," say "can you fix it?", or "can you show me what is wrong?"

5.6 "Would like some help?"

If so, give a verbal cue with one piece of information such as "you have the first part right," or "go from front to back." If that does not help, try pointing out the error. Allow time for the patient to try to figure it out. This is not a timed test. Offer a demonstration if the patient looks lost, frustrated, or in danger of quitting.

"Would you like to be shown how?" If so, continue: "I'll show you how. Watch me carefully. Bring the needle around to the front of the leather. Push the needle through the next hole toward the back of the leather. Don't pull the lace tight but leave a small loop in it. Bring the lace over to the front of the leather again. This time put the needle through the loop you have made and pull the lace through it toward the back of the leather. Keep the lace to the left of the loop. Tighten the lace from the back hole, then tighten the long lace end. Make sure the lace isn't twisted. Now you do 3 stitches.

Encourage the patient to persevere until all twists are removed and tension is correct. Scores between 5.0 and 5.8 cannot be given when twist and tension errors are seen by the patient but not corrected.

An error made by the patient can be identified by pointing and saying "Does yours look like mine?" Ask the patient to fix a recognized error. If the patient does not see the error or chooses not to fix it, you can offer a second demonstration. Score the previous highest level achieved if there is a refusal of a second demonstration, a refusal to attempt to fix an error, or a refusal to attempt to try a stitch.

These guidelines for interacting with the patient during the testing procedures can be followed with the running and whip stitches, too.

## Allen Cognitive Levels Test Scoring Guidelines, 1990

*Note:* There are overlapping scores between the whip stitch and the single cordovan stitch at 4.0 to 4.4. If the scores do not match, score the single cordovan stitch. If the patient complains of visual problems or if the patient can: (1) execute 3 whip stitches, and (2) can fix the cross error, and (3) can identify twist errors but has difficulty fixing; then the administrator should continue the scoring process by scoring the single cordovan stitch. The administration of the single cordovan helps to clarify patient ACL score between 4.0 and 4.4.

### Running Stitch

### Level 3:

3.0 Grasps leather or pushes it away. No attempt is made to grasp the lacing.

3.1 Grasps the leather lacing. Aims the lacing toward a hole or moves the lacing about in a random pattern.

3.2 Pushes needle through at least one hole which can be the wrong location.

3.3 Pushes needle up and down, or back and forth, but ignores left to right direction or skips a hole.

3.4 Completes at least 3 running stitches with one demonstration and additional assistance. More than 3 running stitches are acceptable for this score.

## Whip Stitch

### Level 3:

3.5 Does at least one whip stitch but goes back to doing a running stitch.

3.6 Changes from whip stitch to running stitch but corrects error after 2nd demonstration: other whip stitch errors remain.

3.7 Does more than 3 whip stitches and may continue until out of space. Twists in the lacing are acceptable for this score.

3.8 Whip stitch lacing is crossed in back. Error is not recognized when pointed out and not corrected. Does more than 3 stitches.

3.9 Does 3 whip stitches and asks if that is enough, or "am I done?"

### Level 4:

4.0 Stops after 3 whip stitches are done; does recognize twists, or the cross in back as a error when pointed out.

4.1 Stops after 3 whip stitches are done and recognizes the cross in back as an error but is unable to correct the error.

4.2 Whip stitch is crossed in back and is able to pull it out and do 3 correct stitches. Twists are acceptable for this score.

4.3 Stops after 3 whip stitches are done and corrects by pulling the lacing out and redoing the stitch. A twist in the hole is acceptable for this score.

4.4 Pulls one whip stitch out and untwists at least one whip stitch without pulling it out.

## Single Cordovan

### Level 4:

4.2 Attempts to do the single cordovan stitch are

really a repeat of the whip stitch followed by an error such as not going through the loop, going through the same hole twice, or going on with the whip stitch

4.3 Does running stitch (by alternately inserting lacing needle front to back and back to front through hole) and needle goes through loop before going through next hole. Goes from back to front through the hole.

4.4 Goes from front to back through the hole (like the whip stitch) but inserts needle through loop from the back as if it is one step. (Lacing is under loop but does not wrap around it.)

4.5 Directionality goes front to back through the hole but back to front through the loop or vice versa.

4.6 Goes from front to back through the hole and the loop, but does not tighten. May go through the loop twice or go through the next hole.

4.7 Right/left orientation of lacing and needle are incorrect when going through the loop.

4.8 Lacing is not tightened in sequence (hole then loop), just pulls on needle with no recognition of error.

4.9 Lacing is not tightened in sequence. The error is recognized but not corrected. A third demonstration may be provided but the 3rd response is not scored.

### Level 5:

5.0 Corrects errors in directionality, tangled lace, or tightening in sequence but cannot replicate solutions. Requests a second demonstration but does not improve overall performance. Errors remain.

5.2 Corrects errors in directionality, tangled lace, or tightening in sequence with a second demonstration. If tightening is sequenced the tension may be a little loose but no other errors remain.

5.4 Corrects errors in directionality, tangled lace, or tightening in sequence without a second demonstration but by altering actions two or more times.

5.6 Attempts to do stitch without a demonstration but requires a cue (verbal or pointing to location of error) to do the stitch correctly.

5.8 Completes 3 single cordovan stitches without a demonstration by examining the sample stitches and using trial and error.

## Appendix B: Routine Task Inventory–2

### Routine Task Inventory–2 (RTI–2) Score Sheet

Codes:                                   NA = Not applicable

S = Self-report                          NT = Not tested

C = Caregiver report

O = Observation of performance

Score: The number recorded is the cognitive level. The therapist records the self-report and caregiver report as described.

| | S | C | O | | S | C | O |
|---|---|---|---|---|---|---|---|
| Grooming | | | | Housekeeping | | | |
| Dressing | | | | Getting food | | | |
| Bathing | | | | Spending money | | | |
| Walking/exercising | | | | Shopping | | | |
| Eating | | | | Doing laundry | | | |
| Toileting | | | | Traveling | | | |
| Taking medicines | | | | Telephoning | | | |
| Using adaptive equipment | | | | Adjusting to change | | | |
| Major role | | | | Communicating | | | |
| Spare time | | | | Following instructions | | | |
| Pacing/timing | | | | Family activities | | | |
| Exerting effort | | | | Dependents | | | |
| Judging results | | | | Cooperating | | | |
| Speaking | | | | Supervising | | | |
| Safety precautions | | | | Keeping informed | | | |
| Emergency response | | | | Citizenship | | | |

## Questions for Self-Report based on Routine Task Inventory

### Format

1. What does the activity consist of?

2. Frequency of activity?

3. Assistance required to complete the activity?

4. Social consequences of activity as performed?

5. Patient's awareness of social consequences?

### Physical Scale

#### A. Grooming

1. "What does your grooming consist of?"

2. "How often do you do these things?"

3. "Do others help you with any of these things?"

4. "Does anyone ever complain about your grooming/how you look/smell?"

5. "Do you agree with these complaints?"

#### B. Dressing

1. "How do you decide what to wear each day?"

2. "Are there days when you don't get dressed?"

3. "Does anyone help you decide what to wear or help you get dressed?"

4. "Does anyone ever complain about your clothes?"

5. "Do you agree with these complaints?"

#### C. Bathing

1. "Where do you bathe/shower?" "How do you get soap/towels?"

2. "How often do you bathe?"

3. "Does anyone assist you in any way?"

4. "Does anyone ever complain that you are not clean?"

5. "Do you agree with them?"

(Women only)

1. "What do you do to care for your menstrual flow?"

2. "How often do you change it?" "How often do you bathe during your period?"

#### D. Walking

1. "Where do you walk during the day?" "Do you ever go to new places?"

2. "How often?"

3. "Do you need help in finding new or familiar places?"

4. "Does anyone ever complain about you getting lost?"

5. "Do you think this is a problem?"

#### E. Feeding

1. "What does your diet consist of?" "Are you on a special diet?"

2. "How often do you eat?"

3. "Does anyone have to help you in any way during a meal?"

4. "Does anyone ever complain about your table manners?"

5. "Do you agree with these complaints?"

#### F. Toileting

1. "What do you do about going to the bathroom?" "How do you find a bathroom in a new place?"

2. "Does anyone help you in any way to use the toilet?"

3. "Does anyone ever complain about you failing to flush the toilet/ not making it to the bathroom/ urinating in a public place?"

4. "Do you think these things are problems?"

### Instrumental Scale

#### A. Housekeeping

1. "What do you do (at home/board and care) to keep your place/things clean?" (Transients: "What do you do when your blankets get dirty?")

2. "How often do you do these things?"

3. "Does anyone help you clean your room or straighten your things?"

4. "Does anyone ever complain about how your place/room looks?"

"Have you ever been evicted for not taking care of your place?"

5. "Do you agree with these complaints?"

#### B. Preparing/securing food

1. "How do you get your food?"

(Board and care) "How do you know when meals are served?"

(Cooks for self) "How do you heat things? Have you had trouble with burns/cutting yourself/setting fires?"

(Eat out) "Where do you eat? What is a typical order?"

2. "How often do you eat each day?"

3. "Does anyone ever help you with food preparation?"

(Board and care) "Do you have to be called to dinner?"

4. "Has anyone ever complained about how you cook or prevented you from cooking for any reason?"

5. "Do you think they had good reason for doing so?"

### C. Spending money

1. "Where do you get your money?" (Salary, SSI, Welfare, General Relief, savings, trust funds, insurance, prostitution, stealing, dealing, panhandling, credit cards)
"How much do you get each month?"
"What do you spend it on?"
"How often does your money run out?" "What do you do when this happens?"
"What do you do if your SSI check doesn't come?"
"Have you ever lost your money?"
"Do you have any savings/future securities?"

2. "Does anyone ever help you budget, spend your money, make change, or pay bills?"

3. "Have you a payee? Have you had your money handled by someone else at their request?" "Have people ever complained that you spend your money unwisely?"

4. "Do you agree with people who think that you have problems managing your money?"

### D. Taking medication

1. "What medications do you take?" "What are they for? When do you take them? How do you get refills? Do you have any problems with unwanted side effects? What do you do when this occurs?"

2. "Do you ever stop your medications?" "Why/for how long?" "Do you tell anyone?"

3. "Do you have to be reminded to take your medications? Does anyone help you figure out how many, how often to take your medication? Do you ever use a pill sorter?"

4. "Has anyone ever complained about you not taking your medication?"

5. "Do you agree with their complaints?"

### E. Doing laundry

1. "How do you get your clothes clean?"
"Do you have problems ruining/shrinking your clothes when you wash them?"

2. "How often do you do this?"

3. "Does anyone help you do your laundry?"

4. "Does anyone ever complain about the cleanliness of your clothes?"

5. "Do you think this is a problem?"

### F. Traveling

1. "How do you get places?" What trips have you taken lately?"
"Where do you anticipate going in the near future?"

2. "How often do you take trips?"

3. "Do you need help when you have to go somewhere?"

4. "Have you ever gotten lost/stranded on a trip?"

5. "Do you think these things are problems?"

### G. Shopping

1. "What do you shop for?" "Where do you shop?" "How much do your major purchases cost?" "What is your largest purchase each month?"

2. "How often do you shop?"

3. "Does anyone help you with your shopping?"

4. "Does anyone complain that your purchases are not wise, that you over- or underspend?" "Have you ever been caught shoplifting?"

5. "Do you agree with these complaints?"

### H. Telephoning

1. "What kinds of telephone calls do you need to make? How do you get the numbers to dial? Have you ever made an emergency call?"

2. "Does anyone help you with telephoning?"

3. "Has anyone ever complained that you make too many calls? Has anyone complained that you make unnecessary emergency calls? That you make calls you can't pay for?"

4. "Do you agree?"

### Addendum: Getting Medical Attention

1. "Have you ever had a medical emergency? What do you think is a medical emergency? How would you get help?"

2. "Where/when do you go to an emergency room? How often do you go? Has anyone ever complained that you go too often? Do you agree that this is a problem?"

3. "What symptoms will get you admitted to a hospital?"

4. "What would you do to stop bleeding?"

5. "What would you do to induce vomiting?"

6. "What would you do if someone stopped breathing?"

# Routine Task Inventory-2 (RTI-2)

**Scoring:** Record the cognitive level that best describes the pattern of behavior for each activity.

## 10. Self-Awareness Disability

### .0 Grooming

1. Ignores personal appearance.

May not hold head up or keep head turned to the side to cooperate with the caregiver.

2. Aware of caregiver's help to groom.

May spontaneously move or hold still to assist care giver, or

May actively resist caregiver.

3. Does daily grooming of brushing teeth, washing hands and face. Women may do basic cosmetics (lipstick). Supplies must be placed in front of the patient by the caregiver, or

May quit before completion of the task and require prompting to continue, requiring one-to-one supervision, or

May not be aware of time of day grooming is normally done, or

May be unconcerned about dirty hair, smudged makeup, smeared nail polish, jagged or long nails, or

May not be safe in using sharp instruments for shaving and nail trimming, or

May not be safe in using hot curling irons, hair straighteners, or blow dryers, or

May require removal of dangerous objects.

4. Initiates and completes grooming tasks.

May neglect the back of the head or body, or

May miss spots that are seen when pointed out, or Make-up may be too visibly striking and out of sociocultural context, or

May be concerned about appearance and ask for assistance in selecting and applying standard grooming products, or

May require supervision to avoid damage when using new products or timed products (curling irons, face masks).

5. Initiates and completes grooming without assistance.

### .1 Dressing

1. Generally ignores clothing unless cold or uncomfortable.

2. Aware of caregiver's efforts to dress the patient.

May spontaneously alter position to assist by putting hand in sleeve, foot in pants or shoe when the location is pointed out, or

May not use enough force to get the garment on without further assistance, or

May resist getting dressed, or

May require support for sitting/standing balance, or

May require periodic adjustments of garments throughout the day to keep them on properly.

3. Puts on basic garments, including shirt, pants, skirt, underwear, and shoes.

Clothes may be selected and laid out by the caregiver, or

May require assistance to finish dressing (zippers, laces, bra fasteners, button alignment), or

May be unconcerned about the selection of clothing or how one appears to other people, or

May be unaware of need to change clothes according to time of day, weather, or when soiled and resist requests to change, or

May be unconcerned about errors such as garments that are put on inside out, backwards, or underwear on top.

4. Follows a routine in getting dressed without assistance.

May have errors in button alignment, zipper completion, shirt tucked in the back, or labels showing and corrects errors when pointed out, or

May disregard errors in the back of garments or colors and patterns that are poorly coordinated, or

May disregard errors that are unbecoming because of size or current fashions, or

May avoid errors by following assistance with garment selection.

5. Selects own clothing and dresses without error.

### .2 Bathing

1. Bathed while lying in bed.

May require a Hoyer lift or several people to be lifted into a bathtub.

2. Assists caregiver efforts to bathe.

May stand in shower or sit in bathtub while soap and shampoo are applied and rinsed by caregiver, or

May use transfer board or grab bars when directed by the caregiver and given additional support for balance on slippery, wet surfaces, or

May be frightened by risk of fall and resist entering a tub or shower, requiring bathing elsewhere, or

May stand or sit while dried and toiletries are applied by caregiver.

3. Can get in and out of bath and use bathing articles without assistance.

May require assistance to adjust water temperature, or May require assistance to apply soap, water, and shampoo to all body surfaces and rinse, or

May require assistance to scrub hard enough to remove soil or to avoid pressure to delicate areas, or

May require assistance to dry all body parts and sequence through the use of toiletries.

4. Initiates bathing at usual time, collects supplies, and follows daily routine without assistance.

May need assistance to keep a supply of bathing articles ready for use, or

May be unconcerned about cleaning up bathroom, hanging up towels, putting toiletries away after use, or

May request demonstration when new supplies or new bathroom fixtures are encountered, even after directions are read or given verbally, or

May require assistance to find articles when not in the usual location, or

May need to be checked to be sure that the back of head and body are washed and rinsed and deodorants applied.

5. Bathes without assistance and checks own quality.

### .3 Walking and Exercising

1. Moves about in bed in response to stimuli.

May need side rails on bed to prevent falling, or

May be moved to a wheelchair with physical assistance and a restraining belt to hold in chair, or

May exercise muscles for turning head, rolling over, and holding body against gravity.

2. Spontaneously sits, stands, and walks aimlessly.

May initiate walking through doorways, around large pieces of furniture, and moving between bed, chair, and bathroom, or

May be going to the bathroom without any awareness of where it is, or

May sit in bed or chair without a restraining belt but requires protection for standing, sitting down, or walking, or

May not notice slippery floors, uneven surfaces, stairs, stair railings, or curbs unless pointed out, or

May exercise muscles for trunk stability, walking, stepping up and down, pushing and pulling with arms.

3. Knows how to get to the bathroom and where to go to get food and water in living environment. May

wander out of living environment, get lost, and be unable to retrace steps, or

May wander about, pick up, and manipulate any object that happens to be in plain sight, or

May follow anyone, anywhere, or

May walk slowly and have a brief response to a request to hurry up, and resume slow pace, or

May not understand requests to change amount when doing graded exercises and require one-to-one supervision to sustain change in amount of strength, range of motion, or endurance.

4. Knows how to get to the mailbox and around the neighborhood and recognizes visible landmarks.

May not notice signs and visible activities that require adjustments in pace and walking patterns, or

May require an escort to get to a new location and may need to be taken several times to learn the route, or

May attempt to alter amount in graded exercise but the alteration may not be sustained. The patient may have to be checked every few minutes to sustain graded exercise,

May be trained to follow an exercise program by having the patient go through the program several times.

5. Uses landmarks to get around neighborhood and knows how long it takes to get to ordinary destinations.

### .4 Eating

1. Can chew and swallow a soft diet and drink liquids.

May swallow a soft diet when fed, or

May sit up with hand-over-hand guidance of spoon from plate to mouth, or

May eat soft foods with fingers, or

May drink from a cup when placed in hand.

2. Can pick up and use a spoon or a cup to eat and drink.

May go to table and sit in one location when told meal is ready, or

May start eating as soon as food is served and leave table when done, or

May be very slow to eat and need reminders to finish meal, or

Food may be spilled, dropped, or smeared around eating area and on self without awareness of mess, or

May put nonedible objects in mouth.

3. Can feed self from an ordinary table setting with the exceptions of chopsticks and cutting meat.

May sit at table with others and be unaware of their presence or eat alone without concern, or

May focus attention on food and be unaware of table manners, restricted quantities of food, or a balanced diet, or

May be unable to keep track of meal times and demand meals whenever hungry, or

Pace of eating may be slow or rushed and unable to change upon request.

4. Can eat at the table and recognize the presence of others.

May not eat and talk at the same time, or

May use poor table manners but responds to a request to improve manners, or

May require assistance to season food, serve from communal dishes, check temperatures, or open unusual packaged food.

5. Can eat with others, engage in conversation, and eat with table manners expected.

## .5 Toileting

1. No awareness of need to void or does not communicate need for assistance.

May cooperate with placement of bedpan.

2. Aware of need to void and attempts to go to a toilet.

May not know where the bathroom is or not allow enough time to get there, or

May have trouble opening door, leave door open after entering, or turning around to sit, or

May have trouble adjusting garments and require assistance to get them up and down, or

May need to be handed toilet paper and cued to use or may require assistance with wiping feces clean, or

May require assistance to flush toilet.

3. Recognizes need to void, finds the bathroom, opens ordinary door, turns to sit, lowers lower body garments when loose fitting, voids, wipes self, and pulls lower body garments up.

May leave bathroom door open and forget to flush, or

May require cues to wipe feces clean, wash hands, zip zipper, tuck in shirttail.

4. Cares for self at toilet completely.

May need to have garment errors pointed out, or

May need to be reminded to use bathroom when leaving home or in other conditions of limited access.

5. Can look around for a bathroom in a new setting without requiring the direction of another person.

## .6 Taking Medication

1. May or may not be able to swallow needed pills/liquids.

2. Can swallow medications placed in hand when supervised to check correct amount is taken. May refuse all medications.

3. Can recognize color and shape of daily medications. May not know when or how much is taken, or

May forget to take or that has already taken, or

May have no idea or erroneous ideas about why medications are prescribed that may lead to a refusal to take medications, or

May not understand side effects and refuse to take medications, or

May not recognize adverse reactions and fail to report them to anyone.

4. Can usually remember to take simple dosages at regular times such as with meals or at bed time.

Recognizes color, shape, and amount of daily dosage.

May not recognize a mental reason for taking medications that can lead to a refusal to take, or

May think that side effects are the only effect and refuse to continue taking medications, or

May have erroneous ideas about harmful effects of medications and not understand reasonable explanations when given by physician or loved ones and refuse to take, or

May not recognize adverse effects and fail to report to anyone, requiring regular supervision, or

May have to be coerced or forced into taking medication.

5. Can usually recognize the presence of a mental disorder and consider the effects that medications might have on reducing the functional difficulties. Can usually explain why medication was given and report individual effects with some degree of accuracy. May confuse concepts such as drug effects, side effects, synergies, and tolerance.

## .7 Using Adaptive Equipment

1. No recognition of a physical disability.

May attempt to move in bed in normal manner and may require rails or restraints to prevent falls.

Complications of physical disabilities may be prevented with comfortable positioning devices.

2. No recognition of physical disabilities.

May attempt to sit, stand, walk, and use arms in normal manner, and may require restraint to keep from falling, tripping, removing necessary medical equipment.

Complications of physical disabilities may be prevented with comfortable positioning devices. Uncomfortable devices may be refused or removed.

3. Vague recognition of marked physical disabilities in gross body movements such as paralysis. May not recognize weakness or restricted range of motion.

Accepts adaptations made on objects that allow the dominant hand to be used in a normal manner. May be trained to use these objects in nondominant hand with much repetitive drilling.

4. Recognizes marked physical disability in gross body movements such as paralysis, paresis, or restricted range of motion.

May accept adaptive equipment that can be used with normal movement patterns, or

May learn to use adaptive equipment that produces clearly visible effects and the formation of few new sensorimotor models, or

May require repetitious drilling to learn the new sensorimotor models required to use adaptive equipment.

5. Recognizes physical disabilities and the effects on the individual's ordinary activities as the activity is being done.

May learn to use adaptive equipment to do activities that are important to individual, or

May reject equipment for unimportant activities or when requires too much energy and/or is too time consuming, or

May require assistance with long-term maintenance, adjustment, and repair.

## 11. Situational Awareness Disability

### .0 Housekeeping

2. Does not participate in or is not directed to do any housekeeping activities.

3. When directed may use a broom, mop, dust rag, wash cloth, dish rag, or sponge to wipe a surface.

May unnecessarily wipe in the same spot over and over again or until told to move or stop, or

May do a few wipes and stop before much is done, or

May not cover the whole surface, or do so only with cuing to surfaces not done yet, or

May miss spots and be unconcerned about dirt that remains, even when pointed out.

4. Initiates removing obvious dirt in plain sight on top of counters, tables, desks, and other furniture,

cleans the parts of floor easily seen, removes most food particles from kitchen sink.

May not clean toilet, shower, or bathtub until dirt or mold produces a color contrast.

May empty trash when basket is overflowing but may not take precautions for sharps, spoilage, fires, poisons, or conservation.

May leave streaks on windows, cupboards, woodwork or apply more polish or cleaning agent than is necessary.

May request/need help with anything out of the ordinary.

May have clutter and disarray on open surfaces as well as inside drawers, cupboards, and closets.

5. Tries a new way of removing out-of-the-ordinary dirt or stains, removes streaks and adjusts amount of cleaning agent used according to what is most effective, removes less obvious dirt such as cobwebs, fingerprints, crumbs, and hair or fur.

May not consider precautions on the labels of cleaning agents or consider the long-term effects of use, or

May plug up plumbing by disposing of objects that will not fit, or

May attach objects without considering damage done when removed, or

May overload electrical system and blow fuses or create a fire hazard, or

May put objects away in locations that are inefficient.

6. Organizes home environment for efficient use of objects, anticipates hazards or damage to the home, plans a schedule for completing chores, and considers long-term maintenance.

### .1 Preparing/Obtaining Food

2. Does not participate in obtaining food; eats what is place in front of him or her by others.

3. When directed may assist with meal preparation by setting the table, serving food that is cold or at room temperature, washing or peeling food stuffs, or when directed may pick up a tray or a plate to serve self, or go through a cafeteria line and select dishes to eat.

May not recognize mealtime and need to be directed to eat or told to wait if requesting food at some other time, or

Assistance in food preparation may be very slow and of little real help, or

May not be safe in handling hot food, knives, kitchen appliances.

4. May prepare a simple meal that is cold or at room temperature and has a few ingredients such as a sandwich or a salad; or

May be able to pick up a tray or plate and serving self at mealtime, or

May follow an established routine for obtaining food from a restaurant or other source.

May follow an inflexible procedure for obtaining food and need assistance if anything out of the ordinary restricts access to food, or may go hungry,

May depend on environmental cues to recognize mealtime such as a noon whistle or the arrival of food carts.

May make unreasonable or unhealthy requests for food and not understand explanations, or

May cook hot food with risks of burning self, burning food, forgetting to turn off stove, or starting a fire,

May not handle knives and cooking appliances safely.

5. May bring home the groceries, prepare hot and cold meals, and learn how to make new dishes when shown how, or may eat in restaurants while paying lip service to a budget.

May not do an inventory, make out a grocery list, or may make multiple trips to the store and buy duplicate items, or

May not store food for efficient use or with usual care to prevent spoilage or food poisoning, or

May not follow recipes and may rely on convenience foods for variation in diet.

6. Plans menus for adequate nutrition within budgetary limitations, organizes a system for obtaining food, and develops a contingency plan when something out of the ordinary happens.

## .2 Spending Money

2. Does not handle money, or is given no opportunity to do so.

May not realize that money transactions are occurring.

3. Recognizes familiar currency but not new currency.

May hand cash to another person, or

May not consider the amount of cash given or received, or

May remember old prices and not adjust to current prices, or

May not understand why he or she owes money.

4. Manages daily purchases and may be given a daily allowance, or

May do calculations correctly for small purchases by counting cash, using paper and pencil, or a calculator, or

May be unusually slow in doing calculation, or

May not be able to account for money spent, or

May require assistance to manage money, or

May manage own money but run out of funds, or

May act as if one has an unlimited supply of funds,

May be overwhelmed by the stimuli of a shopping mall.

## .3 Shopping

1–3. Does not shop.

4. Goes to familiar shops and makes familiar purchases.

May be immobilized by changes in shops, prices, or merchandise, or

May not understand any relationship between a purchase and a budget, or

May be slow or require assistance to pay the correct amount, or

May not understand qualitative differences in goods, or

May not protect funds from theft.

5. Does routine shopping for daily/weekly purchases. Examines goods for material properties but may not consider intangible properties, or

May compare prices but not consider secondary affects of purchasing, like distance traveled or warranty, or

May invest in big purchases that place a hardship on budget that exceed understanding of the hardship at the time of purchase, or

May follow an inflexible routine that inhibits taking advantage of bargains or unusual purchases unless assisted by others, or

May require assistance with using checks and credit cards.

6. Shops within a set of individualized priorities, anticipating and accepting the consequences of big purchases, and being flexible in adjusting to the availability of commodities.

## .4 Doing Laundry

2. Dirty clothes/linens are removed by others or does not have the opportunity to remove.

3. When directed, puts dirty clothes in hamper, or

May not realize that clothing/linens are dirty, or

May do repetitive actions for hand laundry but may not judge the effects of actions,

May have no awareness of different methods of doing laundry and not understand explanations, or

May be unaware of ironing, mending, or putting things away, or

May be aware of wet clothing only as affects one's personal sense of comfort/discomfort.

4. Initiates a request for clean clothing, or puts dirty clothes in a hamper, or does hand laundry, or runs clothes through the washing machine and dryer.

May place all clothes, clean and dirty, in the hamper, or

May be unreliable in recognizing a need for laundry, or

May not distinguish between delicate, machine, and dry-cleaning fabrics, or

May not check for stains or a need for ironing and mending without assistance, or

May take laundry to cleaners and forget to pick it up, or lose claim ticket.

5. Understands and usually checks for the difference between fabrics washed in water or dry cleaned, fabrics that shrink in the dryer, or dyes that bleed.

May not allow enough time to get the laundry done prior to an event, or

May require assistance to comprehend and follow instructions or precautions on cleaning agent labels, or

May not anticipate the secondary effects of leaving bleaches and dyes in the laundry area, or

May not check garments for items in pockets, etc., that can be damaged, cause damage, or can get lost during the cleaning process.

6. Understands and usually anticipates the way items can be damaged while getting clothes/linens clean. Reads labels and follows instructions/precautions with flexibility.

Allows enough time for items to be ready for an event.

## .5 Traveling

2. May enjoy riding in a vehicle, looking at the scenery, or

May not have an opportunity to ride in a vehicle.

May require assistance to get in and out of a vehicle, put on a seat belt, open and shut doors or windows, or need restraint to wait for a complete stop and brakes set.

3. Waits for vehicle to come to a stop before attempting to get in or out of the vehicle.

May not know or is confused about destination, or

May try to propel a wheelchair with results that fail to get to destinations, or

May get into a car, bus, train, or airplane without consideration for destination, length of time, or cost.

4. Independently follows familiar routes in vehicles driven by others.

Changes from one vehicle to another when familiar with or trained to by asking for frequent assistance, or

May be inflexible in departing from unfamiliar routes or vehicles, or

May be trained to push a cart along specific routes, or

May insist on driving a car or traveling alone to new places or on new vehicles with negative consequences.

May drive a car slowly on familiar routes without understanding the hazards, or

May travel on public transportation without understanding the hazards.

5. Travels unfamiliar routes with specific directions that include landmarks and street signs.

May confuse left and right turns, or

May be confused by maps and verbal directions, or

May forget where the car is parked, unfamiliar bus stop, or where terminal is.

6. Uses a public map to find present location; anticipates direction to go in a series of turns. Follows verbal directions for 3 or 4 turns.

## .6 Telephoning

2. Does not notice the telephone.

3. Picks up the telephone receiver and may dial one or two familiar numbers.

May pick up the receiver when the telephone did not ring and may leave the receiver off the hook, or

May answer the telephone but not call another person to the telephone on request, or relay a message.

4. Dials familiar numbers, calls information for other numbers, and relays messages in present time.

May forget to deliver messages later on, or

May be slow to write messages down, or

May have difficulty finding numbers in own address book and may refuse to use the telephone book.

5. Uses and updates own address/telephone book and may look numbers up in telephone book where names are listed in alphabetical order.

May not locate numbers listed by classifications such as government agencies or business listings, or

May have trouble learning to use hold buttons, answering machines, and other new technologies, or

May have an overly expensive bill from talking too long or not heeding other factors that influence rates, or

May not consider differences in time zones or amount.

6. Considers external factors like time zones and rates before placing a call and adjusts length of call accordingly. Uses classification systems to find numbers. Can learn to use new technology when so desires.

## .7 Adjusting to Change

1. Withdraws from noxious stimuli.

May not differentiate between temporary and long-term effects.

May not recognize a new physical disability and attempt habitual movements to chew, swallow, drink, roll over, sit, or stand.

2. Moves in accordance with requirements of architecture and furniture such as stairs, doorways, tables, chairs, bed, and bathtub.

May not recognize slippery surfaces on floors or bath, or

May not recognize mobile objects such as chairs on wheels, wall partitions, glass doors.

3. Moves objects that cause discomfort away from self and avoids objects with obvious dangers such as hot enough to burn or the smell of spoiled food.

May perceive a hazard where no hazard actually exists, or

May not perceive less obvious dangers that do exist, or

May harm self or others in efforts to avoid danger and may not realize that harm has been done to other people or that damage has been done to property.

4. Follows routine steps in doing daily activities in a way that avoids ordinary hazards.

May be unaware of circumstances that present unusual hazards, or

May see clearly visible hazards but not be able to alter routine steps to avoid accident or injury, or

May become immobilized when a change is noted, or

May get angry about change.

5. Attempts to alter routine steps in doing daily activities when a change in noted.

May change primary affect without being aware of hazards of secondary effect, or

May do damage while trying to discover a way of responding to change, or

May be swift to act without taking the time to think through the steps and predict negative effects, or

May not consider the pros and cons of different courses of action.

6. Anticipates hazards by thinking through the steps and predicting primary and secondary effects of a hypothetical course of action. If one approach fails, will consider the reason for the failure and try another.

# 12. Occupational Role Disability

## .0 Planning/Doing Major Role Activity

3. Does not produce anything of real value to others. May do a few actions from a previous role when material objects are laid out by others.

May require constant supervision while doing the actions.

4. Can participate in an activity under special circumstances designed for disabled people.

May refuse to participate in activities designed for disabled people, or

May not have access to substitutes for major role activities, or

May choose not to have a major role activity.

5. Can participate in normal major role activities in the community, with supervision. Supervision includes planning schedule of activities, considering the secondary effects that changes in schedule might have on others, and making sure that primary obligations are met on time.

May refuse roles that provide supervision, or see these roles as demeaning, or

May engage in major role activities without supervision and negative social consequences, or

May tolerate major role activities in programs designed for disabled people better than placement in the community.

6. Plans own schedule for doing major role activities according to the priorities set for fulfilling one's primary obligations. Makes sure that obligations are met on time or makes arrangements to minimize secondary effects on others.

## .1 Planning/Doing Spare-Time Activities

3. May spend hours of each day doing nothing.

May show no concern about having nothing to do, or

May lack interest, initiative, and intent for doing activities, or

May engage in actions of an activity when set up and sequenced by others.

4. Expresses interest and desire to do activities. May participate in doing activities when planned and organized by others, or

May pay lip service to wanting to do activities but does not initiate stated activity, or

May not be able to do activities of interest or desire, or

May refuse, reject, or avoid activities within range of ability, or

May do elective activities alone and avoid comparison or discussion of what one did/does.

5. Engages in spare-time activities on a regular basis.
May do elective activities alone and be preoccupied with own interests, or

May engage in group activities and play an inflexible, unreasonable, or ineffective role, or

May blame others or postpone engagement when difficulties arise, or

May avoid planning spare-time activities or be unwilling to make a commitment to do something, or

May make commitments and fail to fulfill them.

6. Plans and follows through in doing elective activities.
May schedule activities with others and follow through on commitments, or

May allow for flexibility in scheduling and type of activity, or

May do solitary activities and be interested in unrelated activities done by others.

## .3 Pacing and Timing Actions

3. Does not change amount of speed or energy or show awareness of a period of time.
Pace may be unusually slow or fast and not modified upon request, or

May repeat actions without awareness of how many times, or

May need assistance to go through a sequence of steps, or

May not know how long it took to do a sequence of steps.

4. Shows awareness of the present period of time but does not change the amount of speed or energy used.
May set a goal to be accomplished within the next hour, or

May sequence self through a series of steps to complete a task, or

May know how long a repetitive action has been done, or

May move slower or faster than usual and not adjust pace upon request, or

May use more or less energy than usual and not be able to conserve less or expend more on request.

5. Shows awareness of present time period within the context of a daily/weekly schedule.
May set own pace within normal limits, or

May not vary pace when time constraints are explained, or

May not anticipate the need to vary pace, or

May adjust the amount of energy expended, or May

ask about the amount of time a task will take, or

May reject tasks that take longer than a week, or

May get bored with tasks that have repetitive actions and accept reduced quality to stop doing the actions, or

May not be able to predict how long it will take to get a task done.

6. Can predict how long it will take to do a task with a reasonable degree of accuracy, or

May vary pace, energy for extended periods of time to meet a deadline or take a test.

## .3 Exerting Effort

3. Does not initiate moving or trying.
May pick up an object that happens to be in front of them, or

May concentrate on a repetitive action, or

May persist in doing a sequence of actions when prompted by another person, or

May not remember doing something shortly after doing the task, or

May refuse to exert effort, or

May be stimulated into a fight or flight response.

4. Looks for, locates, and uses objects that are in plain sight and remembers the storage place for objects that are used frequently.
May not vary the amount of strength, range of motion, coordination, posture, or position while working on a task, or

May concentrate and persist while doing a simple task, or

May be reminded of prior experiences and share the memories, or

May refuse to do selected activities and try to do others for reasons that may not make sense.

5. Varies the amount of strength, range of motion, coordination, posture, or position of moving of one's body according to the effect on material objects.
May not persist with problems that cannot be solved quickly, or

May not persist when verbal explanations and directions are given, or

May not persist long enough to achieve social standards.

6. Understands and accepts cultural norms for standards of performance prior to engaging in a task and persists until the relevant norms are meant.

Persists when verbal or written directions are given.
Persists in attempting to solve a problem after the first sign of moderate difficulty.

## .4 Judging Results

3. Does not check the effects of own actions.

May not look at objects being moved, or

May place objects in a linear sequence but may not look to check for linear placement or notice when objects are out of line, or

May not place objects in groups that are alike, or

May not notice the amount of material used.

4. Notices matching errors, efforts to correct fail, and asks for assistance to solve the problem or leaves the error.

May notice matching errors in the following striking features of objects: color, shape, size, placement in horizontal and vertical lines, and number up to 4, or

May notice that appliances are turned on or off, or

May notice when out of supplies needed to do a task, or

May notice striking changes in customary supplies, or

May not notice errors, changes in material objects that are not a striking feature.

5. Judges the effect of actions after the action is done and evaluates according to personal criteria.

May notice the errors or changes in material objects that the individual can perceive, or

May not notice errors or changes that are not perceivable to one of the five senses, or

May weigh error against a personal desire to correct the error and choose to leave the error, or

May not consider the consequences of leaving an error.

6. Considers the effect of one's actions before acting and weighs personal dislike of correcting errors against the consequences of leaving an error.

## .5 Speaking

3. Speaking is confused.

May invent words, mispronounce words, and alter the sentence structure, or

May not speak at a rate or volume that can be understood, or

May have a slow response time when asked a question, or

Speech content may reflect a situational awareness disability, or

Speech content may reflect an attempt to invent a situation that makes sense to the individual, or.

May be able to name an object and action while holding the object or doing the action.

May not be able to ask for help when needed.

4. Asks for help when need is recognized.

May not be able to describe the problem, or

May not be able to talk and work with hands at the same time, or

Use of simple vocabulary and short sentences may be correct, or

May have trouble with vocabulary that is used seldom and longer sentences, or

May describe the striking features of objects.

5. Talks about self.

May talk and work at the same time, or

May describe the solution to a problem solved by making neuromuscular adjustments, or

May think of a different way of doing something and request the necessary tools and supplies, or

May argue about explanations of the consequences of leaving an error, or

May disagree with social standards for errors.

6. Discusses ways of doing things and inquires about potential errors or hazards.

May make an error and discuss the consequences while considering several ways of solving the problem.

## .6 Following Safety Precautions

3. Unable to retain a sequence of steps for safety procedures.

4. Can be trained to rigidly follow a few safety procedures.

May require drilling to follow procedures consistently, or

May not use hazardous materials and tools safely, or

May require on-site supervision to identify and solve problems.

5. Can learn demonstrated safety precautions and follow the procedure in most instances.

May require assistance to identify hazardous situations and establish safety precautions, or

May deviate from safety precautions in an impulsive manner without considering the consequences, or

May decide that safety precautions are really unnecessary and stop following them, or

May not meet standards of consistency required for tasks of high risk for serious accident or injury.

6. Anticipates hazards, comprehends safety precautions, and can generate protocols when necessary.

## .7 Responding to Emergencies

3. Can recognize an obvious state of emergency and scream for help. May be unable to think of or follow any other response.

4. Can seek assistance by using the telephone or going to get someone.

May not call the most important person, or

May be slow in issuing the call for help, or

May not remember or be able to follow emergency procedures.

5. Can initiate own actions in response to an emergency.

May react impulsively without considering secondary effects or judging priorities, or

May not perceive the need to seek help quickly enough if self is not in danger, or

May not coordinate own efforts with others.

6. Prioritizes actions during an emergency, seeking needed assistance, and attempting to prevent undesirable secondary effects.

## 13. Social Role Disability

### .0 Communicating Meaning

3. Unaware of the listener's needs for volume, rate, or intelligibility.

4. Adjusts volume, rate, and words so that the listener can understand what is being said.

May interrupt what the listener is saying or doing, without apology, or

May not try to keep a conversation going, and be unaware of another's discomfort with silence, or

May limit conversation to personal requests, or

May say unkind things without realizing that the listener's feelings could be hurt.

5. Communicates interesting information from personal experiences.

May not restate/revise information according to the listener's circumstances, or

May not respond to subtle cues to revise a message, or

May not consider an alternative point of view, or

May make the same point over and over again when a disagreement occurs, or

May not take turns in conversation and talk too little or too much.

6. Communications go beyond one's own experiences to consider the experiences of others.

May see a situation from the listener's perspective, or

May change one's point of view, or

May revise messages according to the listener's perspective.

### .1 Following Instructions

3. Imitates a demonstrated action on an object but requires one-to-one supervision to stop and start.

4. Able to follow demonstrated instructions, one step at a time, and may be trained to follow a series of steps.

May require months of repetition to learn a series of steps, or

May not understand verbal or written instructions, or

May not generalize instructions from one situation to another, or

May not apply prior knowledge to immediate situation, or

May require on-site supervision to answer questions, validate procedures, and solve problems.

5. Able to follow a series of demonstrated instructions and can remember a limited amount of new information.

May not understand verbal, written, or diagrammed instructions, or

May attempt to generalize instructions but fail to anticipate errors, or

May not request instruction, or clarification of instruction when needed, or

May take short cuts from instructions to make the task easier without considering the repercussions.

6. Able to follow written, verbal, and diagrammed instructions containing new information.

May request clarification or validation of instructions, or

May request relevant information that may indirectly affect work performance.

### .2 Contributing to Family Activities

3. Efforts to participate in family activities are disruptive or demand constant attention from at least one other person at all times.

4. Participates in a restricted range of family activities.

May play an inflexible role in activities, like it has always been done according to the disabled, but with an "as if" quality that is not quite real to the family, or

May be given simple, limited task by the family to keep patient contributing to family life, or

May refuse to try new activities, or

May need to be reminded to do chores, or

May be perceived as a burden, or as taking more than giving to family life, or

May be embarrassing and/or excluded from activities outside of the family.

5. Participates in full range of family activities.
May not contribute new ideas for future planning and decision making, or
May not place other members' interests ahead of own interest, or engage in give and take gracefully.
6. Dependable in family life according to age, sex, position in household, and sociocultural context.

### .3 Caring for Dependents

3 Does not care for dependents.
May interact with children or pets for a few moments at time, or
May leave or forget about dependent if distracted.
4. Does simple tasks for dependents.
May give food and water to pets, or
May bathe, dress, and feed a child, or
May recognize immediate problems, like a child crying but require help to solve the problem, or
May not protect dependents from hazards, or
May not realize that a dependent is ill or may seek assistance to care for dependent but not follow instructions correctly, or
May give instructions that are unclear or do not account for the circumstances of the dependent, or
May demand obedience, or
May be abusive.
5. Manages routine daily and weekly dependent tasks. May not think to check for unusual needs of dependents such as insects on pets, health check-ups and inoculations, outgrowing shoes and clothes, allergies, food and clothing for special events.
May not encourage the special interests and talents of a child.
6. Protects dependents from hazards and places the welfare of the dependent ahead of own welfare on occasion.

### .4 Cooperating with Others

3. Assists another person in fulfilling personal needs.
May need to be reminded to do self-care, or
May not pay any attention to others most of the time, or
May be unpredictable in making social contacts, or
May become verbally abusive or physically dangerous to others for reasons that are unclear or erroneous.
4. Engages in a narrow range of social contacts with people living in the same space or when contacts are arranged for them.
May interact with others through stereotyped con-versations, only discussing topics of personal concern or repeating the same conversation over and over again.
May be socially ostracized for being belligerent, argumentative, or intrusive, or
May be socially withdrawn and state a preference to avoid contacts with other people, or
May not comprehend requests to consider the rights of others.
5. Makes contacts within sociocultural context but there is often tension in the relationships.
May alienate others through a failure to collaborate, consider the rights of others, or be flexible, or
May be antagonistic toward others who hold a different opinion on a subject, or
May be nervous, irritable, bossy, self-centered, pas-sive-aggressive, taciturn, or solitary, or
May not directly impinge on others but acts in a way that indirectly jeopardizes the overall function or reputation of a social unit.
6. Adapts to others in collaboration to accomplish tasks of mutual benefit. Is flexible in approaching and responding to everyday relationships.

### .5 Supervising Independent People

3. Does not attempt to direct the actions of others.
4. Establishes personal goals and gives orders.
May not establish goals that are realistic or relevant to the situation, or
May not distinguish between personal goals and requirements of subordinates, or
May treat people like subordinates when they are not, or
May demand immediate and unquestioning compli-ance with orders that seem unreasonable to others, or
May avoid supervisory activities.
5. Plans inductively and negotiates through trial and error with subordinates.
May not analyze, evaluate, or synthesize data objec-tively, or
May not recognize significant details or over-value selected information based on personal prejudices, or
May not influence subordinates through negotia-tion, explanation, or persuasion, or
May not be able to anticipate changes that require advanced planning, or
May attack or ignore subordinates who offer evalu-ation or criticism.
6. Objectively plans via inductive and deductive reasoning and influences subordinates and is influ-enced by subordinates.

## .6 Keeping Informed

3. Does not react when new information is presented or may get new information confused with past events.

4 Informed about major world events (war, natural disasters, presidential elections, very famous people) and local events of highly personal interest (changes in family, own support system, or own activities).

May not initiate conversation about current events or contribute any new information to others, or

May lack interest in what is going on in the world, or

May not initiate preparation for seasonal events but relates own activities to the traditional social framework, such as sending Christmas cards.

5. Makes an effort to stay informed about local and world events but may be simplistic in projecting impact on self or others.

May make faulty connections between changes in social context (drought) and need to change own behavior (overly reducing water usage or ignoring conservation), or

May focus on one part of a social context (chemical warfare) and act out of context (buy a gas mask when there is no reason to expect personal danger).

6. Is well-informed about current events, seeking and sharing information and discussing potential impact on self or others.

## .7 Engaging in Good Citizenship

3. Unaware of the effects own actions have on other people or material objects.

4. May live on social welfare or funds of other people and think one has a right to be supported by others.

May protect the public by recognizing dangers to self but may not initiate warning to others in the immediate environment.

May warn others when told to do so, or

May think that one has a right to trespass, loiter, or live on property of others or on public property, or

May make a mess and not think about picking up after one's self.

5. More concern for personal rights than the rights of others.

May use slight care in protecting others and property from injury or damage, or

May give others advice that is misleading or dangerous, with good intentions, or

May recognize a hazard and warn others in the immediate environment.

6. Fulfills duties and obligations as expected by society. Uses ordinary and reasonable care in protecting the public from injury.

# Appendix C: Cognitive Performance Test

*Theressa Burns*

The Cognitive Performance Test (CPT) should be administered by a registered occupational therapist knowledgeable in cognitive disability theory. However, if the test is not being used for clinical purposes or interpretation is not required, another professional might be trained in administration procedures.

Consistent and reliable administration of the CPT requires practice experience with several subjects representing each cognitive level. Subjects will perform to the same task directions in one of several ways. It may be helpful to practice the situations of each task before formally using the test. Before starting the test, give a simple explanation of the purpose for evaluation and nature of the test. For example, "This is a test where I'm going to ask you to show me how you manage everyday activities. This test will allow us to see if you need some help." Higher-functioning subjects may require more explanation, including the reason for referral, or purpose of the research being conducted. Lower-functioning subjects may not attend to an explanation of several statements. Effort should be made to convey to the subjects that they are involved in a test and are asked to demonstrate, rather than describe, their performance of each task. If evaluations are used for clinical assessment, patients should be interviewed about their current living situation and responsibilities, as well as any perceived functional limitations. This allows the therapist to assess insight and orientation by comparing a patient's self-report to the documented functional history, as well as to the level of deficit observed during performance of the test.

If necessary, cooperation can usually be facilitated by providing support throughout the assessment. Reassure anxious subjects that you will help when necessary (this is inherent in the test, as the therapist compensates for performance deficits). Provide support *after* each task, for example, by acknowledging task steps that were executed correctly. It may also be necessary to provide support to subjects who express confidence in their ADL abilities, by acknowledging that the performance of CPT tasks may seem easy or unnecessary. This may be stated by subjects who perform the test without

error, as well as by subjects who demonstrate performance deficits.

Care should be taken to give the subject adequate opportunity to comprehend task directions. Check to see if the subject uses a hearing aid or wears glasses. Speak slowly and clearly. Do not begin giving task instructions until the subject is directly in front of the task props. Each task has an opening statement and often a motion to the task props. These are intended to orient the subject to the nature of the task situation. Task directions can usually be repeated twice (see individual tasks), and confirmation of the subject's questions regarding the *correct* performance procedure usually can be given at any time. For example, when subjects ask if they should do something specific (e.g., "should I butter the toast now?"), tell them yes, if the question reflects the appropriate next step. Use cuing (see below) if the question is vague or reflects the wrong procedure. Be sure to give subjects plenty of time to perform *before* using cuing, additional directives, or demonstration.

Verbal cuing, verbal directions, and demonstration are types of assistance that are *used in progression* depending on the behavior of the subject. Their definitions are as follows:

## Verbal Cuing

Nonspecific verbal assistance could include: "What do you do first?", "What do you do now?", "Do what you think is best," "Finish up." Verbal cuing is used somewhat at levels 5 and 4, and most frequently at level 3.5. (See individual tasks for when to use cuing.)

## Verbal Directives

Specific verbal assistance that actually tells the subject what to do includes statements such as: "Put the bread in the toaster." Verbal directives are used primarily at levels 3 and 2. (See individual tasks for when to use verbal directives.)

## Demonstration

This is physically demonstrating a task step or steps. Demonstration is used primarily at level 3. (See individual tasks for when to use demonstration.)

For each task, the therapist must develop a working knowledge of how and when to use each type of assistance.

## Task 1: Dress

*Equipment:* A wardrobe or rack with the following clothing on hangers:

    1 man's and 1 woman's lined, heavyweight raincoat
    1 man's and 1 woman's unlined, lightweight raincoat
    1 man's and 1 woman's bathrobe

The clothing should be as gender specific as possible (by color and style), and spaced 2"–3" apart.

Hanging on one door of the wardrobe or the wall next to the rack:

    1 man's straw hat
    1 man's rain hat
    1 woman's plastic rain scarf
    1 woman's sheer scarf
    1 umbrella

Each item should be clearly visible. Use the other door or the wall space on the other side of the rack to mount a 3/4-length mirror.

*Bring the patient to stand in front of the clothing.*

*Initial directions:*

*State:*   **This test has to do with getting dressed. I want you to get dressed as if you were going outside on a cold, rainy day. You can use any of the things here.** *(Point across the clothing and items on the wall.)* **There are men's and women's things. Get dressed over your own clothes for going outside on a cold, rainy day.** *(May repeat once.)*

    *If the patient selects and dons only the appropriate coat:*

*State:*   **Would you take anything else from the closet/rack?** *(Don't point.) (Score level 5 if the patient selects/points to rain headwear or umbrella.)*

    *(If the patient makes a selection but does not dress.)*

*State:*   **What did I ask you to do?** *(Score level 5 if the patient has selected the appropriate coat and headwear and dresses with this cue. If the patient does not get dressed after giving the cue, proceed to the specific directions.)*

*Score:*   **Level 5** (does the following):
    Selects and dons gender-appropriate, heavy raincoat and rain hat/scarf and/or umbrella.

*Score:*   **Level 4** (does the following):
    Selects and dons gender-inappropriate heavy raincoat with rain hat/scarf/umbrella

    Selects and dons unlined coat with rain hat/scarf and/or umbrella
    Selects and dons only a coat
    Selects and dons 2 coats
    Selects and dons non–rain headwear and a coat

*Score:*   **Level 3** (does one or both):
    Selects and dons a bathrobe with/without hat/scarf
    Makes gross errors in dressing (clothing inside out or on inappropriate body parts)

    *If the patient does not make a selection [continues to rummage through the clothing or does not perform], give the following specific directions::*

*State:*   **Choose a coat and hat/scarf for a cold, rainy day and put them on.** *(May repeat once.)*

*Score:*   **Level 4** (does the following):
    Selects and dons a coat and hat/scarf/or umbrella

*Score:*   **Level 3.5** (does one or the other):
    Selects and dons only a coat
    Does not dress after selecting without additional cuing.

*State:*   **What did I ask you to do with the coat? Show me.** *(May repeat once.)*

*Score:*   **Level 3**
    Selects and dons a hat/scarf only
    Selects and dons a bathrobe with/without a hat/scarf
    Makes gross errors in dressing (clothing on inappropriate body parts or inside out)
    Does not dress after additional cuing

    *If the patient does not make a selection:*

*State:*   **Put this coat on.** *(Hand coat to the patient.) (May repeat once.)*

*Score:*   **Level 3** (does the following):
    Puts coat on body.

*Score:*   **Level 2**
    Takes the coat but does not put it on.

    *If the patient does not take the coat:*

*State:*   **Let me help you.** (Put the coat on the patient.)

*Score:*   **Level 2**
    Can alter position of the arms to facilitate the dressing process.

*Score:*   **Level 1**
    Does not take the coat when handed.
    Does not alter position of the arms to facilitate dressing.

## Task 2: Shop

*Equipment:* A (woman's) folding wallet (in a dark color) with the following features:

A snap closure

A coin section

A bill section

In the bill section, place 1 5-dollar bill and 2 1-dollar bills. In the coin section, place 2 quarters, 2 dimes, 2 nickels, and 8 pennies.

Twelve belts with buckles, including:

6 women's belts (2 size small, 2 size medium, 2 size large, all in red)

6 men's belts (2 size small, 2 size medium, 2 size large, all in brown)

A small table

*Equipment set-up:* Hang the belts on hooks from the wall at eye level in sets of two (six hooks with 2 belts on each hook). Match the sets by color and size and hang from left to right beginning with the men's (from small to large), then the women's (from small to large). Price and size the belts using tags that adhere to the belts. Mark the six belts on top by size and price them at $9.59. Mark the six belts underneath by size and price them at $6.79. The $6.79 tags should be fairly occluded by the higher priced belts on top, so that the patient must look under the top belt to see the price tag of the belt underneath.

*Bring the patient to stand in front of the belts.*

*State:* **I'd like to see how you do with money when you're shopping. I want you to buy a belt.** *(Point across the belts.)* **Here is a wallet with some money in it.** *(Hand the wallet to the patient.)* **Choose a belt that fits you and one that you can pay for with the money in the wallet.** *(Point to the wallet.)* **Then pay me the exact amount for the belt.**

*(May repeat entire statement or portion once.)*

*At any point during the task, after the patient initiates opening the wallet, suggest that he or she take the money out and put it on the table. If necessary, tell the patient there is change or there are dollar bills in the wallet. If the patient does not take the wallet, set it on the table.*

*Score:* **Level 6** *(does the following):*

Determines the amount of money in the wallet and checks price tags prior to selecting, selects a $6.79 belt that fits (tries it on or makes a statement referring to size, e.g.., "This is my size," or may ask if it is his or her size after payment), pays exactly $6.79.

*If the patient recognizes that there isn't enough money for the top belts but does not know what to do about it, tell the patient to look at the other belts and score level 5 or lower by performance.*

*If the patient selects a $9.59 belt and during payment recognizes that monies are insufficient, direct the patient to look at the other belts on the wall. Score level 5 or lower by performance.*

*Score:* **Level 5** (does the following):

Selects a belt that fits, looks in wallet, locates all of the money (with or without cuing), recognizes that monies are insufficient for the top belts or if the $9.59 belt is chosen, can exchange the $9.59 belt (with or without direction to the wall), pays $6.00 plus some change.

*One or more of the following applies:*

Needs verbal cue to look at belts on bottom

Initially chooses the $9.59 belt

Does not check the wallet prior to selection

Checks the wallet prior to selection but begins selection without determining amount of money available for purchasing

Needs cuing to locate all of the money in the wallet

*(If necessary, tell the patient there is change or there are dollar bills in the wallet.)*

*Score:* **Level 4**

Score here if the patient performs as above but chooses a belt that obviously does not fit (does not make a statement referring to size, does not try on, belt appears too small/large).

*If the patient chooses a $9.59 belt and during payment does not recognize the error in selection (does not make statements referring to not having enough money or is unable to make the exchange when directed to the other belts):*

*State:* **You don't have enough money for that one.** *(Exchange the belt for the patient and continue with next statement.)*

*If the patient does not initiate payment or asks "Now what?", give a verbal directive to pay for the belt.*

*If the patient tries on a belt or belts and then hangs his or her selection back up and does not initiate payment, choose a size-appropriate $6.79 belt and continue with the next statement.*

*State:* **Pay me for this belt. It cost six dollars and seventy-nine cents.** *(May repeat once.) (Point or direct the patient back to the wallet if necessary. Do not hand the wallet.)*

*Score:* **Level 4** (does the following):

Selects a belt, looks in the wallet for money *(Assist in locating all of the money if the patient initiates looking in the wallet but has difficulty)*, pays $6.00. (May also pay some change, but it is not necessary to score here.) (Patient must hand, point out, or separate the $6.00. The therapist may hold out his or her hand for the money.)

One or more of the following applies:
Does not recognize error in price selection
Needs belt exchange done for him or her
Needs verbal directive to pay after making a selection (does not initiate payment without directive to pay)
Pays for a belt on the rack rather than the one selected

*Score:* **Level 3.5** (does the following):

Selects a belt, looks in the wallet, and counts/handles the money but is not able to pay the $6.00 (does not pay at all or pays the incorrect dollar amount with or without change; pays only change)

*Score:* **Level 3** (does the following):

Takes a belt from the wall and works the buckle or ties on. Does not look in the wallet when instructed to pay.

*Payment without selection*
*If the patient is unable to make a selection, select a size-appropriate $6.79 belt, hand the belt to the patient.*

*State:* **Try this on.** *(May repeat once.) (If the patient tries the belt on, have him or her take it off, place it on the table, and point to the price. Proceed with the next statement.)*

*State:* **Pay me for the belt. It costs six dollars and**

seventy-nine cents. *(May repeat once.) (Direct the patient to the wallet again, if necessary.)*

*Score:* **Level 3.5**
Can try the belt on when directed to do so. Looks for money in the wallet. *(Assist with locating the money)*, pays $6.00.

*Score:* **Level 3**
Tries the belt on or works the buckle. Does not pay $6.00 (may look in the wallet and handle money).

*Score:* **Level 2**
Takes the belt when handed, does not try on or work buckle.

*Score:* **Level 1**
Does not take the belt when handed.

## Task 3: Toast

*Equipment:* Supply table with the following:

     Toaster, with the plug placed in front of it
     1 loaf of bread
     Butter in a covered butter dish
     1 jar of jam
     1 jar of mustard
     1 small plate
     Silverware tray containing:
     1 butter knife
     A small whisk or spatula
     A potato peeler
     A spoon
     A set of joined measuring spoons

Set up supplies on table according to the diagram.

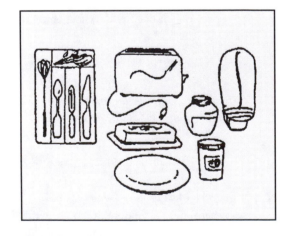

**Equipment set-up:** An electrical outlet should be behind and approximately 10 feet from the supply table so that the toaster must be moved to be plugged in. Have a cleared working space next to the outlet. The supply table should be positioned so that when a patient is standing in front of it the outlet is behind the patient.

*Bring the patient to stand in front of the supplies*

*State:* **This next test has to do with preparing food. Make one slice of toast, then put some butter and jam on it. The supplies are on this table.** *(Point across the supplies.) (May repeat once.)*

*If the patient asks for an outlet, state where it is located or point it out.*

*If the patient appears to be looking for an outlet, ask him or her what is needed.*

*Score:* **Level 5** (does the following):

Locates or asks for an outlet, moves the toaster to the outlet, plugs in the toaster, puts bread in the toaster, pushes the toaster lever down, waits for toast to pop up or pops it up, puts on butter with knife.

Note: Whether or not the patient uses jam is not scored.

*If the patient begins by putting bread in the toaster and popping it down:*

*State:* **You need to actually toast the bread.**

*Score:* **Level 5**

If the patient then proceeds and performs all components listed above.

*If the patient does not ask for/locate the outlet, see the directions for task set-up.*

*If the patient moves and plugs in the toaster, but does not proceed (asks now what or stops), give the initial directions once more or proceed to directions for task set-up and score level 4 or lower by performance.*

*If the patient attempts to put butter or jam on the bread before toasting it, interrupt the patient and tell him or her to toast the bread first and score level 4 or lower by performance. If the patient does not proceed, see directions for task set-up.*

Note: Level 4 patients may have difficulty locating the toaster lever if it is not clearly visible. *Point it out if the patient is attempting to locate it e.g., Are you looking for this? Do not tell the patient what to do with it. Give the verbal cue "Finish up" if the toast pops up and the patient does not proceed.*

*Score:* **Level 4** (does the following):

Puts bread in the toaster, pushes the toaster lever down, waits for the toast to pop up or pops it up, puts on butter or jam with knife or spoon.

*(Also does or needs any of the following):*

Begins with buttering but performs as above when directed to toast the bread

Needs to have the work area set up

Needs the toaster lever pointed out

Needs repeat of initial directions after set up of toaster

Needs the verbal cue to complete the task after the toast pops up

*Score:* **Level 3.5**

*Score here if the patient does not complete the task after the toast pops up, and the cue to finish up has been given.*

**Directions for task setup:** *If the patient does not ask for or locate an outlet or does not perform, move the toaster to the work area and plug it in. Set one slice of bread, the butter with the cover removed, and the silverware next to the toaster.*

*State:* **Make one slice of toast. Then put some butter on it.** *(May repeat once.)*

*Score:* **Level 4** (performs level 4 criteria above):

*If the patient has difficulty performing the toasting sequence, use cuing, verbal directives or demonstration, and score level 3.5 or lower depending on performance and types of assistance.*

*Score:* **Level 3.5** (does the following):

Puts bread in the toaster, pushes the toaster lever down, waits for the toast to pop up, or attempts to pop it up and get the bread out. *(Give assistance with this if necessary.)* Selects a knife or spoon from the tray, butters the toast.

(Needs cuing with one or more of the following):

Initially putting the bread in the toaster

Taking the toast from the toaster

Buttering

*If the patient is unable to complete the sequence with cuing, use verbal directives or demonstration and score level 3 or lower.*

*Score:* **Level 3** (does the following):

#1 Puts bread in the toaster

#2 Takes toast from the toaster

#3 Uses a knife to take butter from dish to toast and butters toast

(Needs one or more of the following):

Bread handed to him or her

Verbal directive to put bread in the toaster

Knife handed to him or her

Demonstration for #1, #2, or #3

*Use your own slice of bread and have the patient follow along with his or her slice.*

**Score:**     **Level 2**

*Score here if the patient performs 1 or 2 of the 3 steps listed above, or does at least one of the following:*

Takes bread when handed

Takes the knife when handed

**Score:**     **Level 1**

Does not take the bread or knife when handed.
Does not take the toast from the toaster.

## Task 4: Telephone

*Equipment:* A telephone, desk style, connected (a large-print, dialing adapter is kept on hand for use as needed)   - telephone

- The Yellow Pages directory
- A small note pad
- A pen

White index cards with different telephone numbers of hardware stores. On each card, print in large black letters and numbers **Hardware Store** (first line), **the telephone number** (second line), and **one gallon of white paint** (third line)

A magnifying glass or pair of reading glasses

*Equipment set-up:* Have the patient seated at a table with the telephone in front of him or her. Place the telephone book to the left of the telephone and the pad and pen to the right. Hold on to the index cards until needed. Different numbers are used to avoid calling the same store repeatedly and for dealing with busy signals, etc. Rotate use of the cards. The pad and pen are there for the patient to use at his or her discretion but suggest that the number be written down when a patient has difficulty following the number from the telephone book. Since scores depend on use or nonuse of the telephone book, tell patients to use the book if they attempt to call information. Before starting the task, ask if the

subject wears glasses and to put them on. Use the magnifying glass or reading glasses as necessary.

*With the patient seated at the table:*

*Initial directions:*

*State:*     **This next task has to do with using the telephone. I'd like you to use the telephone to find out the cost of one gallon of white paint.** *(May repeat one; proceed to specific directions with nonperformance.)*

*Notes: If the patient locates a number and asks if he or she should use it, give a verbal cue such as "do what you think." If the patient has selected an appropriate number, score level 5 if he or she proceeds with the task. If the patient does not proceed after the verbal cue, confirm the choice and level 4 scoring if he or she proceeds with the task. If the patient has selected an inappropriate number, state that you would like him or her to use your number instead. See directions for giving the number below.*

*When a patient makes a successful call, ask him or her how much the store charges in order to score relay of information.*

**Score:**     **Level 6 (does the following):**

Goes directly to hardware or paint in the Yellow Pages. Dials the number without difficulty (may redial once). Obtains and relays the information. If the line is busy or out of service, decides to call another store (without direction).

**Score:**     **Level 5 (does the following):**

Looks up the number of a hardware/paint store in the telephone book. Calls the store. Obtains and relays the information or portions of the information.

One or more of the following apply:

Has some difficulty using the telephone book but locates the number without assistance (does not go directly to paint/hardware section, is slow to select an appropriate number)

Has difficulty going from book to telephone when dialing (dials more than twice; dials once but rechecks the number more than twice)

Needs specific directions give

Needs directive to call another store if the line is busy.

*Score:* **Level 4**

Score here if the patient performs as above but needs confirmation of the selected number

Score here if the patients performs as above but asks the wrong question (i.e., fails to find out cost).

*If the patient does not know whom to call (is not looking in appropriate sections of the telephone book or states he or she does not know whom to call), give the specific directions:*

**Specific directions:**

*State:* **Find the number for a hardware store in the telephone book and call them for the price of a gallon of white paint.** *(May repeat once.)*

*Score:* **Level 5** (performs level 5 criteria listed above)

*Score:* **Level 4**

Is not able to locate a number within a reasonable amount of time (ineffective alphabetizing), and needs the number given. Performs level 4 criteria below.

*If the patient is unable to locate a number, give him or her the number:*

*State:* **Here is the number for the hardware store. Call them for the price of a gallon of white paint.** *(Hand one of the index cards to the patient or hold it for him or her next to the telephone.) (May repeat once.)* May allow 3 dialing attempts. Discontinue with dialing if the patient has major difficulty with the first or second attempt.

*Note: If the patient begins dialing without picking up the receiver, tell him or her to actually make the call and to pick up the receiver. In dialing, the patient may ask if he or she should dial the title (i.e., Ace Hardware) or the hyphen, due to poor use of symbolic information. Help to clarify this (tell him or her to just dial the numbers).*

*Score:* **Level 4** (does the following):

Dials the number. Asks a question related to paint. Relays information or portions of information.

*Note: Give verbal support if the patient has difficulty waiting for the telephone to be answered or with waiting on hold (interpretation of nonvisual events). Reassure the*

subject that someone will answer or that the clerk will come back. Use cuing if the patient has difficulty initiating dialing.

*Score:* **Level 3.5** (does one or the other):

Dials the number but fails to ask a complete question or fails to ask a question at all.

Dials from the card (dials 2 sequential digits and does not complete the dialing or dials the remaining digits incorrectly).

*Score:* **Level 3**

Pushes the buttons but does not dial 2 sequential digits.

*If the patient does not dial:*

*State:* **Dial the telephone.** May repeat once, then use demonstration in conjunction with restating if the patient does not perform. May give 2 demonstrations with interval to observe performance.

*Score:* **Level 3**

Dials the telephone (pushes buttons at random).

*Score:* **Level 2**

Picks up the receiver but does not dial.

*If the patient does not attempt dialing, hand the receiver at mid-line and eye level:*

*State:* **Take the telephone.** May repeat once (rehand the receiver).

*Score:* **Level 2**

Takes the receiver when handed.

*Score:* **Level 1**

Does not take the receiver when handed.

## Task 5: Wash

*Equipment:*

A sink

A table and chair (approximately 10 feet from the sink)

The chair should be placed so that the patient can be seated with his or her back to the sink

A 12" by 6" uncovered box containing:

1 bar of soap (unwrapped)

1 small bottle of aftershave (green or blue)

A toothbrush

Dental floss

A comb

The patient is asked to sit at the table. *Place the box of grooming items in front of the patient.*

*Initial directions:*

*State:* **Here are the directions for the next task; listen carefully. I want you to clean your hands as if you had been working outside in the yard. Take whatever you need from this box** *(point to the box)*, **and use whatever you need in this room.**

*If the patient specifically asks for a sink, tell him or her to find it in the room. If the patient refers to a sink, reiterate that he or she can use whatever he or she needs in the room.*

*Score:* **Level 5** (does the following):

Takes soap from the box, locates sink, turns water on, wets hands, uses soap on hands, rinses hands, turns water off, dries hands.

*Score:* **Level 4**

Score here if performance is as above but one of the following applies:

Needs additional verbal or visual direction *(point the sink out if necessary)* to get to the sink

Leaves the water running

Needs towel pointed out to initiate drying hands

*If patient does not perform or rummages through the box but does not initiate looking for the sink (stop the patient from rummaging), or initiates going to but has difficulty locating the sink:*

**Specific directions:**

*State:* **I want you to wash your hands. The soap is in the box.** *(Point to the box.)* **The sink is behind you.** *(Point to the sink.)* **May repeat once.**

*If the patient initiates looking for the sink and does not take the soap:*

*State:* **Remember to take the soap.**

*If the patient initiates looking for the sink but has trouble locating it:*

*State:* **The sink is behind you/over there.** *(Point to the sink, score level 3.5 if third cue is necessary.)*

*Score:* **Level 4** (does the following):

Takes soap, goes to sink, turns water on, wets hands, uses soap on hands, rinses hands, dries hands, needs more than two directives to get to the sink. (Point to the towels if patient has difficulty locating them.)

*Score:* **Level 3.5** (does the following):

Goes to sink, turns water on, wets hands, uses soap on hands, rinses hands, dries hands, does/needs one or all of the following:

Does not take the soap after given the verbal reminder to do so *(bring the soap to the sink for the patient and set in on the sink)*

Needs third cue to get to the sink

Needs verbal cuing to complete the hand-washing sequence (cuing to use the soap or towels, i.e., **Use this** and point to object)

*If the patient is not able to complete the hand-washing sequence with verbal cuing, use verbal directives and see level 3 scoring.*

*Score:* **Level 3**

Gets to the sink and performs #1, #2, #3 listed below:

One or more of the following applies:

Does not complete the hand-washing sequence without verbal directives (includes stating "wash your hands" if the patient goes to the sink and does not perform)

Perseverates with hand washing (washes/rinses more than twice)

Washes things other than hands (sink, towels, etc.)

Plays with faucets (turns water on/off repeatedly but does not attempt hand washing without verbal directives)

*If the patient continues to rummage through the box or does not perform after specific directions have been given or if the patient is unable to get to the sink with direction:*

*State:* **Come with me to the sink.** *(Escort or have the patient follow to the sink.)*

*State:* **Wash your hands with this soap.** *(Present the soap to the patient.)* **May repeat once.**

*If the patient does not take the soap but begins performing, set the soap down on the sink. If the patient does not perform, see directions for turning on the water.*

*Score:* **Level 3** (does #1, #2, and #3)

#1 Attempts to or turns the water on. *(The patient must initiate to score here but assist with this if necessary.)*

#2 Wets hands.

#3 Dries hands. *(Point out or hand a towel if necessary.)*

Use verbal directives if necessary. The patient may also use the soap and turn the water off, but it is not necessary to score here. A patient at this level may perseverate with any component; use redirection when necessary (i.e., "Finish up" or take the soap away, turn the water off, hand him or her a towel).

*Score:*     **Level 2**

Score here if the patient does not perform the above three steps using verbal directives but performs at least one of them.

*If the patient does not initiate turning on the water, turn on the water.*

*State:*     **Wash your hands.** *(Present the soap to the patient.)* May repeat once.

*Score:*     **Level 2**

Any purposeful motor response to the soap, water, or sink (takes soap, sets soap down or hands back, wets hands, operates faucets).

*Score:*     **Level 1**

No purposeful motor response to the soap, water, or sink (does not take the soap, does not spontaneously wet hands, does not operate the faucets).

## Task 6: Travel

*Equipment:* A simple map that includes the starting point, two intersecting hallways that the patient needs to walk through, and a designated structure (preferably a staircase) at the end of the route.

The staircase or alternate structure should be located approximately 30 yards from the starting point. The patient must be able to make 2 turns to get to the structure (1 turn out of the testing room, 1 turn at the intersection, approximately 20 yards from the starting point). Designate a structure approximately 10 yards from the intersection that will not be clearly visible until the patient gets to the very end of the route (our staircase is just through a Fire Door).

The map should be drawn with several landmarks clearly labeled, including the starting point, a landmark near the designated structure and the specific structure, i.e., stairs.

On a sheet of paper, have concrete, written directions to the selected structure printed clearly in large letters. Keep the sentences short. Have the directions state how to get to the structure but not to **"Find the stairs."** (See written directions included.)

A clipboard.

*Equipment set-up:*

Have the patient stand at the starting point, facing the direction in which he or she is to begin walking. During the test, talk just behind the patient so as not to directionally cue him or her.

*State:*     **I want to see how well you're able to get from one place to another.**

*(Hand the map on a clipboard to the patient, have the map facing in the appropriate direction.)* **This is a map of the hallways in this area. See if you can find this particular set of stairs.** *(Point to the structure on the map.)* **We are standing here.** *(Point to the starting point on the map.)* **Follow the map to these stairs** *(point again to the structure)* **and point them out to me.**

Notes: If the patient does not point out the structure, ask him or her to "point out what I asked you to find."

*If the patient asks for assistance (i.e., Which way do I go now? Do I turn here?), tell him or her to walk several yards before interrupting him or her. Change to the written directions if the patient cannot self-correct.*

*Score:*     **Level 6**

Follows the map to the destination and stops. Points out the structure. Does not ask for help (can *initially* ask for some clarification).

*Score:*     **Level 5**

Follows the map to the destination and stops but asks for assistance along the way and/or makes a wrong turn but self-corrects, or

Follows the map but passes the destination or does not point out the designated structure at the end of the route.

*If the patient initiates with the map but stops performing or makes a wrong turn and does not self-correct, or if the patient does not initiate (hands the map back or continues to look at it but does not initiate walking), exchange the map for the written directions at the starting point.*

*State:*     **I'm going to switch you to the written directions. Follow these to the stairs and point them out.** *(Read through the first sentence to identify the starting point.)*

*Score:*     **Level 5**

Initiates with the map but needs the exchange to the written directions.

Follows the written directions to the destination and stops. Points out the structure.

Does not initiate with the map but follows the written directions to the destination and stops. Points out the structure.

*Score:*    **Level 4**

Score here if the patient follows the written directions but passes the destination (the patient may comment on the structure) or does not locate the designated structure at the end of the route.

If the patient asks for assistance with following the written directions, tell him or her to do the best he or she can. Switch to verbal direction if the patient is not able to get to the destination or makes a wrong turn and does not self-correct or has not initiated to this point.

For verbal directions: *(Walk the patient to a point approximately 5 yards before the intersection [or back up]. Give verbal directions to the destination.)*

*State:*    (This statement will depend on the testing facility.)

**Take a right turn, go through the fire door, and point to the stairs.**

Give the verbal directions twice while pointing.

*Score:*    **Level 4** (one or the other):

Initiates with the map or the written directions but needs to change to the verbal directions. Follows the verbal directions for the shorter distance to locate the structure, or

No initiation with the map or written directions but follows the verbal directions for the shorter distance to locate the structure.

*Score:*    **Level 3.5**

Initiates with the verbal directions and follows the correct route but does not locate or passes the structure.

*Score:*    **Level 3**

Initiates walking with verbal direction but does not follow the correct route.

*If the patient does not initiate with the verbal directions:*

*State:*    **Follow me.**

*Score:*    **Level 2**

No initiation with the verbal directions but follows the therapist to the destination. (The patient may need verbal redirection along the way.)

*Score:*    **Level 2**

Needs intermittent tactile assistance (redirection) to walk to the destination.

*Score:*    **Level 1**

Needs to be taken by the hand to walk to the destination (or is nonambulatory and unable to initiate wheeling or direct being pushed to destination).

# CPT Score Sheets

Name: _____

Date: _____

Tester: _____

Dress: _____/5
Shop: _____/6
Toast: _____/5
Telephone: _____/6
Wash: _____/5
Travel: _____/6
Total: _____/33
ACL: _____

## Dress

### Initial Directions:

(I want you to get dressed as if you were going outside on a cold, rainy day. You can use any of the things here. There are men's and women's things. Get dressed over your own clothes for going outside on a cold, rainy day.)

_____ 5 _____ Selects and dons gender-appropriate, lined coat, with rain hat/scarf and/or umbrella.

_____ 4 _____ Selects and dons gender-inappropriate lined coat, with rain hat/scarf and/or umbrella.

_____ Selects and dons an unlined coat with rain hat/scarf and/or umbrella.

_____ Selects and dons only a coat.

_____ Selects and dons 2 coats (with or without headwear).

_____ Selects and dons non–rain headwear and a coat.

_____ 3.5 _____ Selects and dons a bathrobe with or without a hat/scarf.

_____ Makes gross errors in dressing (clothing on inappropriate body parts or inside out).

### Specific Directions:

(Choose a coat and hat for a cold, rainy day and put them on.)

_____ 4 _____ Selects and dons a coat and hat/scarf and/or umbrella.

_____ 3.5 _____ Selects and dons only a coat.

_____ Needs additional cue to dress (**What did I ask you to do with the coat—show me**).

_____ 3 _____ Selects and dons a hat/scarf only.

_____ Selects and dons a bathrobe with or without a hat/scarf.

_____ Makes gross errors in dressing (clothing on inappropriate body parts or inside out).

_____ Does not dress after additional cuing.

### Task Break down:

(Put this coat on.)

_____ 3 _____ Puts coat on body.

_____ 2 _____ Takes the coat but does not put it on.

### Physical Assistance:

(Let me help you.)

_____ 2 _____ Can alter the position of the arms to facilitate dressing, or

_____ 1 _____ Does not take the coat when handed.

_____ Does not alter position of the arms to facilitate dressing.

# Shop

## Initial Directions

(Choose a belt that fits you and one that you can pay for with the money in the wallet. Then pay me the exact amount for the belt.)

_____ 6 _____ Determines amount of money and checks prices prior to selecting,

_____ Selects a $6.79 belt that fits, _____ pays exactly $6.79.

_____ 5 _____ Selects a belt that fits, _____ looks in wallet, _____ locates all of the money (with or without cuing), _____ recognizes that monies are insufficient for the top belts, _____ if the $9.59 belt is chosen, can exchange the $9.59 belt (with or without direction to the wall), _____ pays $6.00 plus some change.

Also does/needs one or more of the following:

_____ Needs verbal cue to look at bottom belts.

_____ Initially chooses a $9.59 belt.

_____ Does not check the wallet prior to selection.

_____ Checks the wallet prior to selection but begins selection without determining amount of money.

_____ Needs cuing to locate all of the money in the wallet.

_____ 4 _____ Score here if the patient performs as above but chooses a belt that obviously does not fit.

_____ 4 _____ Selects a belt, _____ looks in the wallet for money, _____ pays $6.00. One or more of the following applies:

_____ Does not recognize error in price selection.

_____ Needs belt exchange done for him or her. (**You don't have enough money for that one. Pay me for this belt. It costs $6 and 79¢.**)

_____ Needs verbal directive to pay after making a selection. (**Pay me for this belt. It costs $6 and 79¢.**)

_____ Pays for a belt on the rack rather than the one selected.

_____ 3.5 _____ Selects a belt, _____ looks in wallet, _____ counts/handles the money, _____ does not pay $6.00 (does not pay at all or pays the incorrect dollar amount with or without change or pays only change).

_____ 3 _____ Takes a belt from the wall and works the buckle or tries on, _____ does not look in the wallet when instructed to pay.

## Payment Without Selection:

(Try this on. Pay me for this belt. It costs $6 and 79¢.)

_____ 3.5 _____ Tries the belt on, _____ looks for money in the wallet, _____ pays $6.00.

_____ 3 _____ Tries the belt on or works the buckle, _____ does not pay $6.00.

_____ 2 _____ Takes the belt when handed, does not try on or work the buckle.

_____ 1 _____ Does not take the belt when handed.

# Toast

### Initial Directions:

(Make one slice of toast, then put some butter and jam on it. The supplies are on this table.)

_____ 5 _____ Locates or asks for an outlet, _____ moves the toaster to the outlet, _____ plugs in the toaster, _____ puts bread in the toaster, _____ pushes the toaster lever down, _____ waits for toast to pop up or pops it up, _____ puts on butter with knife.

_____ 4 _____ Puts bread in the toaster, _____ pushes the toaster lever down, _____ waits for the toast to pop up or pops it up, _____ puts on butter or jam with the knife or spoon. Also does or needs any of the following:

_____ Begins with buttering or putting jam on the bread but performs as above when directed to toast the bread first.

_____ Needs to have the work area set up (does not ask for or locate the outlet).

_____ Needs the toaster lever pointed out.

_____ Needs repeat of initial directions after set-up of toaster.

_____ Needs the verbal cue to continue with the task after the toast pops up.

_____ 3.5 _____ Score here if the patient does not complete the task after the toast pops up and the cue to finish has been given.

### With the Work Area Set Up:

(Make one slice of toast. Then put some butter on it.)

_____ 4 _____ (See scoring above.)

_____ 3.5 _____ Puts bread in the toaster, _____ pushes the toaster lever down, _____ waits for the toast to pop up or pops it up or attempts to get the bread out.

_____ Selects a knife or spoon from the tray and puts on butter.

Needs cuing with one or more of the following:

_____ Initially putting bread in the toaster.

_____ Taking the toast from the toaster.

_____ Buttering.

_____ 3 _____ Able to: _____ #1 Put bread in the toaster, _____ #2 Take toast from the toaster, _____ #3 Use a knife to take butter from dish to toast and butter toast. Also needs one or more of the following:

_____ Bread handed to him or her.

_____ Verbal directive to put bread in the toaster.

_____ Knife handed to him or her.

_____ Verbal directive to butter the toast.

_____ Demonstration for #1, #2, or #3.

_____ 2 _____ Score here if the patient performs 1 or 2 of the 3 steps listed above, or does at least one of the following:

_____ Takes the bread when handed.

_____ Takes the knife when handed.

_____ 1 _____ Does not take the bread or knife when handed. Does not take the toast from the toaster.

## Telephone

### Initial Directions:

(I'd like you to use the telephone to find out the cost of one gallon of white paint.)

_____ 6 \_\_\_\_\_ Looks up number in the telephone book, dials without difficulty (may redial 1 time).

_____ asks question, _____ relays information, _____ calls another store if the line is busy.

_____ 5 \_\_\_\_\_ Looks up number in telephone book, _____ dials number, _____ asks question, _____ relays information or portions of information. Also does one or more of the following:

_____ Has some difficulty locating a number but does so without assistance.

_____ Has difficulty going from book to telephone when dialing or dials more than 2 times.

_____ Needs directive to call another store if the line is busy.

_____ Needs specific directions given.

_____ 4 \_\_\_\_\_ Score here if the patient performs as above but needs the therapist's confirmation of the selected number.

_____ Score here if the patient asks the wrong question.

### Specific Directions:

(Find the number for a hardware store in the telephone book and call them for the price of a gallon of white paint.)

_____ 5 \_\_\_\_\_ (Performs level 5 criteria listed above.)

_____ 4 \_\_\_\_\_ Looks in the telephone book but does not alphabetize effectively and needs the number given. Performs level 4 criteria below.

### Give the Number:

(Here is the number for a hardware store. Call them for the price of a gallon of white paint.)

_____ 4 \_\_\_\_\_ Dials the number (up to 3 times), _____ asks a question related to paint, _____ relays information or portions of information.

_____ 3.5 \_\_\_\_ Dials the number but fails to ask a complete question or fails to ask a question at all, or

_____ Dials two sequential digits correctly and does not complete dialing or dials the remaining digits incorrectly.

_____ 3 \_\_\_\_\_ Pushes the buttons but does not dial two sequential digits correctly.

### Dial/Take the Telephone:

(Dial the telephone or take the telephone.)

_____ 3 \_\_\_\_\_ Dials the telephone.

_____ 2 \_\_\_\_\_ Picks up the receiver or takes the receiver when handed but does not dial.

_____ 1 \_\_\_\_\_ Does not take the receiver.

# Wash

## Initial Directions:

(I want you to clean your hands as if you had been working outside in the yard. Take what you need from this box, and use whatever you need in this room.)

_____ 5 _____ Takes soap from box, _____ locates sink, _____ turns water on, _____ wets hands, _____ uses soap on hands, _____ rinses hands, _____ turns water off, _____ dries hands.

_____ 4 _____ Criteria same as above with the following exception(s)

_____ Needs additional verbal/visual direction to get to the sink.

_____ Leaves water running.

_____ Needs towel pointed out to initiate drying hands.

## Specific Directions:

(I want you to wash your hands. The soap is in the box. The sink is behind you.)

_____ 4 _____ Takes soap, _____ goes to sink, _____ turns water on, _____ wets hands, _____ uses soap on hands, _____ rinses hands, _____ dries hands, _____ needs no more than two directives to get to the sink.

_____ 3.5 _____ Goes to the sink, _____ turns water on, _____ wets hands, _____ uses soap on hands, _____ rinses hands, _____ dries hands. Also does/needs one or more of the following:

_____ Does not take the soap after given the verbal reminder to do so.

_____ Needs third directive to get to the sink.

_____ Needs verbal cuing to complete the hand-washing sequence.

_____ 3 _____ One or all of the following applies:

_____ Does not complete the hand-washing sequence without verbal directives.

_____ Perseverates with hand washing.

_____ Washes things other than hands.

_____ Plays with faucets.

## Escorted to the Sink:

(Wash your hands with this soap.)

_____ 3 _____ Does #1, #2, and #3:

_____ #1 Attempts to or turns the water on.

_____ #2 Wets hands.

_____ #3 Dries hands.

(Use verbal directives.)

_____ 2 _____ Does not do all three components above but does at least one.

## Water Turned On:

(Wash your hands.)

_____ 2 _____ Any purposeful motor response to the soap, water, or sink (takes soap, wets hands, operates faucets.)

_____ 1 _____ No purposeful motor response to the soap, water, or sink.

# Travel

## Map:

(This is a map of the hallways in this area. See if you can find this particular set of stairs. We are standing here. Follow the map to these stairs and point them out to me.)

_____6 _____ Follows the map to the destination and locates the structure. _____ Does not ask for help.

_____5 _____ Follows the map to the destination and locates the structure, one or both apply:

      _____ Asks for assistance along the way.

      _____ Makes wrong turn but self-corrects.

_____5 _____ Follows the map but passes destination or does not point out the designated structure at the end of the route.

## Written Directions:

(I'm going to switch you to the written directions. Follow these to the stairs and point them out.)

_____5 _____ Initiates with the map but needs to change to the written directions.

      Follows the written directions to the destination and locates the structure.

      _____ Does not initiate with the map but follows the written directions to the destination and locates the structure at the end of the route.

_____4 _____ Follows written directions but passes destination or does not locate the designated structure.

## Verbal Directions:

(Take a right turn, go through the fire door, and point to the stairs.)

_____4 _____ Initiates with the map or written directions but needs to change to the verbal directions. Locates the structure, or

      _____ Does not initiate with the map or written directions but follows verbal directions to locate the structure.

_____3.5 _____ Initiates following the correct route but does not locate or passes the structure.

_____3 _____ Initiates walking with verbal direction but does not follow the route.

## Follow Me:

(Follow me.)

_____2 _____ No initiation with verbal direction but follows the therapist to the destination. (With or without redirection.)

_____2 _____ Needs intermittent tactile assistance to walk to destination.

_____1 _____ Needs to be taken by the hand to walk to the destination (or is nonambulatory and unable to direct being pushed to destination or unable to initiate wheeling wheelchair.)

# Chapter 5

# Modes of Performance Within the Cognitive Levels

## Claudia Kay Allen, MA, OTR, FAOTA

The modes of performance provide more sensitive measures of cognitive ability. A mode is a designated status for performing a task or solving a problem. To avoid as much confusion as possible, the original delineation of 6 levels is maintained (Allen, 1985). A decimal system has been added to expand the scale to a total of 52 possible modes, ranging from 0.9 to 6.0. The even decimal numbers describe behaviors: the behaviors that are observed, how behavior is timed, and what the person says about behaving. The odd numbers describe the sensory associations required to guide behavior in the next even number. ".1," for example contains the sensory associations for ".2." Because the therapist's assessment of behavior is apt to be more reliable, emphasis is placed on the even numbers. Change can be measured by moving from one mode to another: 4.3 to 4.4 or 4.2 to 4.4.

A behavioral pattern that repeats itself within each cognitive level has been detected. Learning this pattern makes it easier for therapists to learn the 52 modes. The even numbers describe the emergence of the modes within each cognitive level (Table 5.1).

Point zero is an aggregate that is formed by collecting bits of information into a whole. The whole of aggregates is greater than the sum of their parts. The aggregate occurs when the patient is able to spontaneously initiate changes in the information contained in the previous cognitive level. Point zero modes are characterized by fixed attention to the basic or primary components of the level. The patient often appears to be impervious to the therapist's attempts to introduce more information.

Point two modes orient the level to time and place in conformance with the commands of others

or the cultural measures of time and performance. The distinctive characteristics of the level guide behavior, but at .2 people can be easily overwhelmed when given more information than they can process. When people get overwhelmed, their behavior pattern may seem to be inconsistent. Point two modes are open to information from the social context, making people vulnerable to information overload.

The level is consolidated at .4 when all of the information contained in the level can be processed. The consolidation is done by selecting some information and discarding unwanted information. People are busy processing information and usually look comfortable with what they are doing. Their actions are deliberate, fluid, and display a repeated use of the information in the level. They may be absorbed in the challenge of understanding how to use the final bits of information. The therapist's efforts to introduce more information are rejected, and may be stubbornly refused.

Information from the next cognitive level is accepted at .6. Point 6 is a blessing in that patients are curious about information from the next level.

## Table 5.1 Sequence of modes in the cognitive levels

.0 Primary aggregate of the level

.2 Orientation of the level

.4 Consolidation of the level

.6 Open to information in the next level

.8 Composite formation of the next level

Point 6 can also be dangerously unpredictable. Therapists may not be able to predict which bits of information will capture attention. People in the point 6 mode try to work with information without the benefit of an aggregate or a composite. The information is out of context. They will, for example, walk to the bathroom without knowing where the bathroom is. This scattered use of information makes caregiving difficult.

A composite is formed at .8. Bits of information from the next cognitive level are added together into a sum, but a whole is not formed. In the .8 mode people often look hesitant or frustrated. They have all of the pieces of information but cannot understand how the pieces fit together. As a result they appear to be indecisive or dependent on others to tell then how to fit the information together. The information may be used inflexibly, just as it was given to them.

The pieces fit together when the aggregate for the next cognitive level is formed (.0). Once the aggregate for the next level is formed, patients have a more flexible use of the previous level. Patients realize that changes in the previous level can be made. This aggregate seems to give perspective to the previous level. At 5.0 patients realize that they do not have to conform with goal-directed activities and question the need to do an activity. At 4.8 patients conform with directions given.

The observations of behavior described by the modes suggest a sequence for processing sensori-motor information. The sequence is formed by adding bits of information. The natural healing process and psychotropic drugs increase the amount of information that people can process. Overlap between the modes and various tests of impaired perception and cognition is expected. Tests of perception are often used to identify the site of a brain lesion. The validity of these tests can be questioned if no effort is made to process the information. The modes provide a sequence of the added effort to process additional perceptual information. Suggestions are given for where in the sequence of the modes of performance various tests may be introduced. The introduction means that some of the information on these tests, frequently used in practice, may be processed (Siev, Freishtat, & Zoltan, 1986). The tests usually span several modes of performance.

The power of activities to increase the amount of information processed is a basic assumption in occupational therapy. The modes of performance make it possible to test the validity of that assumption. Therapists should test the validity of the assumption within the constraints of doing no harm.

In practice a therapist will probably administer the Allen Cognitive Level (ACL) test first and then observe performance in an activity selected by the patient. The attempt to evaluate performance during any activity that the patient will agree to do is an ambitious undertaking for therapists. To begin the assessment, provide material objects and instructions that match the ACL score. If the patient does that with ease, probe for a higher decimal point. If difficulties are apparent, probe for a lower decimal point. An overall assessment is given for each treatment session, usually lasting about an hour. You score the average quality of performance observed. Activities that have a lot of steps that differentiate between the modes would be expected to provide the most valid evaluation. In some cases an exceptionally high or low step that is out of context with the rest of performance is noted. These exceptions may have prognostic implications, but are not included in the average score. The prognostic implications are often related to medication changes and should be communicated to the physician. Assess improvement or deterioration from 1 day, week, month, or year to the next by recording average response to assistance within a specified time period.

Treatment matches the patient's current ability to the demands of the activity. The decimal system explains the transition from one mode to the next, and the therapist can probe to see if the next mode is emerging. The therapist's probes may or may not be necessary for the emergence of the next mode. Because we are uncertain about the power of activities, therapists are expected to evaluate abilities each time that the patient is seen during the postacute and rehabilitation phases of the illness. A probe for the next mode is done by cuing with information from the mode. If the patient ignores or rejects the information, the next mode is not the just-right challenge. A challenge that cannot be met is frustrating for the patient and the therapist, and should be discontinued. A decline in mode would also indicate a need to reduce the amount of information to match current abilities.

Harm can be propagated by forcing someone to try to process information beyond his or her full capacity. Pushing disabled people to a higher mode provides a disability experience. A disability experience is an encounter with one's limitations, the opposite of mastery, competency, and increased self-esteem. Disabled people are apt to have more of these experiences than they would care to have. Without a better understanding of the validity of the assumptions about the power of activities, there is not adequate justification for making people go through bad experiences. Therapists need to be sensitive to the fact that continuous probing can produce negative experiences that might do more harm than good.

Functional assistance is the need for physical or cognitive help to do ordinary activities safely. While a need for physical assistance is obvious, the largest burden of care is for persons who need cognitive assistance. When physical assistance is the only need indicated, one assumes that there is no need for cognitive assistance. When that assumption is incorrect, long-term goals and plans are also incorrect. To provide an accurate picture of the burden of care, the need for physical assistance must be placed in the context of a need for cognitive assistance when both needs are present.

Modern technology provides a wide range of compensations for physical disabilities, and attendant care is often scheduled for a few hours each day. The burden of care consists of the amount of physical assistance required and the amount of time that another person spends providing that assistance. The need for cognitive assistance is often required 24 hours a day, with a continuous demand on human resources. The burden of care consists of the amount of time and energy required from another person.

The assistance required to do ambulation, self-care, and communication activities is described to facilitate use by physical therapy, occupational therapy, and speech–language pathology. The descriptions are not intended to define the activities done by each profession. The intent is to describe an overall need for functional assistance to do these activities safely.

The modes of performance emphasize the disabled person's remaining abilities in an ordinal scale that is cumulative. A person characterized by 4.4 is thought to have all of the abilities described from 0.8 through 4.4. That person's disabilities would include an incapacity to process the information described at 4.5 and above. A brief description of the social consequences of the disability for each mode is included to help place perspective on the disability.

## Coma

Coma is a prolonged state of being unconscious including a lack of response to stimuli, from which it is impossible to rouse that person.

## 0.8 Generalized Reflexive Actions

These actions are controlled at the level of the brainstem and fail to reach the cortex. A total body response of flexion or extension, or a change in respiration rate may be observed. Startle reactions as well as opening and closing of the eyes, mouth, and hands may occur for no apparent reason or as a general response to a stimulus.

## Level 1: Automatic Actions

An automatic action is a component of the sensori-motor system that shows a meaningful response to an external stimulus. The primary aggregate allows the patient to make an association between a sensory cue and a specific motor action. A change in the level of arousal is a specific response to an external stimulus that produces pain or has instinctive survival value. Meaning may be attached to stimulation of any one of the five senses (see Table 5.2).

*Total assistance* is the need for 24-hour supervision to feed, bathe, and clothe the patient, and maintain the patient's skin integrity.

*Ambulation:* The need for physical assistance is due to a cognitive inability to overcome the effects of gravity. The patient's movements may range from a withdrawal from noxious stimuli to, on command, holding an arm or leg up for a few seconds. While often bedridden, the patient may be secured into a sitting position. Caregivers need to apply bed rails, safety straps, and antipressure cushions, and monitor the fit and position of splints and adaptive equipment. Change in the position of the body must be initiated by the caregiver to maintain skin integrity.

*Self-care:* Eating may range from artificial feeding to picking up finger food and drinking from a cup placed in the patient's hand. The patient may wear diapers or be placed on a bedpan at regular intervals. Bed baths or use of a Hoyer lift to get in and out of the bathtub may be required.

*Communication:* Speaking may range from moans and grimaces to smiles and increased re-

Table 5.2 Level 1: Automatic actions

| | | Behaving | Speaking | Timing |
|---|---|---|---|---|
| 1.0 | Withdrawing | Specific response to noxious stimuli | Moans | |
| 1.2 | Responding to stimuli | Blinks, salivates, sniffs, lick lips | Moans, grimaces | |
| 1.4 | Locating stimuli | Eye tracking. Turns head to find and follow stimuli. Controls mouth and tongue to chew and swallow. | Grunts, grimaces, and smiles | Flicker to a few seconds |
| 1.6 | Rolling in bed | Completes rolling over in bed when initiated by others. | Smiles, grunts, screams | Momentary |
| 1.8 | Raising body part | Raises extremities. Pushes away. With cue, raises buttocks. | Increased response to loved ones. "No." | Hold against gravity is brief and unreliable. |

sponse to loved ones. Communication can also include the word "no" and pushing away feared objects. Efforts to communicate are initiated by pain or external stimulation. Caregivers must initiate and fulfill the basic needs for survival.

## 1.0 Withdrawing

A specific withdrawal from a noxious stimulus is usually the first response when coming out of a coma. Noxious stimuli are often tactile and may include pin pricking or icing. Visual stimuli may include a flash of lights shown in the patients eyes. The patient may or may not moan.

## 1.2 Responding to Stimuli

A general response to stimulation of one of the five senses occurs. Opening and shutting eyes may occur in direct response to visual/auditory stimuli that are not noxious. Visual stimuli may include mirrors and faces, followed by tracking of visual stimuli and watching mobiles. Auditory stimuli may include looking in the direction in which the patient's name was called or a bell was rung. Olfactory stimuli may include responses to odors that are pungent such as mustard, garlic, onions, vanilla, or peppermint. Gustatory stimuli may be sweet, sour, or salty. Licking lips, salivating, or sniffing in response to smells and tastes may be observed. Memories of familiar stimuli may be evoked but cannot be verified; orientation is to present stimulus. Patient is

bedridden and requires tube feeding. Communication may be limited to moans and grimaces. Twenty-four-hour nursing care for artificial feeding and turning to maintain skin integrity is required.

## 1.4 Locating Stimuli

Turning the head to locate a stimulus may be observed. Locating a stimulus is often associated with enough awareness to begin eating a soft diet of pureed food. With abnormal adults, pureed food precedes the introduction of liquids. Control of lip and tongue movements, swallowing, and chewing may be elicited. Hand-over-hand feeding may be effective in improving posture; the caregiver guides the patient's hand to the mouth. An automatic action of lifting the head to the spoon may help clear the passageway. Food preferences may be expressed through grunts, grimaces, or smiles. The attention span may be a flicker to a few seconds; continuous cuing to eat may be required

Therapists testing for ocular pursuit, saccadic eye movements, visual field, or visual neglect must consider this tendency to turn the head. The direction to hold the head still may not be understood until level 4, making the test results invalid until the direction is understood.

## 1.6 Rolling in Bed

When rolling is initiated by someone else, the patient may complete the turn. Momentary attention to external stimuli may last as long as 10 seconds. Rocking and moving to a sitting position may be initiated by others and continued by the patient. The patient may smile, grunt, or scream to communicate pain or pleasure. Increased responses to own name may occur.

## 1.8 Raising Body Part

The patient may hold an arm or leg up against gravity with continuous cuing. Holding the buttocks up for a few seconds may be elicited with cuing. The patient may cooperate with a sponge bath given in bed and roll to ease placement of a bedpan. The patient may push objects away if viewed as noxious or say "no." Increased responses to loved ones may occur. Favorite objects from home and pictures of home may evoke responses of recognition.

## Level 2: Postural Actions

Postural actions are self-initiated gross motor movements that overcome the effects of gravity and move the body in space. Common actions that overcome the effects of gravity include sitting, standing, walking, and preventing falls. Other associated actions include clapping hands, waving, nodding head, and voluntary blinking. The purpose that seems to make sense to the patient is comfort. Comfort is a state of ease or satisfaction of bodily wants, with freedom from pain or anxiety. Comfort is noted in efforts to move body parts voluntarily in response to internal sensations or external commands. To follow exter-

nal commands the patient must think that the commands are benign (see Table 5.3).

Therapists use vestibular, tactile, and verbal cues to elicit gross body movements. Essential objects such as bed, chair, table, sliding board, or grab bars may be used.

*Maximum assistance* is the need for 24-hour supervision to prevent falls as the patient sits, stands, walks, and grabs onto objects for postural stability.

*Ambulation:* The patient has enough trunk stability to sit up and will spontaneously push self up in a chair to overcome the effects of gravity. Standing may be with or without physical assistance. A major physical disability, like paralysis, may not be recognized, requiring restraint for those who try to stand when unable to bear weight. Walking may be aimless or directed within a familiar environment; an escort outside of the home or institution may be required. Caregivers may need to lock the doors or install alarms to prevent wandering off and getting lost. The need for physical assistance is due to a lack of awareness of hazards that could contribute to falling.

*Self-care:* Toileting assistance may range from needing to be placed on the toilet to help with wiping and adjusting garments while holding onto grab bars. Food must be precut, with temperatures and seasonings checked and placed in front of the patient. Caregivers must be nearby to assist with spills, choking, opening containers, and ensuring

Table 5.3  Level 2: Postural actions

|  |  | Behaving | Speaking | Timing |
|---|---|---|---|---|
| 2.0 | Overcoming gravity | Holds trunk stable for sitting | Reocgnizes own name; "Bed" | Holds trunk in chair until tired |
| 2.2 | Righting reflex/standing | Puts out arm to prevent falling; Stands | Says own name | Stands/sits on command |
| 2.4 | Walking | Aimless walking through doorways, around objects | Perseverative words ("Thank you;" swear words) | Walks until tired |
| 2.6 | Directed walking | Steps up, over; Pushes, bangs on closed doors | Asks for, identifies locations ("bed," "bathroom") | Walks until gets there |
| 2.8 | Using grab bars/railings | Grabs objects or people to stabilize the motion he or she is doing | Gestures, uses short phrases | Holds until postural stability achieved |

adequate food intake. The patient may cooperate with grooming, dressing, and bathing by moving body parts in response to cues; response times may be very slow and impractical in some settings.

*Communication:* The patient may recognize and say his or her name, use perseverative words, identify locations such as bed and bathroom, or use short phrases and gestures. A few vital needs may be expressed but most must be initiated and fulfilled by the caregiver.

## 2.0 Overcoming Gravity

Overcoming gravity is the first self-initiated motor action, providing enough trunk stability to stay seated in an upright position. The patient may stay seated until tired and indicate a desire to go to bed when asked. The patient may feed self finger food and drink from a cup without physical assistance. Recognition of own name and discrimination between yes and no may occur. All response times are very slow, without awareness of intervening stimuli or the passage of time. Twenty-four-hour nursing care to change position, provide food, and do bathroom activities is required.

## 2.2 Righting Reactions/Standing

A righting reaction is a spontaneous and effective use of the arms to keep from falling over to the side or backwards. A righting reaction requires a conscious awareness of the effects of gravity. The patient may stand, take a few steps with physical assistance, or do a pivot transfer with standby assistance. Standing may be sustained as long as endurance allows. The patient may be able to say his or her name when asked.

## 2.4 Walking

Walking is on flat surfaces without being aware of a destination. Walking around large pieces of furniture and walking through doorways shows some awareness of the environment. Some patients persist in walking to the point of pacing and continue to walk as long as endurance allows. A few perseverative words may be spoken ("thank you," swear words). Twenty-four-hour nursing care to initiate and assist with all activities of daily living and prevent wandering into dangerous locations is required.

## 2.6 Directed Walking

The patient may be walking with a destination in mind, like going to the bathroom or to bed, but not know where the destination is. Patients may continue to walk until they get to their destination or until tired. Stepping up a curb, lifting feet over the edge of the bathtub, or placing feet on the wheelchair may occur. If doors or gates are closed, the patient may push, bang, or shake the obstacle. Imitation of gross body movements of the upper extremities and trunk may be elicited. Words related to vital needs may be spoken, usually bathroom or bed.

Some cooperation with pointing to body parts may begin at level 2.6, suggesting the possibility of reliable results for tests of somatognosia. Understanding body relationships such as left/right, above/below, behind, between, and so forth, would not be expected until level 4.

## 2.8 Using Grab Bars

The patient may spontaneously reach out and grasp grab bars, railings, or any other object that is handy to keep from falling. Objects that will not hold the patient's weight should be removed, and objects on wheels should have the wheels locked. The patient's grasp may not be tight enough to support him or her, or too tight for too long. A caregiver may have to pry the patient's hands off a grab bar. The patient is apt to hold on until a sense of postural stability is achieved, which is apt to be processed very slowly. The patient's use of gestures and short phrases may be out of context. Twenty-four-hour nursing care to initiate activities of daily living and ensure postural stability is needed.

## Level 3: Manual Actions

Manual actions use the hands, and occasionally other parts of the body, to manipulate material objects. The objects are picked up, moved, and set down, but the effect of these actions is not noted. A sequence of actions required to achieve a goal is not initiated but may be imitated or followed when cued. The quality of the actions may be too fast/slow, weak/strong, short/long, or too much/too little. The action seems to be done because it is interesting to the patient. Interest is in the action suggested by the object (see Table 5.4).

Therapists should provide objects that can be grasped in one hand and used in a classic manner. Grooming supplies may include: wash cloth and soap, toothbrush and paste, comb and hair brush, towel, deodorant, lipstick, shampoo and condi-

Table 5.4 Level 3: Manual actions

| | | **Behaving** | **Speaking** | **Timing** |
|---|---|---|---|---|
| 3.0 | Grasping objects | Grasps or throws objects; Walks away | Names a few objects | Slow response; Sustains grasp a few seconds or holds on until removed |
| 3.2 | Distinguishing objects | Uses associated action of object; Random placement of object | Names objects; Names home/ hospital | Starts and stops on command |
| 3.4 | Sustaining actions on objects | Repetitive actions; May follow left to right | Names actions; Speaks without considering comprehension of listener | Duration of sustained action; Distractible |
| 3.6 | Noting effects on objects | Notes shape; Linear or perimeter placement | Names shapes; Message related to vital need | Will wait for effect when cued |
| 3.8 | Using all objects | Covers space or uses all supplies | "I'm done;" May not ask for help in discomfort; May accept discomfort or abandon task | Sense of completion; Duration of sustained action determined by available objects |

tioner. Other objects may include a spoon, fork, food that has been cut up, liquids that have been poured, toilet paper, paper and pencils, paint brushes, sand paper, needle and thread, mosaic tiles, string and beads, carrot/potato peelers with vegetables, green peas in shells, string beans, linens to be folded, brooms and mops, and dust rags. These objects tend to be cross-cultural, with a universal way of handling these objects.

*Moderate assistance* is the need for 24-hour supervision to remove dangerous objects, restrain misuse of common objects, and guide the patient through the steps of an activity.

*Ambulation:* In the absence of a physical disability, ambulation is slow but within normal range and endurance. Wheelchairs may be used for ambulation difficulties when pushed by caregiver and assisted with locks and foot pedals. The patient may be able to push the wheelchair forward and back, but may not be able to turn corners. Walkers, canes, and crutches may not be used safely. The patient may need to be restrained from weight bearing due to an inability to understand a physical disability. Other wandering preventions and escorts may be required.

*Self-care:* Caregiver assistance is required to place familiar objects in front of the patient and sequence the patient through the familiar steps of bathing, grooming, dressing, eating, toileting, and taking medication. To achieve an acceptable level of hygiene or adequate intake of food, a caregiver must be present to check results, prompt continued actions, interrupt perseverative actions, and prevent unfavorable effects. Adaptive equipment, such as built-up spoons and wash mitts that resemble unadapted objects may be used. Dangerous, nonedible, and valuable objects may need to be removed from plain sight.

*Communication:* Messages concerning vital needs may be communicated and familiar objects and actions may be named. The patient may not ask for help when in mild discomfort or may speak or write without considering the comprehension of the listener or reader. The patient may not distinguish between day, date, or time but may differentiate between home and hospital. In some cases, the patient may insist on going home, or make an attempt to go home and require restraint when not possible.

## 3.0 Grasping Objects

The patient reaches for, grasps, holds, or throws objects placed in front of him or her. These responses are apt to be very slow and may be sustained for a few seconds or until the object is removed. An object may be rejected by walking or turning away. Objects should be offered at eye level or placed on a table about 6 inches in front of the patient. Response time to pick up the object may be delayed for a few seconds. Grasp may be sustained for a few seconds or until the object is removed. The patient's posture is apt to be hunched over, gazing at the table. The patient may be able to name the object in his or her hand.

## 3.2 Distinguishing Objects

Distinguishing between objects is separating the actions associated with one object from another, such as making a distinction between a hairbrush and a toothbrush. The patient picks up an object and goes through the associated motion correctly. Movements indicate that the characteristic actions associated with the object are recognized. These actions can be started and stopped on command. The patient may act without looking at the object, and the object may be laid down in a random location.

Some parts of constructional apraxia tests include these movements. The patient may not understand that the movements are supposed to be pretend or may be unable to do the action in the absence of the object.

The patient may be easily distracted. Assistance may be required to stop an action, to move an action to a different location, or to introduce another action. The quality of the effects of the actions are not judged and demonstrated modifications are ignored. The patient may distinguish between home and the hospital and name the objects used. Twenty-four-hour nursing care is required to restrict access to dangerous objects as these patients are apt to pick up and manipulate anything that they find. One-on-one supervision is required to complete the self-care activities with an acceptable result.

## 3.4 Sustaining Actions on Objects

Sustained actions are actions that change the location of a bunch of similar things, like mosaic tiles, or change the exterior surface by adding something to it or removing something from it, like sanding and staining. One action on one object is repeated over

and over again for a minute or longer. The actions may move from left to right in response to internal organization if the person has learned to read and write in a left to right sequence. The duration of the action may be brief or prolonged and may be easily interrupted by distractions.

The patient may be able to identify the action being done but is not apt to speak with consideration for the comprehension of the listener. The patient may restate a goal given by the therapist but forgets the goal within minutes. Interest is in the repetitive action and the effects are poorly understood. The patient may not differentiate between objects being used, trash, samples, or patterns. Some objects, like sandpaper or pencils, may be used upside down.

Twenty-four-hour supervision is required to place objects needed for activities of daily living in front of the patient and sequence the patient through the necessary steps to achieve acceptable results. One person may supervise three patients at a time. An escort to help the patient avoid getting lost is needed outside the living environment.

## 3.6 Noting Effects on Objects

Noting the effects on objects is starting, stopping, and placing objects according to a feature of the object. The feature is usually the perimeter of the object, and objects are often placed in a row. The shapes of objects may be named. The naming of shapes may not be adequate for obtaining reliable results on tests of visual perception and tactile agnosia. An understanding of the testing situation is also assumed by these tests. Test administration needs to make explicit modifications to account for this deficiency at levels 3.6 and 3.8.

Cooperation with finger agnosia tests may begin by imitating finger movements or pointing to a hand chart. Responses are apt to be very slow and require considerable redirection of attention. During activity performance, the patient may stop a repetitive action when errors in the shape of the object or in linear placement are noted. Imitation of manual actions for changes in duration and location may occur when a clear functional reason is given, like shaving missed spots. The patient can wait for an effect when cued, for example will wait for the water to get warm. The patient may realize that a message is being conveyed to another person; the content usually contains a vital, personal need.

Twenty-four-hour supervision is needed to provide the materials needed for activities of daily living, remind to finish necessary steps, check results, and remove access to dangerous objects. The patient must be watched while awake because of impulsive and unpredictable actions that can be dangerous.

## 3.8 Using All Objects

Using all of the objects is covering all space, using all supplies, or recognizing the task is done upon completion. The patient systematically covers the interior space of an object, or uses all available supplies and stops when this is done. The concept of being done is generated after the task is completed and is not part of the process of doing the task. The patient says "I'm done." Surprise that a project has been made or that the job is done may be expressed. The patient may not be depended on to request help when needed and may accept discomfort or abandon a task when help is needed. Timing is determined by the number of objects available or the size of the surface to be covered; social conventions for measuring time have no meaning.

Twenty-four-hour supervision is needed to get materials out that are needed for activities of daily living, check results, and remove access to dangerous objects.

## Level 4: Goal-Directed Activity

Goal-directed activities sequence the self through a series of steps to match a concrete sample or comply with a known sequence for getting a task done. The purpose that seems to make sense to the patient is compliance. The task is done in the customary manner and complies with standards of performance set by or accepted by the patient. The effects of the patient's actions are judged, and the patient requests help when mistakes are noticed (see Table 5.5).

The information processed while doing an activity is from the striking features of objects. Striking features are the prominent or conspicuous qualities of objects, and all of these qualities can be seen. Striking features include shape, color, size, horizontal and vertical axes, sequence, and number up to 4. The shape of the object should be about 3 to 16 inches long and two-dimensional. Use shapes of classic objects such as flowers, trees, butterflies, vegetables, animals, clothing or furniture. Use black and white, and primary and secondary colors; strong

colors are more conspicuous. Parts of objects should be lined up on a horizontal and/or a vertical axis. Parts of objects may be of a different size, shape, or color; limit the number of each feature to four.

The easiest standard of performance is a sample of a craft project or work task that concretely exhibits the expected outcome. Both the therapist and the patient share the stimulus for what is expected. The standards for many activities of daily living are located in the stored sensorimotor models in the patient's and the therapist's mind. When the patients say that they want it that way, the therapist must accept that standard of performance. For evaluation purposes, a physical representation of what is to be reproduced is recommended.

*Minimum assistance* is the need for daily assistance to remove access to dangerous objects and solve any problems occurring through changes in the patient's environment.

*Ambulation:* Recognition of a physical disability exists, along with a need for physical assistance. Bathroom safety may require assistance to recognize hazards produced by flooding or slippery floors. The patient may learn to use a wheelchair or walker after repetitive training but require assistance to lock the brakes of a chair or adapt to uneven surfaces. The patient may not be able to learn to use a walker with wheels, crutches, or canes safely.

*Self-care:* Familiar routines for doing self-care activities may be done along as long as nothing out of the ordinary happens. The pace may be slow and invariant. Caregiver assistance may be sought when something unusual happens but no distinction between a minor change and a major emergency may be made. Caregiver supervision may be needed when using objects that are sharp, hot, toxic, chemical, electrical, or harmful in any other way. Medical complications caused by adaptive equipment, splints, medication compliance, wound care, and following a restricted diet may require daily supervision. The patient may insist on doing activities with potential harm (driving) and restricted access may be required.

*Communication:* The conversations of others may be interrupted with personal demands or the needs of the listener may not be considered. Speech is self-centered, immediate, and concrete. The patient may not produce a new idea or consider future possibilities. The patient may fall back on previously learned social formalities but miss nonverbal cues or current context. Assistance may be required

Table 5.5  Level 4: Goal-directed activity

| | | Behaving | Speaking | Timing | |
|---|---|---|---|---|---|
| | | | | Orientation | Sequence of Events |
| 4.0 | Sequencing | One way to do an activity. Redirects self. Arm's length. Accept/reject actions. | Asks for next step/ help; No problem identification | Disoriented to day/date | Actions |
| 4.2 | Differentiating features | Recognizes matching error. Looks to side or 24 inches in front. | Identifies features/ problems | Asks for day/ date; One hour increments | One activity at a time |
| 4.4 | Completing goal | Contrasts/compares to conform. Plain sight with 3 to 4 feet. | Requests matching supplies | Knows day/date | Follows routine sequence of activities |
| 4.6 | Personalizing | Scans environment. Stands/retrieves supplies. Varies amount, depth, pressure. Notices others. | Requests past supplies; Comments on others' nonconformity | Knows two concurrent schedules exist | Initiates change in routine sequence |
| 4.8 | Rote learning | Rotates objects when done. Slow visual inspection. No choice in activity. | Asks for verification | Knows how two concurrent schedules fit together | Fits daily routine into schedule of others |

to limit personal demands to an acceptable time and place. Assistance with or limited access to money management may be required. The need for assistance may not be recognized and the assistance offered may be rejected unless legal actions are taken.

## 4.0 Sequencing

Sequencing is directing the self through known steps to complete a task or seeking instruction with the next step when a new task is being done. The patient may know one way to do an activity and follow the sequence of steps without assistance. The patient may be distracted while doing the task, but redirects self back to the task. The patient may work until done, out of time, told to quit, or exhausted. Spontaneous attempts to move through a familiar sequence of steps may be incorrect, but the patient may not comply with a demonstration to correct the sequence.

The patient moves within the spatial proximity of arm's length. For tabletop activities, the space can be measured by placing one's elbows at the edge of the table, arms at the side, and bending fingers across the top. Objects located within that space are noticed and used. The patient may be unable to shift attention to any other person, material object, or external event outside of working space. If distracted by external or internal stimuli, the patient may stop working to shift attention. After the distraction, the patient may redirect his/her own attention back to the task.

In an unfamiliar sequence the patient may ask what the next step is and may be expected to ask for assistance when something out of the ordinary happens. The request is a general "help me," usually lacking a clear identification of the nature of the problem. On-site assistance is required to clarify the problem and demonstrate the solution after a call for help.

Time is measured by the immediate goal and does not usually extend beyond an hour. A few very important goals can be prioritized and maintained over the course of a month, like a monthly source of income. Otherwise the patient is disoriented to the day and date, measuring time as a sequence of actions.

Twenty-four-hour supervision to remove dangerous objects and solve any problems occurring through minor changes in routine is needed. The patient may engage in simple habits like making a sandwich or going to the corner store to buy cigarettes or chewing gum.

## 4.2 Differentiating Features

To differentiate is to point out the difference between two things according to one of the following features of objects: linear measure, shape, color, or linear direction. The patient matches features one feature at a time. A matching error is recognized as a problem, which is usually followed by a request for help. No attempt, however, may be made to solve the problem.

Matching is an implicit expectation of tests of tactile agnosia, constructional apraxia, and visual perception such as figure ground, form constancy, and position in space. The initiation of activities, memory of prior activities and how to do them, and topographical orientation may be more reliably tested when the patient understands that he or she is asked to match a sample of behavior.

Attention may be totally focused on the task while working, with no attention paid to other people or other activities. The visual field extends about 24 inches beyond the space described at 4.0, usually looking toward the dominant side or in front. The patient may look at a sample of a completed project and try to replicate the sample.

The patient may remember doing similar tasks and familiar sequences of events, but may not bring experiences to present task to suggest changes. The comparison with the past is concrete, usually mentioning the physical properties of objects. An incorrect sequence for a familiar task is not self-corrected, but the patient will comply with a corrected demonstration.

The patient may be fixed on a task or goal that is most important to him/her. The sequence of events that leads to achieving that goal may be remembered with repetition. Attention may become fixated on valued goals, making it difficult to direct attention to other tasks. The patient may be disoriented to clock and calendar but may ask about the day and date. Time may be measure in 1-hour increments, one activity at a time.

Protection from hazards outside of the patient's visual field is required. The patient needs 24-hour supervision to remove dangerous objects and solve any problems arising from minor changes in the environment. The patient may spend a daily allowance, walk to familiar locations in the neighborhood, or follow a simple, familiar bus route when trained to check for visible hazards. The patient may go to the drug store or a medical clinic and may state a medical problem that has been present for a period of time.

## 4.4 Completing a Goal

Completing a goal is complying with the steps to match a standard of performance according to the 4.2 properties with the addition of number up to four and simultaneous consideration of horizontal and vertical axes. Two features are considered simultaneously, but only one pair at a time. Attention may shift from one pair of features to another pair. Tests for spatial relations and form constancy often require matching for two features at a time and may start to be reliable. Demonstrations to solve problems involving a pair of features may be followed. Compliance may aim for an exact match of a sample, or a stored model may serve as a standard of performance. The patient may be unwilling to deviate from the sample or solve any other problems but matching for visual/tactile features.

The patient may lift his or her head to look around and may notice objects located at eye level, or 3 to 4 feet in front of him or her on a counter or a table. Changes in posture in response to the location of an object may be observed, but the patient may not rotate material objects to make working easier.

The patient may ask for supplies needed to match a standard and concretely compare present task to tasks done in the past. Interruptions of others to ask for assistance with own goals may occur, with the expectation of being waited on immediately.

The patient may follow a set routine for doing daily activities, which may not be guided by the clock. The patient may be oriented to the day and date.

When able to read, the patient may not apply the ability to read labels on products, signs of warning, precautions, or instructions. Reading is not functional.

The removal of hazardous objects from visual field and restricted access to dangerous objects may be required. Frequent safety checks of environments in which daily activities are done may be recommended. The patient may need to be reminded to put trash in the trash can, take out the garbage, and put tools and supplies away. The patient may need to be told that he or she can get a desired object for himself or herself.

The patient may live with someone who does a

daily check of the environment and removes any safety hazards and solves any new problems. The patient may be left alone for part of the day with a procedure for obtaining help by telephone or from a neighbor. The patient may have a daily allowance and go to familiar places in the neighborhood when trained to check for visible hazards. The color, number, and time of day for taking medications may be stated, but not necessarily followed without assistance.

## 4.6 Personalizing

Personalizing is done concretely by changing one of the features or changing tools according to past experience. The patient may remember similar tasks and individualize the present task by changing a striking visual feature. The patient may ask for supplies used in the past that are not seen in his or her visual field. These requests may or may not fit with the present task. Compliance with an exact match of the sample is no longer required. The patient may overcome a difficulty with a primary effect on a striking feature of an object, but secondary effects are not understood when they are pointed out. The primary effect is the patient's intended effect on the object. The secondary effect is caused by the primary effect. The secondary effect is a change in the object that is caused by the properties of the object rather than the intent of the patient. Examples of the primary effect include gluing objects, polishing nails, or curling hair with a curling iron. The secondary effects might be sticking projects to the work surface when glue spills over the edge, smearing nail polish that is not dry, or burning fingers or forehead with a hot curling iron.

Scanning is looking around the immediate environment and noticing objects and people that are in plain sight. People hold their head up and turn their head at 4.6. Searching on countertops, tables, open cupboards, and in top drawers for an object needed to achieve a goal may be observed. The patient looks across a table to see what others are doing or to locate a supply. Once a desirable object is seen, the patient may get up and go get it, without being told to do so.

The patient may make comments about what he or she sees that is embarrassing to others, like negative comments about someone's appearance. These statements may be an observation of nonconformity with a standard, or a comparison to a standard.

Attempts to use the distinguishing properties of objects from the next model may be observed for a short duration of time. Neuromuscular adjustments of short duration may be successful. Neuromuscular adjustments are changes in the amount of strength or range of motion applied to improve effects on material objects. The adjustments made at 4.6 tend to rely on brute force, pressing harder to change the effects or realizing that too much force was applied.

Demonstrations of spatial changes in the parts of objects may be imitated, such as moving a piece higher, lower, or upside down to increase efficiency or effectiveness. Variations in the amount of a supply used may be tried with some success. A beginning awareness of the third dimension may be seen when gouges or dips in the surface are noted. Actions may be varied according to the top or bottom of an object: stirring stains at the bottom of the can, scraping the bottom of the bowl, or putting on a second coat of nail polish or paint. Awareness of features from the next model may be spotty, of short duration, or unpredictable.

These patients may follow their own routine for doing activities and initiate a change in their schedule. The patient may follow a routine for a restricted diet. Recognition of their daily schedule and awareness that another person has a concurrent schedule may occur. When a scheduling conflict occurs, the patient may not be able to fit the two schedules together. Patients may expect others to make changes in the sequence of events for them or require assistance to conform with the schedule of others. The patient may need to be taken to a physician's appointment.

The patient may live alone with daily assistance to monitor personal safety and provide a daily allowance. Bills and other money management concerns require assistance. The patient may require reminders to do household chores, attend familiar community events, or do anything in addition to daily household routine.

## 4.8 Rote Learning

Rote learning is memorizing a new sequence of steps by adding one step at a time. The memorization may be slow and rigid, requiring frequent verification. The patient may not talk and work at the same time. Performance may be characterized by frequent stops to examine the object, seek verification, or talk to others. During performance, patients may note the primary effects of their actions on the striking features and correct any errors without assistance.

After the task in completed, the patient may detect and correct errors in the secondary effects on striking features. A slow and careful examination may be done when the patient stops acting on the object or when the task is done. Patients may rotate the object and inspect the effects of their actions.

Use of information from the next model is apt to be most successful in adjusting the amount of a supply to be used and correcting spatial location difficulties without assistance. When instructed in use of neuromuscular adjustments, surface properties, and spatial properties, efforts to follow instructions are apt to be done laboriously.

The clock may be used for periods of about 15 minutes, with great effort. The patient may understand how two schedules fit together and fit his or her daily schedule into the schedule of others. Assistance with activities that are not done daily may be required.

Living alone may be possible with daily assistance to monitor safety and check for secondary effects. The patient may go to a regularly scheduled community activity or succeed in supportive employment with a job coach. The patient may be compliant with medical routines or not consider the possibility that medications could be changed.

## Level 5: Exploratory Actions

Exploratory actions are discoveries of how changes in neuromuscular control can produce different effects on material objects. The patient detects the best effect by exploring the distinctive properties of objects and trying different actions. The determination of what is best may be made according to personal preferences or social standards. The purpose that seems to make sense to the patient is learning a new way of doing things. Learning is recognized and repeated during the process of doing an action. The aggregate for new actions allows the patient to estimate the effects of his or her actions during the process of doing the action (see Table 5.6).

An estimate of the effects of actions takes prior experience into account and makes a rough guess of what the effects will be on present objects. While the action is being done, the patient can check the accuracy of the estimate. An unexpected or unwanted effect can be detected, and the action can be varied to produce a different effect. Varied actions and effects allow the patient to learn which is the best effect.

Estimates of effects can be characterized as primary, secondary, and potential secondary effects. The primary effect is the intended change in the material object that the individual estimates will happen by varying actions. Secondary effects are the natural and inevitable consequences of following a course of action, given the properties of objects. Potential secondary effects are natural but not inevitable and depend on a combination of conditions for occurrence.

*Standby assistance* is the need for supervision while learning to do new motor actions or activities to prevent unfavorable secondary effects and ensure compliance with safety precautions in hazardous situations.

*Ambulation:* New movement patterns may be demonstrated and practiced until refinements are learned. Continuous adjustments in new motor learning may be made and corrected during the process of moving with verbal and demonstrated directions. The application and use of new movement patterns and mobility aids must be monitored until well-learned. Assistance in judging distance, space, pace, endurance, and pain may be required. The accuracy of self-report and understanding of functional limitations may improve when discussing the performance of new movement patterns.

*Self-care:* Assistance with selecting and scheduling daily activities according to changing physical cognitive abilities may be required. Discussions of hazards in using adaptive equipment are understood when dangerous objects are present or during the process of performance; abstract discussions of possibilities may not be understood. The patient may act impulsively after hazards seem to be understood and safety precautions are learned. When frustrated, the patient may question the need to do the activity, insist on an ineffective or inefficient way of doing things, ignore safety precautions, or stop working to talk.

*Communication:* Conversations that employ new information may be concrete and self-centered. Abstract reasoning may not be understood or followed in an inflexible manner. Assistance may be needed for the patient to follow written directions, plan future activities, establish priorities, and anticipate needs and safety hazards.

**Table 5.6  Level 5: Exploratory actions**

| | | Behaving | Speaking | Timing | | Pacing |
| --- | --- | --- | --- | --- | --- | --- |
| | | | | Orienting | Sequencing | |
| 5.0 | Making neuromuscular variations. | Continuous neuromusbular changes with difficulty. Rejects activity in process. | Stops working to talk. Questions need to do activity. | Knows need to make appointments and to schedule infrequent events. | Apt to forget or miss. | Invariant. |
| 5.2 | Discriminating. | Explores tangible properties. Rotates objects while working. | Talks and works. Seeks tools/ material to alter methods. | Uses watches, calendar, appointment book, alarms, memory aids. | Depends on tangible reminders to keep schedules. | Impulsive. |
| 5.4 | Self-directed learning. | Alters tools, sequences. Acts on spatial properties. Adjusts posture. Reorganizes work space. | Insists on own methods. | Chooses to follow/ disregard schedules. | Plans spare time around own priorities. | Argues with requests to change. Requests more time. |
| 5.6 | Considering social standards. | Compares instructions. Substitutes methods. | Discusses pros and cons of methods. | Considers conventional schedules, cultural trends, politics, fashion. | Internal awareness of passage of time. | Adjusts on request. |
| 5.8 | Consulting. | Assumes activities have potential for unwanted secondary effects. | Describes possible effects. Seeks advice to avoid. | Seeks opinions of secondary effects of schedule changes. | Future effects of properties of objects. | Varies own pace. |

## 5.0 Comparing and Changing Variations

Comparing and changing variations are differences in the amount of strength, pressure, or range of motion applied to a material object that produces different effects. Continuous comparison and change require full attention while working. Talking and working at the same time do not occur. The patient may compare directions for doing a sequence of steps with prior experience to identify similarities and differences. Similarities may be retained and differences may be highlighted.

The patient may cluster this information to learn a sequence of new steps. The patient may watch a sequence of steps and replicate the process but may not form a new sequence independently.

The patient may estimate the internal adjustments of actions needed to produce a different effect. Neuromuscular variations may be made throughout the process of performance. Neuromuscular variations are self-initiated alterations in motor actions made to detect the relationship between changes in motor actions and effects on objects. The relationship between actions and striking effects is estimated, and the patient may eventually learn how to produce the effect consistently. Materials that offer resistance are more difficult to do conceptually. Inconsistent variations in the amount of strength and range of motion may be observed, with considerable change in actions and effects. The effective variations are not repeated consistently, suggesting that new models are formed but not stored. After several variations are explored, the patient may stop to talk or do something else. The persistence required to learn at 5.0 may consume a lot of time and energy.

The patient may recognize a choice in continuing or discontinuing an activity. Compliance in doing the activities identified by others is not required. The patient may have a schedule for daily activities and may make appointments and try to schedule infrequent events. With unusual frequency, the patient may be late, miss, or arrive at the wrong time for appointments. The pace of movement and the rate of speech may not be altered on request.

The patient may live alone with weekly checks to monitor safety and problem solving. Comparisons between prior and new medical procedures may be made and may cause confusion. The patient may succeed in supportive employment with a job coach and get self to a regularly scheduled community activity.

## 5.2 Discriminating

Discriminating is estimating the significance of a primary effect that actions have on the outward appearance of objects while in the process of producing the effect. Objects may be rotated while working on them to inspect effects, and surface properties are taken into consideration. Surface properties are the sheen, texture, evenness, smoothness, and highlights of objects that are a part of outward appearance. Tests for stereognosis that use materials of different textures may begin to be meaningful to the patient.

The patient may estimate the primary effects actions have on the outward appearance of objects. Secondary effects on surface properties are noted and corrected after they occur including small scratches, streaks, stains, tarnish, highlights, and uneven edges. The patient may not anticipate these secondary effects while working. Assistance to improve surface property effects may be needed.

Postural adjustment may be made according to the primary effects on objects, such as standing up straight to saw a straight line. Tests for motor apraxia that require postural adjustment for imagined actions may not begin to be reliable until level 5.2. A

consideration of the horizontal and vertical axes may occur simultaneously. The patient may follow a diagonal line with close scrutiny of the sample. Groups of two or more objects may be put together to form a functional unit such as bundles, stacks, or kits. The patient may throw trash in the wastepaper basket without being prompted to do so. Initiation of actions to find tools and materials to alter effects are apt to be made quickly without consideration of secondary effects, making many mistakes. Behavior may appear to be impulsive because the patient may consider primary effects without estimating secondary effects.

The patient may talk and work simultaneously but may not stop to think. Conversation may extend beyond what the patient is doing at the moment. The patient may make remarks that are irreverent to social standards by being facetious, flippant, or unduly familiar. The patient may have trouble adhering to a schedule or changing pace. Watches, calendars, appointment books, alarms, and other memory aids are used, with a reliance on these and other reminders to keep to a schedule.

The patient may live alone with weekly checks to monitor safety, medical compliance, and examine potentially dangerous effects of impulsive behavior. Success in supportive employment with a job coach and participation in community events may occur.

## 5.4 Self-Directed Learning

Self-directed learning is initiating changes that improve the effectiveness of efficiency of performance and may include alterations in tools, sequence of steps, linear measure, or work space. Fine-motor adjustments may also be observed. When a different tool or supply is needed, the patient may search around all of the work area for the desired item. A new solution to a problem may be formed and remembered.

The spatial properties of objects are taken into consideration. *Spatial properties* are the parts of objects in relation to the whole and include the spaces between objects, the space between parts of objects, negative spaces, overlaps in parts of objects, over and under for weaving, and small parts such as joints, corners, angles, arcs, and pieces smaller than one quarter of an inch. Different arrangements for better balance or harmony in the overall appearance are considered.

Patients may prevent inevitable secondary effect but not recognize or be inflexible about potential secondary effects. Insistence on their own method of doing things may occur, and extra precautions may need to be taken for errors that are unaffordable or too dangerous.

The patient may not persist if the task is tedious. Requests to change pace, be on time, or follow a schedule may be followed by a request for more time. Spare-time activities follow personal priorities and may be done on the spur of the moment.

The patient may live alone and work in jobs permitting a wide margin of error.

## 5.6 Considering Social Standards

Considering social standards is adjusting performance of the task outcome according to conventional expectations. Cultural trends, fashions and fads, politics, seasons, and holidays may be considered and discussed. Changes in the correspondence among parts of a whole can be made to improve symmetry, balance, proportion, and harmony according to current cultural values. The patient may harmonize, coordinate, or blend shades and patterns according to current fashions. Changes in the pace of actions may be made on request.

Estimating how the volume of an object can fit into a three-dimensional-object space may occur such as moving furniture, organizing closets, parking a car, or opening a door while seated in a wheelchair. The patient may see these interrelations between parts and the whole in three-dimensional space with assistance.

The patient may describe the properties of objects and discuss ways of adjusting the primary and secondary effects of the properties of objects. Two sets of instructions may be compared, and one method may be substituted for another after comparison. Unfortunately, potential secondary effects, including medication side effects, may not be understood. An internal awareness of the passage of time may allow the patient to adjust his or her pace on request. The patient may have an unusually high tendency to get busy doing things and forget about the passage of time.

## 5.8 Consulting

Consulting is seeking opinions about the expected effects on task outcome and unwanted secondary effects. To consult, one must assume that activities have the potential for unwanted secondary effects, and seek advice to avoid hazards. The future effects on the properties of objects are discussed and understood in the presence of material objects.

The patient may form a chain or sequence of effects on objects when the objects are present. The patient may anticipate inevitable secondary effects, but potential secondary effects may need to be explained by others. The expected effects may be described, and advice may be sought. The needs of others may not be anticipated. The patient may form chains of possible effects but cannot reverse the chain to imagine how a new effect was achieved by another person.

Variations in pace may be made in accordance with the properties of objects, secondary effect, and the clock. These variations are self-initiated. Consideration of the immediate future of about a week may occur. Advice about the secondary effects of schedule changes may be sought.

## Level 6: Planned Actions

Planned actions estimate the effect of actions on material objects, but the objects do not have to be present for the estimate to occur. The significance of sequence of effects is that an imagined sequence of steps permits the anticipation of secondary effects. Two sequences of effects can be compared before the performance process begins.

Speculation is the act of imagining actions in order to make a decision based on an evaluation of anticipated outcomes and secondary effects. Speculation is observed when people pause to think to consider potential errors before they occur and in verbal discussions of the pros and cons of potential courses of action.

An assumption is self-initiated that one's actions can produce unwanted secondary effects. Estimates of the speed and trajectory of moving objects may be made. Synchronizing the various parts of an activity, like getting dinner, so that events occur at the same time may be considered.

The patient may reverse a chain of events done by others when the material objects are present to formulate a plan of action. The patient may change a course of action by forming an alternative plan based on a speculated problem. Speculated problems are derived from the tangible properties of present objects. To be considered new problem solving, the speculation must be new to the individual, not one generated by the individual in the past. Past speculations are modified according to current circumstances by inductive reasoning, one speculation at a time. The patient may consider the safety of others to prevent injury or negligence.

*Independent of cognitive assistance* is the use of consultation to adjust to a physical disability to that new motor learning can be done safely and consistently. Hazardous situations are anticipated and avoided or help is sought when needed. Maintenance of adaptive equipment, mobility, and communications is self-monitored. Self-report of functional limitations is accurate and the patient initiates discussions of what might happen and how to avoid complications. The patient understands abstract explanations of complications and requests clarification of concepts when needed.

The need for physical assistance can be reported as a separate assessment when there is no need for cognitive assistance. The readers of rehabilitation documentation tend to make that assumption. When a cognitive disability is present, the need for physical assistance should be stated within the context of the cognitive disability, which is a more severe and pervasive need for assistance.

## Reliability and Validity

The task that needs to be done right away is establishing the interrater reliability of the modes of performance. The amount of training one needs to get reliability should be investigated. Some questions can be suggested: What is the interrater reliability in your current treatment sessions? Does it improve after studying chapter 5? Does it get any better after studying chapters 6 and 7? Does changing your activities improve your reliability? Many therapists are working in situations where interrater reliability cannot be established. The confidence that these therapists have in their assessments could be clarified if therapists who can investigate interreliability would publish their results. To be truly reliable the modes must be scored the same way by the average people in practice. The amount of experience and knowledge required to be reliable needs to be investigated. If therapists are going to assume the burden of responsibility for making recommendations about major changes in legal status, they and the judiciary system must have confidence in the reliability of their evaluations.

Therapists who are beginning to use the modes of performance and the cognitive levels could help us all by doing descriptive studies of the experience and study required to achieve interrater reliability. Interrater reliability on the ACL should be established first, and I assume without much difficulty. Then investigate your interrater reliability with the activities you are using in practice. Interrater reliability is being stressed here because the usual trade-off in developing a more sensitive measure is a decrease in reliability. The modes of performance can be expected to be vulnerable to this problem. Reliability must be established before one can consider validity. Interrater reliability is a check on the therapist's understanding of the modes of performance.

Predictive validity is what therapists need in practice, but most of the research has been done on concurrent validity. What we need to know is how well our observations in the clinic predict performance in the community. A major question is does performance in doing a craft predict performance in self-awareness and situational awareness activities? Therapists working with the physically disabled need to know if an improvement in self-care activities is a reflection of training to do the activity or an improvement in cognitive ability. A training effect would not be expected to predict performance in other activities, but an improvement in ability would. Therapists working with children need to know how normal growth and development compare to the modes of performance. And writing treatment goals would be a lot easier if we knew more about the course of the diseases we see. A treatment goal is a prediction of what is going to happen, part of which is beyond the control of the therapist. Longitudinal descriptive studies would be a big help in predicting what is beyond the control of the therapist and what unfavorable events might be prevented.

## Activity Analysis

A theoretical discussion of what has been learned about activity analysis during the development of the modes of performance follows. Performance occurs within the context of doing an activity. The activity has social, cultural, and historical features that have meaning for individuals. The meaning must be dealt with first, before performance is observed.

At any time that the meaning of performance comes into question, the therapist must stop and clarify or change the activity to one that does have meaning. When an activity is meaningless, so is performance. There must be an acceptable reason for doing the activity (Allen, 1987).

The analysis of universal activities seems to be reasonable. There are a limited number of self-care and housekeeping chores that most people do all around the world. These same activities are found on many functional inventories, enjoying general acceptance. Chapter 7 analyzes these activities according to the modes of performance. The meaning of life is obviously not covered by self-care and housekeeping chores. To consider all of the spare-time and major role activities that people do, one needs to think about writing an encyclopedia, which we were not interested in doing. Another approach to activity analysis was needed and is referred to as task analysis. Task analysis assumes that an acceptable reason for doing the activity has been established.

Activities can be divided into actions and operations. Actions are the sequence of steps one goes through to do an activity. Operations are the quality in which the actions are done. Sanding, staining, and gluing are actions used to complete many different craft projects. The amount of pressure, rate of movement, surface covered are operations that describe the quality of performance. Activities can be analyzed according to the actions required or the operations performed (Allen, 1987). Because the quality of performance is restricted by a cognitive disability, the modes of performance describe operations.

Task analysis aims at maximizing remaining abilities by avoiding disabilities and using abilities. Each mode of performance is described by the information that can be added to the information-processing system. Added information is thought to be associated with an improvement in the medical condition. The reverse is also expected; information is subtracted from the information-processing system with progressive conditions. Task analysis can be used to measure changes in the medical condition, but that is not regarded as the primary benefit of task analysis. Task analysis can be used to find and use remaining abilities without getting tangled up by the patient's limitations.

Anyone who knows a cognitively disabled person can provide a long list of problems. As soon as the person moves or speaks, other people know that something is the matter. The modes of performance tell therapists what kind of information is apt to

cause problems because it cannot be processed. The modes also tell therapists what kind of information can be processed. When information can be processed, the patient can function successfully. When information that cannot be processed is eliminated, problems can be avoided. Therapists maximize remaining abilities by avoiding limitations and providing opportunities to use abilities.

The patient is in control of the quality of performance. The therapist can provide the opportunity by supplying the information in the next mode of performance. The patient can choose to ignore or reject the information. The therapist cannot force the patient to process the information. In that sense, the therapist follows the patient's lead.

The correct sequence of the modes is very important. The sequence suggested is based on clinical experience that needs to be examined. Rasch analysis tools hold promise for being able to investigate the validity of the sequence as well as the distances between the modes. The modes make it possible to sequence physical, social, work, and spare-time tasks according to the information that needs to be processed and evaluate the relative difficulty of the tasks.

The most productive use of Rasch analysis may come by sequencing actions that are used in a wide range of activities. Chapter 6 provides an analysis of actions according to the modes of performance. An action like cutting can be used to do a lot of activities. The modes describe different qualities of cutting that include both physical and mental abilities. One Rasch analysis of cutting might be useful with a wide range of patient populations and activities. The actions selected for chapter 6 actions that would be the most useful in clinical practice need to be developed.

## References

Allen, C.K. (1985). *Occupational therapy for psychiatric diseases: Measurement and management of cognitive disabilities.* Boston: Little, Brown.

Allen, C.K. (1987). Eleanor Clarke Slagle Lectureship—1987; Activity: Occupational therapy's treatment method. *American Journal of Occupational Therapy, 41,* 563–575.

Siev, E., Freishtat, B., & Zoltan, B. (1986). *Perceptual and cognitive dysfunction in the adult stroke patient.* Thorofare, NJ: Slack.

# Chapter 6

# Analysis of Performance Actions

## Catherine A. Earhart, OTR

## Introduction

While cognitive disabilities are manifested in the performance of day-to-day activities, therapists may not have the opportunity to view these difficulties as they occur in the home environment. Identifying a disability is often done in an artificial setting, such as a hospital or an outpatient rehabilitation center. Therapists are often faced with the need to select tasks that provide the opportunity to view and measure a potential cognitive disability.

The processes in the following analysis are encountered in a variety of craft, work, and self-care activities. Careful observation of the performance of these processes in a specific task context may assist the therapist in detecting the presence of a cognitive disability.

Processes were selected for their common use and generalizability to other activities. For instance, sanding to produce a smooth surface in woodworking is essentially no different than filing fingernails. Polishing surfaces, a finishing step in lapidary, copper tooling, and jewelry making is the same process used in cleaning floors, polishing silverware, washing windows, and waxing cars.

Gluing, cutting, staining, and sewing have wide applications in both crafts and activities of daily living: trimming and polishing nails, cutting hair, sealing envelopes, tying shoelaces, and securing packages. Measuring amounts and mixing are essential components of cooking and many craft activities.

Each process is first defined, and the tools and materials typically used are described. The qualities of actions used and important properties of material objects and tools are then identified. A general discussion of the performance of the process at various levels of disability is offered, and advantages and disadvantages of use for evaluation are noted. Finally other activities in which the process is encountered are identified.

A list of tools is suggested to facilitate evaluation set-up. The analysis that follows provides key observations and examples of behavior that attempt to provide a high degree of specificity. These lists are not inclusive as it is impossible to list all potential behaviors that reflect disability.

## Sanding

Sanding is the action of rubbing surfaces with sandpaper or other abrasives in order to produce changes in texture or shape. Objects that are sanded include wood, ceramic greenware, and plaster. Sanding tools include sandpaper graded from fine to coarse; files; sanding blocks; and power sanders. Sanding is often the first step in a finishing process (such as in woodworking or ceramic glazing).

Tool selection is based on properties of the surface to be sanded, including roughness, hardness, size, and shape (flat, curved, irregular) as well as desired smoothness. The actions of sanding are varied in direction, pressure, angle, and duration. Effects are judged by visual inspection and feeling.

The repetitive action of sanding is successfully performed at level 3. Higher abilities are demonstrated in the neuromuscular adjustments required by more complex tools and in consideration of less tangible properties of objects such as wood grain and density. Sanding by hand is safe and requires a minimum of supplies.

The disadvantage of sanding includes its relatively restricted application to craft tasks, whose content may not be agreeable to some persons being evaluated. Sanding may be difficult for persons with limitations in hand mobility or strength or with allergies to dust.

Applications in other daily activities include filing nails and cleaning with abrasives.

## Suggested Tools and Supplies for Evaluation Using the Action of Sanding

### 3.0 to 3.4

Sandpaper precut to fit in hand

Flat wooden surfaces, such as plaques

Small wooden boxes

All objects within 6 inches

### 3.6 to 4.4

Sandpaper of various grades and sizes

Sanding blocks

Flat surfaces with visible edges (3/4 inch)

Objects with inner surfaces, such as boxes

Objects with several parts, such as unassembled wood kits

Exact samples of completed sanding

All objects within view

### 4.6 to 6.0

Sandpaper of various grades and sizes

Sanding blocks

Files, rasps

Power sanders with appropriate safety equipment

Objects with difficult-to-access inner surfaces, such as boxes, or greenware cups, vases

Objects with several parts, such as unassembled wood kits

Objects of varying hardness, including wood, plaster, ceramic greenware

Various samples, need not be exact

Objects may be stored in hidden locations

## Analysis of Sanding

3.0    Picks up sandpaper or object to be sanded when placed within 6 inches or puts/throws it down when placed in hand. May say "sandpaper."

3.2    Spontaneously picks up sandpaper and initiates back and forth movements through 3- to 6-inch range of motion randomly on the object. May not apply enough pressure to produce smoothness, may sand in one place, may not look at object being sanded, may need to be stopped. Can resume stopped actions when requested.

3.4    Picks up sandpaper and imitates repetitive back-and-forth actions. May not consistently look at the object being sanded. Moves sandpaper when new location is pointed out. Does not check for smoothness; may hold sandpaper upside down.

3.6    Moves sandpaper around the perimeter of object while looking at the object. May check for smoothness by feeling inconsistently. Fails to sand inner or hidden surfaces. Imitates demonstrated actions that change duration and location of sanding. May sand too vigorously or impulsively. May sand the biggest object only.

3.8    Spontaneously sands exterior surfaces of all available objects within immediate grasp and this suggests completion (not smoothness). Stops when highly visible error is noted, such as a broken piece of wood, but may not ask for help.

4.0    Sands all pieces within arm's reach, redirecting self back to task if distracted. Checks for smoothness by looking and feeling. May work slowly but still misses edges, interior, or hidden surfaces and ignores grain of wood. Works until done or told to stop. Asks for help when a problem is encountered (such as sandpaper being too large to fit a space) but can't identify the problem or a solution. Does not refer to a visible sample.

4.2    Sands to match a sample's smoothness and spontaneously seeks out and uses sample within 24 inches to front or side. Recognizes and names a visible or tactilely perceptible problem differing from sample (such as a knothole, split in wood, or big splinter), one feature at a time. Misses interior, edges; if accidentally discovers an interior space, asks if surfaces require sanding.

4.4    Sands all visible and discovered surfaces,

checking for smoothness, but misses small edges. Recognizes highly visible errors or departures from a visible sample and may attempt a simple solution, such as asking for a replacement part or sanding longer in one spot. Compares previous sanding experience with the present task.

4.6    Asks for supplies used in past (such as different grades of sandpaper) without regard for appropriateness to present task. Attends to edges when cued. May attempt to alter pressure or angle of sanding actions, but does not sustain or has poor results. May attempt to fold or tear sandpaper to reach a smaller area. May choose to sand for a visibly different result from the sample (a rounded edge).

4.8    Sands all visible surfaces and rotates objects to check at completion for errors. Can learn a sequence of proper sanding techniques slowly by rote (i.e., changing sandpaper grades, changing position of objects for better results, or cleaning work space between steps), and uses these procedures inflexibly.

5.0    Initiates changes in strength, pressure, direction of sanding, and repeats improved methods. May note but then fail to dispose of sawdust in work space. Sets own pace but can't vary it.

5.2    Rotates objects while working to examine results. Notes small scratches or other surface qualities. Considers grain of wood to guide direction of action. Removes sawdust from surface of project and working areas spontaneously. May note worn sandpaper surfaces or sandpaper grades.

5.4    Makes successful motor adjustments to sand in tight spaces, in corners, around irregular edges. Alters tools, sequence of tool use, sequence of sanding in relation to other steps. Sets own standard for completeness, which may not conform to suggested quality. Searches for tools in closed areas. Questions need to consider potential secondary effects (such as fragility of ceramic greenware).

5.6    Discusses ways of varying methods to achieve different effects and may substi-

tute methods when these are suggested. Varies work pace on request.

5.8    Asks about potential problems (i.e., hardness or softness of material sanded) when selecting tools. Varies pace of work to conform to a time constraint.

6.0    Speculates about properties of material objects to be sanded and plans methods based on awareness of all properties of these objects. Can generate alternative plans based on imagined difficulties. Potential hazards are considered. Tool condition is checked before beginning to sand. Attends to safety considerations when using power tools.

## Staining

Staining is the action of applying liquid pigment to wood surfaces in order to produce changes in color. Stain products penetrate the wood surface and leave natural qualities of the wood grain exposed.

Most stains require stirring before use. Stain can be applied with a brush or rag, then wiped or rubbed to remove excess. Increased time between application and wiping usually intensifies color as will repeated applications. Stains may be water or oil based. The latter require solvents for clean up and precautions for adequate ventilation and flammability.

Working with liquids can be messy at level 3 due to inattention to amounts, the effects of gravity, and potential spillage. Immediate and striking color changes are noted at levels 4.0 to 4.8. Surface qualities of wood grain, sheen, variations in application procedures, and neuromuscular adjustments during application are observed at levels 5.0 to 6.0. Precautions for working with volatile products must be taken by therapists at levels below 6.0.

While staining has fairly narrow applications to woodworking, difficulties observed in working with the properties of liquids, gravity, amounts, and absorption can be generalized to other daily activities. The action of painting is used in applying fingernail polish, glazing hams, frosting cakes, applying make-up, and shining shoes.

## Suggested Tools and Supplies for Evaluation Using the Action of Staining

*3.0 to 3.4*

Water-based stain, one color
Brushes, 1-inch-wide

Rags, cut to fit comfortably in hand

Flat wood surfaces, such as plaques

Small boxes

All objects within reach

Protect work surfaces

### 3.6 to 4.4

Water-based stain, different colors

Brushes, various sizes

Rags, various sizes

Series of objects, or objects with more than one color

Boxes with hardware

Plaques with small (less than 1/4-inch) edges

Exact samples of finished objects

All objects within view

Protect work surfaces

### 4.6 to 6.0

Water- and oil-based stains, various colors

Solvents for clean-up

Brushes, various sizes

Rags, various sizes

Objects with hard-to-access surfaces

Samples need not be exact

Objects may be stored in hidden locations

Protect from harmful effects of volatile materials

## Analysis of Staining

3.0    Picks up a brush placed within 6 inches or puts/throws brush down when placed in hand.

3.2    Spontaneously picks up brush or rag and initiates back and forth movements through 3- to 6-inch range of motion randomly on object in front of them. May not remember to dip brush in stain before painting, may not look at object being painted or wiped, may paint or wipe over and over in one spot, may need to be stopped. Can resume actions when requested.

3.4    Picks up brush or rag and initiates repetitive back-and-forth actions. May not look at objects consistently. Dips brush and paints without awareness of too much or too little stain. Moves brush or rag to new location when this is pointed out. May miss spots on flat surfaces and does not stain or wipe hidden surfaces (bottom, back, inside of a box.) Fails to note color/part correspondence from a sample. When told, "washes" brush by holding it under water for a few seconds.

3.6    Moves brush or rag around the perimeter of an object while looking at the object. May miss smaller pieces entirely. May change location or duration of action, such as wiping or painting longer in one spot. May imitate a change in actions, which solves a problem (wiping edge of brush on can to remove excess stain before applying stain) but does not understand reason for these changes.

3.8    Paints or wipes all strikingly visible surfaces of available objects within immediate grasp. No awareness of color/part correspondence. A highly visible error may be noted (paint overlapping hardware) but does not ask for help or attempt to problem solve. Senses completion after all pieces have been stained and wiped. May forget to wipe after painting on stain.

4.0    Spontaneously paints and wipes all strikingly visible surfaces of objects or series of objects within arm's reach. Asks for the next step. May miss hidden or interior surfaces, small edges, or hard-to-reach areas. May apply too much stain and be reluctant to wipe off, dabbing instead. May not wash brush before changing colors.

4.2    Applies stain to all visible surfaces except small edges and notes striking deviations from a sample located within 24 inches, one feature at a time. Asks for help with problems (such as a piece stained wrong color) rather than attempt a solution. "Dabs" instead of wiping off stain. If hidden surfaces are discovered by chance, asks if they require staining.

4.4    Attempts to replicate a sample by matching color of stain, and by color/part correspondence. Recognizes effect of unstirred stain but fails to understand cause. May attempt a simple solution such as asking for a new can of stain. Compares past experience with painting and may refuse to wipe off stain, thinking it is the same as paint. May refuse to wipe off stain because the darker color is preferred. Initiates washing brush at end of task but rinses only until exterior surface of brush is clean. Recognizes but cannot correct or anticipate contamination from puddles, sawdust, dirty fingers, or unwashed brushes.

4.6 Requests a preferred color of stain that may differ from the sample, and can scan the visible environment for it. Attempts to correct drips on one side and be unaware of effects on other side of object. Attempts to vary amount of stain but may still use too much. Attempts to vary pressure of wiping but may not sustain. Paints small edges (less than 1/4 inch) when cued.

4.8 Rotates stained object and examines for errors when finished. Learns correct amounts of stain, pressure for wiping, methods for avoiding contamination, and prestirring stain by rote when these are demonstrated; follows these procedures inflexibly.

5.0 Varies direction and length of brush strokes, and duration and pressure of wiping to achieve uniformity of color. May not be aware of surface qualities, such as wood grain or sawdust.

5.2 Understands grain as a decorative surface quality of wood and notes color variations on different types of wood and on end cuts. Notes streaking, sheen. Rotates objects and catches drips as work proceeds. Can use stain samples.

5.4 Paints and wipes in corners and hard-to-reach interior spaces successfully. Alters tools, methods of staining, mixes or dilutes stains to achieve new effects. Searches for tools in closed storage areas. May understand that hidden surfaces such as joints do not need to be stained. Uses nailboards to increase access to edges. Reorganizes work space.

5.6 Asks for opinions of others or compares instructions before deciding on new course of action. Color selections reveal aware-ness of coordination with current fashion or social convention (room decor or other relevant factor). May make estimates of quantity of stain required to cover areas.

5.8 Asks for assistance to avoid errors or undesirable secondary effects such as contamination or waste before beginning to work. When all materials are present, can plan out actions. Consults regarding potential hazards such as working with volatile materials.

6.0 Speculates about best tools and plan of action based on awareness of primary, secondary, and potential secondary effects and properties of objects. Anticipates hazards. Can plan to minimize waste of time and material.

## Gluing

Gluing is the action of attaching objects together by means of a liquid adhesive material. In crafts, gluing is used to attach parts and affix surface coverings.

Effective adhesion requires selection of the appropriate type of glue, and consideration of correct amount, pressure, drying time, and positioning of parts. Common household white glue, a synthetic resin adhesive, is a strong, fast-setting, nontoxic glue that can be used with wood, paper, ceramics, and fabric. Applied by squeezing, dabbing, or spreading, it is quite suitable for evaluation purposes.

Persons who work with glue at level 3 create messes resulting from inattention to amounts, drying time, the effects of gravity, and secondary effects. Gluing small parts or using exact amounts is usually difficult at all levels below level 4.8. Precautions for proper ventilation and avoiding skin contact for toxic or flammable glues must be taken by therapists for persons under level 6.0.

White glue is commonly used for mending or repairing such diverse items as furniture, shoes, toys, or ceramic dishes in the home. Related tasks involving adhesion principles include affixing postage stamps, sealing envelopes, applying bandages, taping packages, masking surfaces before painting, and splicing or repairing electrical cord.

### Suggested Supplies for Evaluation Using the Action of Gluing

*3.0 to 3.4*

White glue in squeeze bottles

Flat surfaces such as paper or tile trivets

Ceramic tiles (5/8- to 1-inch square)

Ribbon cut into small pieces (1/2 to 1 inch)

All objects within 6 inches

### 3.6 to 4.4

White glue in squeeze bottles

Tile trivets with straight edges

Recessed top wood boxes for tiles

Round and vertical surfaces, such as 1-pound coffee cans

Ceramic tiles (5/8- to 1-inch square)

Stiff decoupage paper prints

Precut strips of ribbon, cloth, rick rack

Objects requiring assembly of several different parts such as wood kits

Exact samples of completed objects

All objects within view

### 4.6 to 6.0

White glue in squeeze bottles

Rubber cement

Two-part epoxy glues

Irregularly shaped trivets for tiling

Irregular shaped tiles, shells, other mosaic materials

Thin papers or porous material

Leather

Objects requiring consideration of gluing sequence, overlapping of parts, angled joints, or partially hidden surfaces

Objects of varying weight, absorption, texture, surface contact area

Small objects, sand, glitter

Various samples, need not be exact

Objects may be stored in hidden locations

## Analysis of Gluing

3.0     Picks up glue bottle or object to be glued when placed within 6 inches or puts/throws it down when placed in hand. May not invert bottle or move it towards surface to be glued. May not squeeze or squeezes ineffectively when told. Does not distinguish between objects or surfaces to be glued.

3.2     Spontaneously picks up glue bottle and squeezes. Moves bottle randomly on the objects to be glued. May not look at the objects to be glued, may stop actions before glue comes out, or may apply excessive glue until stopped. Can pick up an object, dip in a puddle of glue, and place on a surface when so directed but placement is random.

3.4     Picks up, inverts, and squeezes glue bottle while looking at objects, then stops. Repeats over and over or until distracted. Moves bottle back and forth. May use too little or too much glue; does not note if objects are adhered. May not differentiate between objects and puts glue on any available surface. Places objects such as ceramic tiles next to each other; may proceed from left to right.

3.6     Squeezes glue around the perimeter or along the edge of objects while consistently looking at objects. May use too much or little glue. Placement of objects such as tiles follows the perimeter or edge. May imitate a change in the location of placement of glue or placed objects. Is not aware of completion or problems with adhesion.

3.8     Spontaneously covers a surface with glue and then stops. Places objects on surfaces until surface is covered (such as ceramic tiles on trivet, or ribbons around a coffee can, or collage parts on paper) or until all available supplies are used up. Recognizes completion based on coverage or use of all objects.

4.0     Spontaneously applies glue to a sequence of objects or surfaces and places in predetermined arrangement until finished. May use too much or too little glue; recognizes an adhesion problem, but cannot think of a solution to the problem.

4.2     Application of glue and placement of parts attempts to replicate a sample's length, shape, direction, or color. Usually matches one feature at a time, can recognize a highly visible placement error, and asks for assistance. Drips, bumps from excessive glue, or poorly adhered edges are not noted. The effect of time on adhesion is poorly understood, and parts are repeatedly moved before adhesion occurs. May attempt to glue on vertical surfaces without regard for effects of gravity.

4.4     Applies glue to particular surfaces, and placement of parts attempts to replicate, in addition to features in 4.2, size and number up to four. Usually attends to two features at a time. May lean or bend over to view effects of actions, but usually does not rotate objects in space. Does not note dripping glue on hidden surfaces or check for these errors. Identifies highly visible placement errors, and can initiate a simple placement change to match a sample. Tends to use excessive amounts of glue, thinking more is better. Does not distinguish between types of glue. Unaware of secondary effects, such as need to move glued objects to prevent adhesion to work surface.

4.6     Turns or rotates objects to reach surfaces to be glued. May use too much or too little glue but recognizes effects and attempts to alter actions, such as squeezing bottle with more or less pressure, pressing surfaces together with more force to promote bonding, or wiping away excess glue. Results of such adjustments may be ineffective. May apply past experiences with gluing to present task, such as wanting to use a C-clamp or a vise. Such applications are often ineffective.

4.8     Rotates glued object when finished to check for drips or adhesion of parts. May not check for glue on work surfaces as he or she works. Can learn a new gluing procedure slowly by rote, including glue amounts, drying times, the use of rubber bands or C-clamps to promote bonding, and mixing two-part glues. Follows these procedures in an inflexible manner. Unable to adjust pace to account for fast-drying glues.

5.0     Initiates changes in strength and pressure to improve bonding with effective results. Retains several demonstrated steps of a new procedure, such as working with two-

part epoxy glues. Has difficulty adjusting pace for fast-drying glues.

5.2     Notes effects of glue on surfaces, including dulling wood or ceramic finish, interfering with absorption of stains, and causing adhesion to work surfaces. Understands effects of drying on the appearance of glue (opaque and white to transparent.) Rotates objects to check for drips or adhesion as he or she works.

5.4     Changes tools and methods of gluing to gain a desired effect. Considers spatial relationships between parts to be glued to determine the sequence of assembling parts. Considers spaces, overlaps. Discovers effects of properties such as weight, surface contact area, or absorption of glue as he or she works and alters methods. Can glue small objects in tight spaces.

5.6     Compares various adhesives and their uses with particular objects (white glues, paste, epoxy, rubber cement, etc.). Seeks information about new methods. On request can adjust work pace effectively to use fast-drying glues.

5.8     Can vary pace as needed to accommodate fast drying times of glues. Seeks opinions of ways to avoid potential hazards or undesirable secondary effects, or to clarify intangible properties of glues (e.g., acetone-based glues dissolving plastics).

6.0     Speculates about best materials and methods based on awareness of all properties and potential secondary effects of objects. Anticipates hazards and plans to minimize waste and contamination. Includes passage of time in planning.

## Polishing/Cleaning

Polishing is the action of rubbing an object with a cloth or other tool to produce changes in the surface quality of the object. In this discussion, polishing includes dusting, cleaning, waxing, and drying. Objects that are polished include wood furniture, glass, tile, silverware, brass, mirrors, windows, floors, shoes, leather goods, and copper tooling pictures.

Effective polishing requires selection of the appropriate types of cleaning agents (water, soaps, metal polishes, rust removers) and tools (cloths, brushes, mops); as well as variations in actions in direction, pressure, and duration of actions.

Wiping without cleaning or polishing agents (drying dishes or dusting), can be performed levels 3.0 to 3.8, with varying degrees of success. The addition of water, soaps, polishes, or other agents provides the therapist with the opportunity to observe sequencing at 4.0 and above. Higher abilities are demonstrated in the neuromuscular adjustments required by hard-to-remove dirt or tarnish, hidden or hard-to-reach surfaces, or more complex tools. Higher abilities are also required to consider surface properties such as streaking, scratching, and uniformity of sheen as well as secondary effects and intangible properties of various cleaning agents.

Advantages of using polishing or cleaning in evaluation include direct applicability to a variety of household tasks and cross-cultural familiarity. While cleaning is often perceived as a valuable, relevant, and constructive activity, cultural and personal values vary widely in this regard. Individuals may refuse to do this process. If toxic cleaning or polishing agents are used, precautions for proper ventilation and avoidance of skin contact must be taken by therapists at all levels below 6.0.

## Suggested Supplies for Evaluation Using the Actions of Polishing/Cleaning

### 3.0 to 3.4

Dish cloths, dust cloths

Wet dishes or silverware

Small flat surfaces, such as ceramic trivets

Shoes in need of polishing

Objects within reach

### 3.6 to 4.4

Cleaning cloths

Hand-held brushes

Cleaning agents such as soap, detergents, glass and metal cleaners

Polishing agents such as shoe and furniture polish

Tarnished silverware or other metal

Copper tooling

Shoes in need of polishing

Furniture with dirty surfaces not at eye level

Flat surfaces such as tabletops, counters

Exact samples of cleaned objects (polished silver)

All objects within view

### 4.6 to 6.0

Cleaning cloths of various sizes, absorption qualities

Various brushes, steel wool, mops, sponges

Cleaning and polishing agents of various types including those with toxic properties

Floors, furniture, metal, chrome, leather, tile surfaces in need of cleaning or polishing

Irregular or hard-to-access surfaces, as in copper tooling or furniture

Small objects such as jewelry

## Analysis of Polishing/Cleaning

3.0    Picks up cloth when placed within 6 inches or puts/throws it down when placed in hand.

3.2    Spontaneously picks up cloth and initiates back-and-forth movements within a 6-inch range of motion randomly on the object to be polished/cleaned. May not look at the object, may stop actions when distracted, or may continue in one place until stopped.

3.4    Picks up cloth and wipes it across object; may not look at the object consistently. Repeats this over and over. Subtle visible effects such as removal of dust or silver tarnish are not noted or forgotten when pointed out. Tactile effects such as achieving dryness when wiping dishes or silverware may be understood.

3.6    Follows the shape or perimeter of an object as he or she wipes it and will imitate a change in the duration or location of his or her action. The need for these modifications (i.e., to remove all smears or achieve a shiny finish) is not understood. If given cleaning or polishing agents, applies these without awareness of appropriate use, amount, and manner of application.

3.8    Wipes all available objects (silverware) or the entire surface of an object (small tabletop or front of a television). Usually neglects less visible parts (sides, back, legs of a table). A highly visible effect such as the removal of thick dust or dirt is noted when pointed out. If given cleaning or polishing agents, may cover the surface of the object without awareness of appropriate amounts or manner of application. A sense of being done may be expressed when all objects have been used (drying all the dishes).

4.0 Moves through a familiar sequence of steps to completion such as applying polishing agent to cloth and then wiping or rubbing. Wipes surfaces of all objects within arm's length and notes highly visible effects consistently. Misses hidden surfaces and less visible features, such as smears on glass. Demonstrated corrections or variations in a familiar sequence are not imitated.

4.2 Attends to one visible feature at a time when polishing or cleaning and attempts to replicate a sample of performance, such as removal of dark tarnish on silver or dirt on shoe. Fails to change posture to reach surfaces such as backs of furniture, and may not note objects outside immediate adjacent space when cleaning. Sees a highly visible error or problem (a spot that won't respond to rubbing) and asks for help.

4.4 Wipes all visible and easily accessible surfaces to achieve a result that matches a sample such as a polished spoon, a finished copper tooling picture, or clean shoe. Fails to see less visible dirt (i.e., in corners). Modifications in strength or fine-motor movements to produce desired results may be attempted but abandoned. May change posture but fails to rotate objects for easier access to surfaces. May use excessive amounts of polish or cleaner, thinking more is better. Fails to take into account the secondary properties of such agents (soap film, irritating fumes, combustion potential).

4.6 Rotates objects for better access to surfaces when wiping. Makes a spontaneous adjustment in pressure or location of action to produce better results, but this may not be effective or sustained. Requests supplies or tools used in the past. Scans immediate environment for needed supplies. In cleaning, will neglect surfaces that

are not at eye level unless cued. Secondary properties of agents are ignored, as in 4.4.

4.8 Polishes, cleans, or dusts all visible surfaces and checks results by rotating objects at completion. Can learn to use a new product slowly by rote and uses in an inflexible manner. Follows safety precautions by rote, but does not note secondary effects or properties spontaneously.

5.0 Initiates changes in strength, pressure, and range of motion when polishing or cleaning to achieve a uniform color or cleanliness. Fails to attend to surface properties such as streaks created by the direction of application of polish, or small scratches created by abrasives on chrome or other polished surfaces.

5.2 Notes and considers tangible surface effects created by polishing process, including shine, streaking, removal of fine dust, removal of tarnish, or highlighting (as in copper tooling or antiquing). Rotates objects to check effects as he or she works. Discriminates between cleaning agents and tools based on tangible properties (various metal polishes, plastic versus leather cleaners, soft versus stiff scrub brushes).

5.4 Varies methods, sequence of steps, posture, amounts of cleaning agents while cleaning and polishing. Considers spatial properties in planning sequence of actions, such as polishing from top to bottom on a vertical surface to catch drips, or starting in corner and working toward door when waxing floors. May consider how to avoid an inevitable secondary effect, but may not anticipate all potentially harmful secondary effects when experimenting with new methods.

5.6 Compares various methods (instructions, advice) and selects procedure for polishing or cleaning. Notes effects of cleaning or polishing objects on their context (cleaning only a spot on carpet or polishing one piece of brass will expose otherwise inconspicuous dirt). Uses conventional or cultural standards for cleanliness to judge outcomes. Hazards of new materials or cleaning agents or combinations of agents are not anticipated.

5.8      Aware of potential for harm to objects or people from improper use of agents and seeks opinions to avoid undesirable effects. Follows verbal or written explanations of safety hazards associated with use of various polishing and cleaning agents.

6.0      Speculates about best materials and methods for cleaning or polishing new objects. Anticipates hazards. Plans to conserve energy. Generates alternative plans based on imagined difficulties.

## Cutting

Cutting is the action of using various tools to change the size, shape, or length of objects. The many ways this action is applied can be inferred from the multitude of terms that further define it: trim, carve, incise, slice, chop, clip, pare, mow, shave.

Effective cutting requires proper tool selection based on properties of materials and desired outcome. Neuromuscular adjustments are required to some degree with most cutting tools for accurate results.

The use of any sharp instrument entails some risk of injury, and this risk increases when a disability is present. From levels 3.0 to 3.8, immediate supervision of scissors is recommended; the use of straight-edge razors, knives, and other tools with exposed blades can be dangerous. At levels 4.0 to 4.8, the awareness of primary effects usually engenders some degree of exercised caution, but secondary effects predisposing patients to injury must be anticipated and controlled by the therapist. Errors at 5.0 to 5.4 are apt to result from impulsivity, failure to anticipate consequences, or failure to follow advice.

The advantages of using cutting for evaluation include its familiarity and direct generalizability to a variety of common activities. Such applications include cutting hair and fingernails, shaving, preparing food, cutting food while eating, cutting fabric for sewing, mowing lawns, trimming bushes, and chopping wood.

Cutting usually requires a certain degree of visual acuity and the use of two hands. The presence of vision or hand impairments (strength, mobility, joint pain, tremors, one-handedness) or suicidal or homicidal impulses will limit use of this action in evaluation.

## Suggested Supplies for Evaluation Using the Action of Cutting

Items with (*) should be closely supervised.

### 3.0 to 3.4

Scissors with 6- to 8-inch blades that have two different-sized finger grips, such as Fiskars*

Lightweight paper such as construction paper or felt, on which is drawn simple shapes, such as a circle or square

Stiff ribbon

### 3.6 to 4.8

Above materials

Prints on lightweight paper with straight and curved edges

Papers that differ in weight and resistance

Fabrics that differ in weight, texture, and slippery qualities

Fingernail clippers or fingernail scissors*

Toenail clippers*

Straight razors*

Small paring knife*

Serrated knife*

Small, long vegetables or fruit to be cut crosswise, such as celery or bananas

Vegetable and fruits that require a series of different cutting strokes, such as tomatoes or apples

Cutting boards

Lightweight metals, such as copper-tooling foil*

Samples of cut objects

Series of objects to be cut

### 5.0 to 6.0

Above materials

Prints requiring trimming around irregular shapes or cuts in interior spaces

Scissors of various sizes and weights, including pinking shears and wire cutters, which may be unfamiliar*

Straight-edge cutters, such as Exacto knives*

Two-handed cutters, such as hedge clippers*

Paper cutter machines*

Large pieces of material requiring awareness of waste and planning for placement of patterns or locations of cuts

Tools of varying quality, especially sharpness and dullness*

Power tools*

## Analysis of Cutting

3.0 Picks up tool placed within 6 inches or puts it down when placed in hand. May grasp sharp edge of tool and cut self.

3.2 Spontaneously picks up scissors, positions them in hand, and opens and shuts them in a snipping motion. Scissors may be held upside down. Action may be sustained only a few seconds, may lack normal strength; range of motion may be limited to 3 to 6 inches. Actions may need to be stopped by others. May not look at objects to be cut. May cut self.

3.4 Picks up scissors and attempts to cut along a line while looking inconsistently at the object to be cut. Scissors may be held upside down. Snips or chops at material, may use tearing motion if resistance is encountered. Scissors are opened partially. May not turn material if cutting a curve or changing direction of cut. No attempt is made to alter methods or evaluate results. May grossly approximate a line. May cut self with knives or other straight-edge tools.

3.6 Cuts with scissors along a line or around perimeter of a simple shape while looking at the object. Turns material when cutting a curve or changing direction but effects are jagged or uneven. Gross errors at perimeter may be noted. Imitates a change in the location of a cut, or in the location of an action (as in shaving) but does not understand the problem that such a modification solves. Modifications in positioning cutting edge of scissors on material, angle of cut, or pressure, or in the position of the hand holding the material are not understood or imitated. If allowed to use a knife for chopping, does not keep the hand holding the material a safe distance from the knife.

3.8 Cuts around a perimeter or along a line and recognizes completion when all available materials or objects have been used, such as cutting all fingernails. Recognizes

a visible error in shape—for instance, a carrot cut too long—when this is pointed out. Modifications in positioning the material being cut, angle of cut, or pressure applied for better results are not understood as in 3.6. Tools requiring such adjustments are not used effectively or safely.

4.0 Cuts along a line or in a specific location to produce a particular shape or length. Attends to strikingly visible changes in objects. Sequences spontaneously a series of cutting actions on objects within arm's length (cutting apple in half, taking out core, slicing into quarters). Objects that are not visible may be neglected. For instance, fingernails may be cut but not toenails. May attempt to use tools requiring adjustments in angle, width of opening, pressure, or stroke length but cannot modify tool use and may abandon task.

4.2 Cuts along a line or in a specific location to produce a length or shape and recognizes highly visible deviations from a sample. Coordination of hands is clumsy. Asks for assistance to replicate effects as seen in a sample. Attends to one striking feature at a time, such as length of a fingernail, ignoring other salient features (angle of the cut). Secondary effects and potential hazards are not anticipated, such as needing to protect working surfaces from cuts, cutting too close to a nail bed, or positioning hands or tools to avoid injury.

4.4 Concentrates on producing an exact match to a sample or previous performance (length, shape, other striking feature). Coordination of hands may be clumsy. Attends to a pair of striking visible features (dark line, edge as defined by color change.) Less striking features, such as a penciled cutting line, or a sharp edge at the corner of a clipped nail, or hair at back of head, are not attended to. Tools requiring continuous neuromuscular adjustments in pressure, angle, positioning of materials in hands (clippers, Exacto knife, two-handed shears, straight razor) are not used effectively or safely. Past cutting methods are assumed to work with novel material objects.

4.6 Attempts to make a neuromuscular variation in tool use such as the amount of pressure applied or the angle of cutting edge, but efforts are usually not successful or sustained. Can imitate a placement change to produce a better effect, such as placing a fingernail clipper closer or farther away from a nail bed, or positioning hands on fabric to control angle of cut when using scissors, or pressing harder with razor on soft-tissue areas when shaving. Remembers past cutting experience and may request previously used tools that are not in the visual field. Attempts to individualize results of cutting by purposefully producing a striking effect different from a sample.

4.8  Turns or rotates objects to check for effective results when finished (turns head and neck after shaving). Notes all striking visible effects on objects being cut. Can memorize a series of new steps with a cutting tool or follow demonstrated safety procedures (protecting work surfaces from cuts, cutting on the waste side of a line in case of an accidental slip when using an Exacto knife). Neuromuscular adjustments in strength, range of motion, or positioning of tools are imitated laboriously and induce fatigue, which may lead to errors.

5.0  Initiates changes in strength, pressure, range of motion, or angle of tool for better effects. Cutting in small spaces is done very slowly and may be abandoned as too tedious. May ignore surface or edge qualities and is not aware of secondary effects or potential hazards.

5.2  Aware of qualities of cut surfaces and edges; trims edges to achieve uniformity of shape or smoothness or height (e.g., trimming a bush or beard). Rotates objects as he or she works to check effects. Discriminates between cutting tools based on tangible properties (toenail clippers versus fingernail clippers; shears versus scissors). Use of tools may be appear impulsive as potential secondary effects are not considered.

5.4  Alters tools, sequence of actions, angle of cutting, and posture to produce better

effects. Spontaneously attends to spatial properties (negative spaces, overlaps, or waste generated by cutting). May not anticipate but can discover ways to save material by cutting near the edge or using an existing edge of a large piece. May blame properties of materials (dull tools, etc.) for poor results. May resist following recommended safety precautions to avoid injury.

5.6  Compares cutting methods (instruction guides, advice of therapist) before proceeding; alters tool selection or substitutes methods. May judge result by social standards (hair cuts, length of fingernails) or esthetic criteria.

5.8  Consults others to clarify possible harmful secondary effects, such as damage to working surfaces, proper storage and use of tools to avoid damage to tools, safety precautions with power tools. Plans out a course of action when all material objects are present.

6.0  Speculates about material objects to be cut, including best tools, best plan of action based on awareness of all properties of objects. Can generate alternative plans based on imagined difficulties. Potential hazards are considered. Tool condition is checked before cutting is attempted. Can do cutting that requires continuous high level of care for safety reasons, such as professional hair cutting, or little tolerance for error, such as operating power cutting tools.

## Sewing

Sewing is the joining or fastening together of fabric, leather, plastic, or other material by thread, string, yarn, or other tying material.

Sewing methods and tools vary greatly, but basic hand sewing can be accomplished with a needle and thread, pins, and scissors. More complex construction often involves use of patterns and machines. Activities that may involve sewing as actions include embroidery, braiding, basketry, weaving, knitting, crocheting, and macrame. Results are usually judged by effectiveness of sewn joints and aesthetic appearance.

At levels 3.4 to 3.8, a running stitch can be performed, but effectiveness of joints is not judged.

Sequencing of actions and awareness of functional joints are observed at levels 4.0 to 4.8. Construction of parts into new wholes, awareness of surface, spatial, and other properties allows for variation and new learning at levels 5.0 and above.

Most persons are willing to attempt a familiar task such as braiding, tying, or sewing. Cultural and individual preferences are usually accommodated with a large selection of materials to choose from (a person may agree to sew on leather but not on fabric). The presence of visual or hand impairments may limit use of sewing for evaluation.

## Suggested Supplies for Evaluation Using the Action of Sewing

### 3.0 to 3.4

Running stitch

Leather with prepunched holes

Leather needle threaded with waxed thread

Felt or other semi-stiff material

Threaded sewing needle

Ribbon, rope, or lacing to tie bow or knots

### 3.6 to 4.4

In addition to above

Whip stitch

Leather with prepunched holes

Leather needle threaded with leather lacing

Felt, fabrics of different weight

Thread

Sewing needles

Hand sewing requiring turning seams inside out

Bargello

Yarn

Plastic mesh/scrim

Weaving with table loom, tabby only, pre–set up

Weaving with ribbon

Braiding with yarn

Simple embroidery, designs printed on fabric

Mending with running, whip stitch

Buttons, other fasteners

Exact samples of projects that can be completed within 1 hour

All materials in view

### 4.6 to 6.0

In addition to above

Sewing from patterns

Sewing involving turning, stuffing

Patchwork

Needlepoint

Counted cross-stitch

Weaving, floor loom

Basketry

Macrame

Knitting

Crochet

Sewing machines

Exact samples not necessary

Materials can be stored away from view

## Analysis of Sewing

3.0    Picks up a string, threaded needle, crochet hook, or other tool placed within 6 inches or puts/throws it down when it is placed in the hand.

3.2    Spontaneously picks up string or tool and initiates back-and-forth movements through 3- to 6-inch range of motion. For example, pushes a threaded needle in and out, or up and down while ignoring length, tension, or direction of stitching; or grasps a shoelace and attempts to tie it. May not look at objects as he or she works.

3.4    Pushes a threaded needle back and forth through a series of prepunched holes to complete a running stitch. Usually proceeds left to right. Looks at object inconsistently; stops and starts actions spontaneously. Does not attend to visible effects such as stitch length or tension, or judge effectiveness of joint. Ties a knot or bow when string is visible and within easy arm's reach, but does not attend to tension. Unties a bow but not a knot in a shoelace or drawstring.

3.6    Pushes a threaded needle back and forth through a piece of cloth following a line or next to an edge. Imitates a demonstrated change in the placement of the needle without understanding the problem that such a modification solves (i.e., making a particular stitch length or sewing through a hidden layer of cloth). Sews until out of thread, without awareness of need to tie knots or allow extra thread for tying knots. May braid or crochet if familiar, when task is started by others. Actions are repetitive (such as crocheting in a circle) and tension is ignored. Does not initiate a sequence of actions or show awareness of completion.

3.8    Sews with a running or whip stitch completely around a perimeter, or fills in a space (as in bargello or embroidery) and stops when space is filled, or supplies in immediate vicinity are used up. Sense of completion is determined by filling space or using all available supplies. Does not attend to features of thread or string such as tension, or twisting. Does not attend to hidden surfaces, or to errors or effects on such surfaces.

4.0    Sews with a running, whip, or a previously learned stitch until an immediate goal is achieved. Sequences a series of familiar actions such as cutting thread, threading a needle, and sewing, without assistance. May forget to allow extra thread to tie knots. Uses materials within arm's reach. Sequence of actions may be incorrect; corrections in sequence are not imitated. A highly visible error, such as a badly misplaced stitch, may be noted but is not corrected. May be able to reverse a simple familiar action (backing out of a crossed whip stitch). Fails to attend to hidden surfaces (back of fabric).

4.2    Refers to a sample within arm's reach or to a previously completed standard (i.e., a sewn button) and tries to replicate it by matching one feature at a time, with materials provided. Stitches may include running, whip, blanket, or previously learned stitch. Features noted include linear measure (discerned by placing objects side by side), shape, color, or direction. Recognizes a matching error and asks for help. Appears confused by hidden surfaces and spatial properties, including over and under relationships in weaving, or turning sewing inside out to hide seams.

4.4    Looks at and attempts to replicate exactly a sample located within 3 to 4 feet. Notes striking visible features, including shape, color, size, horizontal and vertical arrangement, sequence, and numbers up to four. Considers two features at a time. For example, notes alternating colors on a simple woven piece, or different stitch types and color changes on embroidery. May recognize a striking error and make a simple correction such as untwisting leather lace or removing a stitch. Abandons problems requiring awareness of secondary effects, such as moving a macrame knot up or down, or moving a drawstring or shoelace to change the length of the tying ends. Does not search for supplies or materials but may request a previously used tool. Fails to consider hidden surfaces; may tie knots on the front of a sewing surface instead of hiding them on the back or inside. Secondary effects (influence of thread weight, stitch length, and number of stitches, on seam strength) are not understood when explained.

4.6    Refers to samples located in plain sight and purposefully varies one or more of the striking visible features listed in 4.4 to produce an individualized goal. Recognizes an error and attempts a variation in action, such as removing a stitch or pulling it tighter, with careful attention to results. Such variations are done one at a time, without awareness of the effect on the rest of the task. For instance, an error in a tabby weave may be pulled out and corrected without awareness of effects on the preceding row. Attempts to untangle a simple knot or reties a bow for a better effect.

4.8    Memorizes a series of demonstrated new actions slowly and by rote, such as the actions of right and left half hitches in macrame. Attends to all striking visible effects as he or she works, and turns or rotates objects when complete to check for errors on hidden surfaces. Corrects spatial location difficulties without assistance, such as the location of a knot. Neuromuscular adjustments in strength or range of motion or positioning of a tool may be imitated laboriously, one at a time, for more effective results. New processes requiring continuous neuromuscular adjustments, such as knitting, may be abandoned as too stressful. A visible secondary effect, such as making stitches that are smaller than the stuffing material in a bean bag, are understood when pointed out. Untangles knots. Checks knots by pulling on them when done.

5.0    Varies range of motion and strength as he or she works, for better effects. For instance, pushes or wiggles needle through resistive material, varies force used to pull knots tight, and varies methods of passing weaving shuttle through shed. May forget new solutions discovered in this process. A new activity requiring continuous adjustments such as knitting or crocheting may be done slowly and with difficulty.

5.2    Considers tangible surface qualities of materials, such as the straight grain of the fabric, the appearance or pattern on the reverse side of an embroidered or woven piece, or the pattern formed by the stitching of a coiled basket. Considers qualities of edges, such as the tendency of loosely woven fabric to unravel. Notes warp and woof effects in weaving, understanding diagonal pattern formation (as in twills). Discriminates between specialized sewing tools.

5.4    Considers and manipulates spatial properties of materials, including negative spaces, interior and exterior spaces, overlapping. Lays out pattern pieces flexibly. Understands need for seam allowances for construction or extra fabric for easing. Remembers solutions. Can make fine-motor adjustments in small spaces. Can successfully sew on small fasteners such as hooks and eyes or small buttons. Two-handed novel tasks requiring continuous fine-motor adjustments, such as knitting or coiling a basket, may be learned without undue stress. Searches for needed tools and materials. Alters tool use, stitching methods, and sequences of actions to discover new effects. May not seek or heed advice to avoid potential undesirable secondary effects.

5.6    Considers creating a balance or harmonious appearance between parts and whole by coordinating colors, patterns, fabric types. Considers context of use and social convention or current style or fashion in making selections. Instruction books or samples may be referred to for examples of coordination or good taste. Estimates amounts of materials but seeks verification. Can adjust work pace on request. Compares methods of sewing before proceeding.

5.8    Plans a new sequence of actions when all materials are present; invents a new weaving pattern, or new method for assembling a sewing project. Asks for assistance in identifying potential undesirable secondary effects to avoid. Sets own work pace.

6.0    Speculates about methods of accomplishing a new sewing project. Considers available materials, time requirements, expense, methods, potential effects to avoid to achieve desired results.

## Measuring

Measuring is the action of determining amounts such as extent, volume, or duration according to a unit of measure. The purpose of measurement is to ensure a functional outcome in a task. A functional outcome is that quality of outcome that avoids error, waste of materials, and hazards; it also ensures conformity to social requirements for product appearance, function, and punctuality.

Most properties of material objects can be measured in some fashion, with numerical values assigned to a conventional unit of measure (inches, pounds, degrees). Properties that are frequently measured and the tools of measurement include: length (rulers, yardsticks, tapes), weight (scales), volume (teaspoon, cup, other liquid measures), heat and cold (thermometers, temperature gauges). Duration is measured by marking the passage of time (standard clocks, digital clocks, calendar). Numbers are used throughout measuring to quantify amount. This discussion will focus on those measurements frequently used in day-to-day activities and will not include little-used or highly technical forms of measurement.

Measurement appears to be ignored at level 3, and disorientation to clock and calendar is common. Striking visual characteristics form the basis for comparison at moderate levels of disability (4.0 to 4.6), and rigid use of conventional measuring devices usually occurs at 4.8. Flexible use of some devices such as rulers seems to begin at 5.4, but intangible factors affecting measurement (such as the angle of eye gaze) may not be considered consistently until 5.8 or 6.0.

Familiarity with units and tools of measurement varies widely according to educational and cultural background. As with all other actions, previous experience should be ascertained. The failure to measure, when this is a specified requirement in a particular task, can often be excused by the disabled person as an individual preference. Hence, the selection of tasks where measurement is critical to functional outcome is preferred.

The variety of daily activities requiring measurement includes cooking (determining liquid and volume, heat, considering the passage of time), doing laundry (determining amounts of soap, bleach, water, passage of time in hand washing and drying), cleaning (mixing correct amounts of cleaning agents with water), following medication prescriptions, determining water and food amounts for plants and animals. Awareness and measurement of time can be considered a critical factor in overall social adjustment.

## Suggested Supplies for Evaluation of the Action of Measuring

### 3.0 to 4.6

Clocks in view

Rulers

Clearly marked volume measures

Objects that can be matched by comparison to an exact sample

Recipes requiring measurement of specific quantities, heat, duration for functional outcomes (macaroni and cheese)

Materials requiring awareness of passage of time (facial masks, hair dyes, nail polish, glues, paints)

Thermometers

### 4.8 to 6.0

Conventional measuring devices with or without striking markings

Recipes or tasks requiring use of several different units

of measure and passage of time concurrently

Measurements in three dimensions

Tasks requiring estimation of linear, volume, weight, or other measurement

Tasks with time constraints

## Analysis of Measuring

3.0 to 3.6    Measurements of amounts are ignored. Passage of time appears to be marked by the duration of actions. A visual or other perceptible cue (such as a smell, or the appearance of a person) signals time for a familiar event (such as dinner or a daily group activity).

3.8    Measurements of amounts are ignored. Passage of time may be marked by completion of a specific task. Usually disoriented to calendar, clock.

4.0    Measurements of amounts are ignored. A well-learned amount (such as 2 teaspoons of sugar in coffee) can be invariantly used in a habitual sequence. Time passage is measured by an immediate goal; usually not more than 1 hour is anticipated. May be aware of the date of regularly occurring and highly valued events, such as a monthly check. May otherwise be disoriented to date, clock.

4.2    Aware of length of objects and measures by placing objects next to each other to establish equivalence. May not use a ruler or other linear measuring device. Aware of numbers up to two by scanning; may need to count to determine small amounts greater than two. Measurement of liquid volume is grossly approximated (putting in "what looks right"); may ignore markings on measuring cup or fill it to the top. May have no clear awareness of "too much" or "too little" of such materials as glue or paint. Weight and heat are understood in relation to a personal criteria such as "too heavy for me to lift," or "too hot to pick up." Makes gross comparisons of size (small, medium, or large.) Asks for the date, or the time of day; may have trouble remembering this information.

4.4    Measures by matching linear distance with an exact sample. Prefers not to use rulers or other measuring devices if matching is possible. May not estimate distance or perceive small length or size differences (such as the difference between 6 and 7 inches) by visual scanning. May use a clearly marked liquid measure such as a glass Pyrex measure, to measure marked amounts only. Awareness of excessive amounts of such materials as glue or paint is usually limited to a judgment that "more is better." May follow a known sequence of actions including measurements (such as making a pot of coffee) but cannot vary amounts. May read instructions to determine amounts but not follow them. Aware of a few well-learned quantities, such as personal clothing and shoe size, height, and weight. May be aware of numbers up to four by visual scanning. For large numbers, can establish equivalence by counting, but may be frustrated by this. May divide things into a limited number of equal parts, such as halves or quarters, but may estimate and divide into thirds with difficulty (folding a letter into thirds.) May not time actions (such as waiting 15 minutes to remove a facial masque) even when cued. May not estimate the time required to complete an activity or use such estimates to plan use of a block of time. Follows a set routine of daily activities that may not be guided by the clock. May know the time of day and the date.

4.6    May detect small differences in linear distance (such as between 6- and 7-inch lengths) by visual scanning, not matching. May recognize an excessive amount of glue or stain and attempt to remove excess. May rotate a liquid measure to gain access to the markings on the other side or may rotate a glass thermometer to see the mercury. May alter a measured amount from a sample, one amount at a time, with a cue. May confuse different units of measurement used concurrently. May note passage of time with a cue, but usually does not maintain awareness for more than 15 minutes.

4.8    May consider two measurement quantities at a time such as width and length. Three or more amounts or different units

of measurement may be considered slowly and with difficulty (such as time of day, intervals, and amounts of medication in a prescription). May use a ruler to measure a quantity equal to or less than the ruler. May have difficulty modifying use to measure longer lengths. May use liquid measures by close examination of all markers. May learn a new measurement procedure by rote, following it inflexibly (such as taking a temperature with a glass thermometer or monitoring glucose levels with dipsticks). May follow a series of measurements, such as a recipe, rigidly. Closely watches the clock to monitor the passage of time for short periods (5 to 15 minutes). For longer periods, may ask for verification or require cuing. May follow a weekly schedule of regularly scheduled events set up by others.

5.0    May vary placement of rulers or other linear measures to measure a length longer than the device but may fail to consider overlapping. May be able to associate three measurements with the correct unit of measure at one time (such as a medication prescription). May generate own schedule of regularly scheduled events for a month period but may have trouble adhering to it.

5.2    Discriminates between various types of measurement devices and makes selections based on awareness of tangible properties of objects being measured. Aware of small differences in amounts. Relies on watches, calendars, appointment books, and alarms to keep on schedule.

5.4    Uses rulers effectively, including considering overlapping width of the measuring device, empty spaces. Parts or fractions of a whole may be understood in linear measure better than in volume, or area measures. Can calculate distances on a map. Applies own criteria for strictness and consistency in use of measurement. Fails to anticipate effects of deviation from strict measurement in a particular task. May argue with requests to change pace, adhere to a schedule, or to be on time. Can speed up pace for short periods to meet a deadline. Has trouble estimating time needed for a particular activity, though may recall similar activities' time requirements from past experience.

5.6    Seeks out and follows measurements suggested by recipes or other standard practices, compares methods of measurement, substitutes new tools or methods when benefits are understood. Understands the importance of exact measurement and may use measurement to achieve balanced or visually pleasing proportions. May make accurate estimates of volume or time.

5.8    When all materials are present can plan out new methods to accomplish measurements. Considers all inevitable secondary effects and properties of measuring tools and material objects. Estimates of three-dimensional space, volume, and time requirements for an activity are made but require verification. Varies pace of work, taking into account the tangible properties of objects, past experience, and the clock. Understands an indirect measure of volume when demonstrated (such as the displacement of water). Considers future effects of particular properties on measurement.

6.0    Measurements are used to formulate plans in new activities when material objects are not present. Many different units of measurement may be considered concurrently to generate a plan. Complexity of activities ranges from planning a meal to planning production costs of a motion picture.

## Mixing

Mixing is the action of combining material objects in order to alter their character or appearance for a particular purpose. Elements combined include solid edible foodstuffs, nonedible materials such as paints or make-up, chemicals, liquids, air, water, and heat. The effects of combinations may be strikingly tangible (mixing dry ingredients with water, heating water to boiling, whipping air into cream), or less tangible (chemical changes, use of subtle seasoning).

Tools used for mixing include hand-held spoons, eggbeaters, whips, or sticks; as well as power-driven machines such as electric mixers and food processors. Heat is added by using appliances such as stoves, toasters, microwave ovens, or by exposure to sunlight. This discussion will focus on those tools and objects commonly combined in day-to-day activities.

At levels 3.0 to 3.8, objects are mixed without awareness of the effects of the combination. Undesirable and hazardous results must be anticipated and prevented by others. From levels 4.0 to 4.8, objects are combined to produce a particular goal. Selection of combinations is based on familiarity and visibility. Awareness of the need to measure amounts varies from no awareness (4.0) to rigid application of prescribed amounts (4.8). Mixing methods preferred are well-learned and conventional. Effects noted are visible or otherwise tangibly perceptible. Secondary or intangible effects may not be noted. Potentially harmful combinations are not anticipated. At levels 5.0 to 5.8, material objects are combined in new ways to produce variations. Awareness of properties expands as do the neuromuscular adjustments applied during the mixing process. Hazardous or potentially harmful combinations may not be anticipated until level 6.0.

Tasks that involve mixing frequently require the need to measure amounts; in addition, some require time awareness. Cooking is highly valued, essential to daily survival, and provides an excellent context for viewing mixing as well as measuring. Familiarity as a confounding variable can be minimized by providing new recipes and less familiar tools or equipment. Tasks with clear functional outcomes are preferred (i.e., rice can be judged to be under- or overcooked; toast can be burned; but tuna salad can be made a number of ways).

Daily activities in which mixing and combining are encountered include: applying make-up; preparing hair colors or conditioners; preparing prescriptive solutions for injection or oral administration; cooking and baking; mixing or reconstituting drinks; preparing cleaning solutions; mixing paints, plaster, cement, and glues with water or solvents.

### Suggested Supplies for Evaluation of the Actions of Mixing

Items with (*) should be used with supervision.

*3.0 to 3.8*

Nontoxic materials

Hand-held mixing tools such as spoons

Water colors or tempera paints

Frozen juice for reconstitution

### 4.0 to 4.8

Nontoxic materials

Toxic materials*

Short recipes requiring measurement of time and amounts

Cake mixes

Macaroni and cheese mix

Hamburger helper mix with ground beef

Tacos with ground beef

Potato salad with hard boiled eggs

Pancakes

Stove, toaster, microwave oven*

Electric mixer, food processor*

Electric coffee maker*

Acrylic paint

Water-based stains

Oil-based stains and solvents*

Plaster of Paris*

Clay slip

Clocks within view

All materials in view

### 5.0 to 6.0

Above appliances*

Kilns*

Unfamiliar recipes, implements, processes

Meals consisting of several dishes

Dishes requiring subtle seasoning

Recipes from scratch

Yeast bread making

Candy making

Wedging clay

Plaster of Paris*

Oil-based paints and solvents*

## Analysis of Mixing

3.0    Picks up a spoon or stick placed within 6 inches or puts/throws it down when it is placed in the hand.

3.2    Picks up a spoon or stick and begins a mixing action back and forth for a few seconds without looking at the objects or effects.

3.4    Performs a mixing action (back and forth or around in a circle) with a common tool or hands while looking at the objects inconsistently. Stops actions when distracted or mixes over and over without noting effects. Does not attend to amounts of materials combined nor to passage of time.

3.6    Picks up a spoon or other stirring implement and performs a mixing action while looking at the objects. Notes a striking effect (such as color change or disappearance of big lumps). May continue to stir when told until a particular effect is achieved (frozen juice is melted) or until told to stop.

3.8    Mixes all visible objects within reach, without awareness of amount, passage of time, or outcome. "Done" when all objects are used.

4.0    Spontaneously sequences well-known actions to combine objects (placing cake mix in bowl, adding water, stirring). Well-known amounts only are used; other measurements are ignored. Stirs or mixes while watching for a visible change, such as mixture becoming moistened, or mixes for a period of time idiosyncratically determined. No recognition of an error. Uses objects within arm's length.

4.2    Moves through a well-learned sequence to combine objects and recognizes a highly visible deviation from an external sample or a personal standard (pancake batter is very runny, or soap bubbles are overflowing from dishwashing pan) but cannot identify reason for the problem or suggest a remedy. Approximates liquid measurement with errors resulting. Prefers hand-held tools (versus appliances). Hidden properties (unmixed ingredients at bottom of bowl) are not attended to.

4.4    Combines objects to replicate exactly an existing sample or personal standard. Uses amounts that are standard for him or her and will not deviate from these. Uses objects located within 3 to 4 feet. May use a clearly marked volume measure to measure marked amounts only. May use an appliance if familiar with it, but may attend to the primary effect and neglect secondary effects (splattering, safety concerns). May not vary mixing actions to produce different effects or rotate bowls. Attends to highly visible effects and features (big lumps, changes in color, gross texture, or consistency changes) but may miss more subtle changes in texture, consistency, or sheen. May fail to scrape bottom of bowl, or mix bottom of can of paint. May neglect to shake bottles of liquids that separate (salad dressing, catsup) before use. When heating water, may attend to striking change (boil) but neglect more subtle change (simmer). May not attend to the passage of time as he or she works. May be unaware of intangible effects (burning at bottom of saucepan; contamination by dirty hands, working surfaces, or tools; heat transfer from one object to another) or hazardous combinations (combustible chemical combinations; combustibles near flame, gas, or solvent fumes; toxins in proximity to edibles; harmful medication combinations; electricity and water; etc.).

4.6　　Scans visible environment for objects used in combinations. May attempt to change the rate, location, or duration of mixing actions one at a time to alter an effect. May alter an amount or substitute ingredients to produce an individualized outcome. May rotate a bowl or can while stirring or push a spoon to the bottom of bowl or can to mix all ingredients.

4.8　　Learns a new method of combining (such as folding in ingredients in cooking, or using a mixing appliance, or kneading bread) slowly by rote and asks for verification. Determines amounts or methods by rigid adherence to prescriptions (recipes) and does not vary from these. Closely watches the clock to time actions while working for periods of up to 15 minutes. Needs cuing for longer periods. Checks for completeness or conformity with a prescribed method at end of task. Can learn by rote harmful combinations or procedures to avoid for safety reasons.

5.0　　Varies strength, range of motion, pressure applied in mixing process (kneading bread,

wedging clay, stirring stiff dough) to produce better results.

5.2　　Notes surface properties including textures (as in bread), sheen (as in candy, sauces, paint, make-up), consistency of color or texture; attempts to produce changes in these features by adding or subtracting amounts without awareness of effect on final product. Distinguishes between mixing implements and methods on the basis of specialized function (whips versus beaters, whipping versus folding in ingredients). Relies on clock to time mixing process.

5.4　　Considers spatial properties when combining including container sizes, tool sizes, and needed work space. May not consider secondary effects of properties that may affect space requirements, such as expansion from heating or adding air (cooking spaghetti, whipping cream). Measurement of ingredients is consistently considered but idiosyncratically applied. Varies combinations of ingredients or sequence of combining to see what happens. Requests tools used previously in a new context. Alters mixing methods, postural alignment, rearranges immediate work space for better results. Does not consider potential secondary effects, and can be dangerous in exploratory combinations as a result. May ignore advice.

5.6　　Combinations are varied to achieve a perceived subtle effect that is pleasing to the eye and palate such as blending herbs and spices in cooking, diluting a perfume, or blending paint tints. Alters small amounts. Estimates volume. Considers convention or cultural standards in selecting combinations as in meal planning, or follows recipes or guidelines of others to ensure a socially acceptable result. Aware of the passage of time while mixing.

5.8　　Plans new combinations and methods of mixing when material objects are present. Considers future effects of properties of objects combined, such as the continued cooking of a turkey after it is removed from the oven. Varies work pace and times actions according to the clock and the tangible properties of material objects (can mix quick-setting materials). Asks for assistance in identifying potential secondary effects to avoid. Speculates about best mixing methods and amounts in making new combinations. Imagined problems may be identified and considered to avoid undesirable results.

# Chapter 7

# Analysis of Activities

## Catherine A. Earhart, OTR

The impact of cognitive disabilities on daily activity performance varies from minimal disturbance requiring little assistance to profound disruptions necessitating continuous supervision by caregivers. The bottom line in deciding which activities should be attempted by the disabled person is usually safety. Ironically, many a therapist or caregiver has been forced to withhold assistive devices that increase functional independence, such as walkers, because they increase the disabled person's risk of accessing potentially dangerous objects or situations. Weighing the risks against benefits is a clinical judgment based on predictions of performance ability.

The following analysis describes various modes of performance of 15 activities commonly used in practice according to the typology described in chapters 2 and 4. The format of the analysis is intended to assist therapists in predicting behavior, assistance, and reasonable treatment goals for those individuals with stable cognitive disabilities. The specific behaviors described within each mode are not comprehensive or inclusive descriptions of all possible behaviors within that mode.

It has been noted by clinicians that the performance of eating does not parallel other self-care activities. Perhaps because of its life-sustaining import, persons at level 2 have been observed to pick up and place food in their mouths when unable to grasp or manipulate other objects successfully. The analysis for eating has been shifted down one level to reflect this empirical evidence.

A column of warnings has been included, recognizing that a cognitive disability predisposes an individual to error and possible harm in the process of doing an activity. A warning is a prediction of what might happen, but does not imply that an undesirable consequence is inevitable.

Therapists need to be aware of their responsibility to warn patients and caregivers of potential harmful consequences of undertaking particular activities. Furthermore, therapists should clearly document when specific warnings have been issued. This is especially needed when patients or caregivers insist on pursuing activities that place them at risk for harm.

## 10.0 Self-Awareness Disability: Grooming

Grooming includes care of the hair (combing, brushing, setting, arranging, curling, and straightening); teeth (brushing, flossing); face (washing, shaving, tweezing, applying make-up or lotion); and the hands (applying lotion, trimming, filing nails, applying nail polish).

| Level | Behavior | Assistance | Goal | Warnings |
|---|---|---|---|---|
| 1.0 | Unable to comb hair, shave, care for teeth or nails. | Caregiver does all tasks. | Caregiver will meet all hair, teeth, facial care needs. | Inspect for dental problems. Remove dentures. |
| 1.4 | May turn head or open mouth on command or with tactile cue. | Provides water to rinse mouth after meals; lifts and holds head. | Same as 1.0. | Same as 1.0. |
| 1.8 | While seated, may open mouth and keep open with continuous tactile cue to allow brushing. May drink rinse water. May rotate head to cooperate. | Caregiver brushes teeth, holding mouth open with hand or verbal commands. Provides rinse water, bowl near face to spit in. | Same as 1.0. | Same as 1.0. |
| 2.0 | While seated, may hold mouth open with verbal cues. May swish water, lean to spit into adjacent bowl. May lean forward or back to allow for combing or shaving. | Caregiver initiates all grooming tasks. Gives verbal commands to rinse, spit, lean, turn head, open or close mouth. | Caregiver will maintain dental hygiene, initiate hair, face, and nail care. | Watch for discomfort that may result in striking out. |
| 2.4 | Holds mouth open while standing next to a sink. Leans over at waist to spit when cued. May stand while shaved or combed. | Caregiver leads to basin, gives verbal cues to open mouth, drink, rinse, bend, spit. | Same as 2.0. | Watch for discomfort that may result in striking out. Watch for loss of balance while bending, standing. |
| 2.6 | Walks to bathroom on request for grooming activities. | Caregiver tells patient to go to bathroom for grooming. | Same as 2.0. | Same as 2.4. |
| 2.8 | Maintains stability during grooming activities by using grab bars or railings. | Caregiver provides grab bars near sinks. Removes movable furniture. | Caregiver will maintain dental hygiene, hair, and nail care. Patient will use grab bars as needed. | Same as 2.4. |

| LEVEL | BEHAVIOR | ASSISTANCE | GOAL | WARNINGS |
|---|---|---|---|---|
| 3.0 | Grasps brush, comb, toothbrush, offered at eye level. May do back and forth action in one place briefly with cuing only. | Caregiver offers or places tools within 6" (comb, brush, toothbrush with toothpaste). Cues to begin action associated with object. | Patient will grasp grooming objects. Caregiver will provide familiar safe objects and will cue with associated action. | Restrict access to harmful objects (hot water, razors, hot combs, curling irons). |
| 3.2 | Spontaneously initiates brushing and combing when objects are in close proximity. No awareness of effects. May attempt to squeeze toothpaste, turn on water, pick up bottles. | Caregiver places objects in visible close proximity. Cues to start and stop actions with verbal commands. Checks results. Does missed locations. Caregiver does tasks requiring sequencing of actions, or precise results. | Patient will initiate familiar actions of brushing, combing. Caregiver will supervise and provide assistance to avoid harmful effects, ensure effective results. | Same as 3.0. |
| 3.4 | Spontaneously sustains actions of combing, brushing, shaving with electric razor, applying lotion or makeup. Looks at objects but fails to note effects. Uses too much/little toothpaste, lotion, make-up. Misses obvious dirt when washing face or hands. May start actions when objects are seen. | Provides necessary, safe tools at appropriate time of day. Sequences through actions. Stops excessive actions. Checks results. Does hard-to-reach spots and corrects errors. Arranges hair, trims nails, flosses teeth, applies makeup, and shaves with straight razors. | Patient will maintain grooming actions and cooperate with caregiver assistance. Caregiver will provide tools and objects and appropriate supervision to avoid harmful or undesirable effects. | Restrict access to harmful or undesirable objects (see 3.0). Monitor for excessive use of materials or action. Do not leave alone when using water. |
| 3.6 | Combs, brushes hair while looking in the mirror. May miss back, sides, or under chin (shaving). May initiate tasks based on a familiar association (end of meal for brushing teeth, washing face in morning). May wait for water to get warm before using. Imitates change in location or duration of action (washing in one place longer). Alters amounts of make-up. | Provides necessary, familiar, safe objects at appropriate time of day. Sequences actions, demonstrates changes in locations, amounts for more effective results. Checks for and corrects socially unacceptable results. Does flossing, denture care. Assists with use of hair dyes, fingernail clippers, or other harmful tools or products. | Patient will note effects of actions and will imitate changes in location and duration of actions. Caregiver will supervise, provide appropriate assistance to avoid harmful effects. | Restrict access to potentially harmful objects. Watch for impulsive or unpredictable actions. Do not leave unsupervised for long periods. May be able to schedule short dental visit. |

| LEVEL | BEHAVIOR | ASSISTANCE | GOAL | WARNINGS |
|---|---|---|---|---|
| | toothpaste, hair products, lotion only with assistance. May engage in impulsive actions (shaving off eyebrows). | | | |
| 3.8 | Combs, brushes hair, or shaves face or legs until all area is covered. Recognizes completion (all nails are trimmed). May miss back of head, sides of face, or other hidden surfaces. May attempt to style hair; uses clips in front only. Brushes front surfaces of teeth. May forget a step in a customary sequence (using mouthwash, or rinsing mouth) and think they are done. May use all available lotion, shampoo. | Caregiver provides necessary safe objects at appropriate time of day. Provides correct amounts of shampoos, lotions. Assists with styling back of head, cutting nails, correcting socially unacceptable results. Patient can be left alone for short periods if hazards are removed. | Patient will recognize completion of grooming tasks. Caregiver will supervise and provide appropriate assistance to avoid harmful effects. Caregiver will arrange for long-term or special dental care. | Restrict access to dangerous or undesirable objects. Do not leave unsupervised with any sharp, toxic, or hot materials. Check every few minutes if left alone. |
| 4.0 | Initiates and completes a familiar sequence of actions (combing, shaving, nail care, washing face) when all necessary tools are visible and within reach. May not initiate consistently or at correct time of day. May miss back or sides of head when shaving or combing. May miss small particles of food when brushing. May request a straight razor to shave but may cut self. Follows routine sequence without variation. | Caregiver provides necessary safe objects. Objects should be in visible locations, within arm's reach. Provides familiar products and tools. Checks results. Suggests corrections for socially unacceptable results (heavy make-up). Supervises use of straight razors or chemicals (hair or nail products). Assists with new hair styles, procedures, or tools. | Patient will complete familiar routine of grooming with assistance in setup and to avoid harmful effects. Caregiver will provide familiar tools in accessible locations; will supervise use of new and potentially dangerous tools and materials. Will schedule dental check-ups. | Same as 3.8. Allow ample time for task completion (2 to 3 times average rate). Expect cuts with straight razors. |
| 4.2 | Initiates and completes a familiar routine of grooming. May ask if time of day is appropriate. May collect own supplies from | Caregiver provides familiar, safe objects and products for hair arrangement, shaving, teeth, and nail care. Stores objects in | Patient will complete familiar routine of grooming tasks with assistance to avoid harmful effects. | Same as 4.0. May argue with corrections of heavy make-up application. |

| LEVEL | BEHAVIOR | ASSISTANCE | GOAL | WARNINGS |
|---|---|---|---|---|
| | familiar, accessible locations. Stops when a highly visible error is made (i.e. cutting self with razor) and asks for help. Notes one feature at a time. Prefers striking effects of make-up and may not consider social appropriateness. | familiar and visible locations. Supervises use of new, sharp, or harmful tools or products. Checks results and suggests corrections for errors. Well-lit area and large mirrors assist with judging effects. | Caregiver will assist with error correction and supervise use of harmful materials. | Patient may be upset if usual materials are not available. Hazards are not anticipated. |
| 4.4 | Initiates and completes a grooming routine at the usual time of day. Combs, brushes, styles hair, or applies make-up to match a particular previous performance (i.e. a particular hairstyle). May insist on familiar products/supplies/time of day for tasks. Works at invariant pace, slower than average, and can't alter pace. Finds supplies in familiar locations. May be unable to master use of new tools requiring neuromuscular adjustments (curling iron). Misses hidden spots and may prefer striking effects in make-up, perfume ("more is better"). | Caregiver provides familiar, safe objects and supervises use of new or potentially dangerous supplies: hot combs, hair dyes, depilatories, sharps. Supervises timed procedures (facial masks, hair dyes, hot curlers). Checks heat settings on hot curlers. Does tasks involving attention to back of head (hair cuts, home permanents, some hair styles). | Patient will complete familiar routine of grooming with assistance to avoid harmful effects.<br><br>Caregiver will assist with error correction and supervise use of harmful materials and new procedures and products. | |
| 4.6 | Initiates grooming tasks, and varies one aspect of typical procedure or one feature (hair style, make-up) on his or her own. May be willing to try new products or tools. Makes attempts to make neuromuscular adjustments (mastering use of dental floss, curling iron) but may not be successful. May want to cut or color hair but fail to | Provides supplies in accessible locations or inside drawers if familiar. Explains consequences of variations or product substitutions. Supervises use of potentially harmful products. | Patient will complete familiar grooming routines with some variations from his or her standard performance with assistance to avoid harmful or undesirable effects.<br><br>Caregiver will assist with error correction and supervise use of new or potentially harmful products. | Vigilance is recommended to anticipate consequences of changes in actions, products for patient. Actions may be impulsive. |

| LEVEL | BEHAVIOR | ASSISTANCE | GOAL | WARNINGS |
|---|---|---|---|---|
| | consider consequences. Scans environment for needed tools and supplies. | | | |
| 4.8 | Checks results of grooming, hair styling, application or make-up by close examination when done. Corrects all striking errors one at a time. Learns new grooming procedures slowly by rote. May rigidly follow prescribed routines such as care of dental appliances. | Demonstrates new grooming procedures slowly, one step at a time. Provides explanations of secondary effects. | Patient will correct perceived errors one at a time in grooming tasks and will follow explanations of harmful secondary effects to be avoided in shaving, dental, nail, hair care. Caregiver will monitor use of new supplies and provide explanations of potential hazards. | |
| 5.0 | Initiates and completes routine grooming tasks independently. Solves a problem by varying pressure or range of motion. May forget newly learned solutions. May fail to anticipate need to purchase grooming supplies and make appoint-ments for dental check-ups, haircuts. May not blend make-up or consider coordination of make-up with clothes, occasion. Fails to anticipate secondary effects or intangible properties (allergies, chemical interactions) of new products. May not read directions before using new product. | Caregiver assists with problems involving attention to surface properties (blending make-up), spatial properties (cleaning teeth with water pik). Explains secondary effects and points out dangers to be avoided in new tasks. Reminds to check grooming inventories, makes appointments. | Patient will complete routine grooming care independently with assistance to avoid harmful effects in new tasks. Caregiver will explain secondary effects and provide assistance with spatial and surface properties. | May question need to conform to the expectations of others for grooming. May miss scheduled dental/hair appointments. |

| LEVEL | BEHAVIOR | ASSISTANCE | GOAL | WARNINGS |
|---|---|---|---|---|
| 5.2 | Initiates and completes routine grooming tasks independently. Blends make-up, aware of surface properties (closeness of shave, smoothness of skin, uniformity of nail color). May not coordinate make-up with clothing, occasion, or current styles. | Caregiver assists with problem solving requiring awareness of spatial properties or sociocultural considerations. Explains secondary effects in new tasks. Reminds to check supply inventories and make appointments. | Patient: same as 5.0. Caregiver will explain secondary effects and provide assistance with spatial properties. | Same as 5.0. |
| 5.4 | Initiates and completes routine grooming tasks independently. Makes successful fine-motor adjustments with new grooming tools (curling irons, clippers). Varies routines, products, and methods to produce new results. Applies own criteria for judging appropriate grooming outcomes and may not consider social consequences of this. | Caregiver points out consequences of selections that deviate markedly from social standards of grooming. Points out potential harmful secondary effects of new procedures or products. | Patient: same as 5.0. Caregiver will explain secondary effects and consequences of failing to consider social rules governing appearance. | May argue with requests to alter pace or need to consider social standards. |
| 5.6 | Independent in all grooming tasks. Harmonizes combinations of clothes, make-up, hairstyle. May consult magazines or other sources for current make-up or grooming products. May adjust pace of work on request. | Caregiver discusses various standards for comparison. Identifies potential secondary effects of new products, procedures to avoid. | Patient: same as 5.0. Caregiver will explain potential harmful secondary effects of new procedures/ products. | May get busy doing routines and forget about the passage of time. |
| 5.8 | Independent in all grooming tasks. Plans out new actions when all materials available. Requests clarification of potential harmful effects of new products or routines (hair dyes, allergic reactions, etc.). May read instructions on home permanents, etc. Varies pace when needed. | Caregiver clarifies potential harmful effects of new products or procedures. | Patient: same as 5.0. Caregiver: same as 5.6. | |

## 10.1 Self-Awareness Disability: Dressing

Dressing includes selecting and putting on clothes with a consideration for the time of day, temperature, season, comfort, and how garments go together. Dressing includes obtaining clothing from storage areas, dressing and undressing in a sequential fashion, fastening and adjusting clothing and shoes, and applying and removing assistive or adaptive equipment, prostheses, or orthoses.

| Level | Behavior | Assistance | Goal | Warnings |
|---|---|---|---|---|
| 1.0-1.6 | Unable to select, obtain, or don clothing or adaptive equipment. | Caregiver selects garments and dresses patient. Puts on adaptive equipment (splints, posy belts). Uses loose-fitting, easy-to-remove garments. | Caregiver will dress patient, apply adaptive equipment to avoid medical complications. | Inspect for signs of binding, skin redness from ill-fitting garments or adaptive equipment. |
| 1.8 | Patient may move arm or leg to assist with donning garments, and equipment when cued. | Caregiver selects garments. Verbally gives commands or tactilely cues to elicit cooperative postures. Loose-fitting garments preferred. | Caregiver: same as 1.0. | Same as 1.0. |
| 2.0 | Sits while dressed by caregiver. Moves extremities or trunk to assist with donning. | Caregiver selects garments. Verbally commands or tactilely cues to move trunk or body part. Loose-fitting garments. | Patient will move arms, legs, trunk, in response to cues to assist with dressing. Caregiver: same as 1.0. | Same as 1.0 Ensure stability (chair with back or wheelchair). May resist dressing. |
| 2.2-2.4-2.6 | Stands while being dressed. Pushes arm or leg through garment when held next to body part. May remember and initiate familiar dressing movements (raising arms overhead). | Caregiver selects clothes. Positions garments next to body part and cues patient to move when appropriate. Works fasteners, laces; applies adaptive equipment. Monitors clothing for periodic adjustment. | Patient will push arms and legs through garments when cued to assist with dressing. Caregiver: same as 1.0. | Same as 1.0. Don pants while seated, to avoid falls. Avoid loose shoes or slippers. Watch for needed readjustment. |
| 2.8 | Stands, sits, grabs onto bars, railings, or other support for stability while being dressed. Usually moves slowly. | Caregiver provides assistance as in 2.4. | Patient will use grab bars or other objects for stability while dressing. Caregiver: same as 2.4. | Same as 1.0. Dons shoes, pants while seated to avoid falls. |

| LEVEL | BEHAVIOR | ASSISTANCE | GOAL | WARNINGS |
|---|---|---|---|---|
| 3.0 | Grasps garment offered at eye level or puts/throws it down. May walk away. | Caregiver provides assistance as in 2.4. Hands garments to patient and cues to move. | Patient will grasp garments when these are handed to him/her. Caregiver will select and assist with donning clothes and adaptive equipment. | May reject offered garments. |
| 3.2 | Picks up garment in close proximity and begins to don it. Associates action with garment type. May stop before completion, but may resume on command. May pick up any nearby garment. May be unable to don tight-fitting garments, hosiery, or do fasteners. | Caregiver selects and hands garments to patient, one at a time. Redirects attention or cues to move as necessary. Does fasteners, laces. Applies adaptive equipment. Periodically checks for correct adjustment of clothing and equipment. Velcro closures recommended. | Patient will grasp and begin correct actions of donning familiar garments. Caregiver: same as 3.0. | Avoid unfamiliar, tight-fitting apparel. |
| 3.4 | Selects from items laid out and begins donning garments. If allowed to select from many alternatives, may pick several items of one type or be unable to decide. Dons all familiar items but may quit before finished or may don several layers or may dress and undress. Actions usually slow. Errors not noted include misaligned buttons, inside-out garments, mismatched socks or shoes, torn or soiled garments. Can't do unusual fasteners or fasteners in back. Ties a bow but fails to note tension. | Caregiver selects and lays out appropriate items of clothing on bed or in other visible location. May provide limited (2) choice between appropriate items. Reminds when to commence and monitors progress. Assists with unusual fasteners; adjusts undergarments. Restricts access to undesirable garments. Checks results and corrects errors. Puts on adaptive equipment. | Patient will complete dressing with caregiver assistance. Caregiver will provide appropriate assistance, check results, and correct errors. Caregiver will monitor for correct adjustment of donned items. | Garments selected by patient may be inappropriate to time of day, temperature, season, occasion, or may not be in proper condition (repair, cleanliness). May put on many layers or not cover body. |
| 3.6 | Selects one top and one bottom garment from dresser/closet to cover all body | Caregiver groups clothing items in drawer or closet to assist proper selection or | Patient: same as 3.4. Caregiver: same as 3.4. | Same as 3.4. May argue with caregiver suggestions to |

| LEVEL | BEHAVIOR | ASSISTANCE | GOAL | WARNINGS |
|---|---|---|---|---|
| | parts. May choose same items over and over or use idiosyncratic criteria. Associates time to dress with events such as breakfast. Dons common clothing items without assistance, except for unusual or hidden fasteners, sticky zippers, small buttons, or ties. May layer clothes incorrectly. May note a visible error at perimeter of garment (crooked hem or misaligned buttons). May imitate a modification of a habitual action (pulling on shoes). | provide corrections to poor selections. Assists with small, hidden, unusual fasteners. Demonstrates simple modifications in habitual actions that increase effective donning, but expects to repeat such instruction next time. Puts on and adjusts adaptive equipment. | | change selections. Monitor all adaptive equipment for proper fit to avoid medical complications. |
| 3.8 | May be trained to initiate dressing at a particular time of day. Dons all common articles of clothing slowly with some errors in sequence. Recognizes when dressing is completed (all body is covered). Stops when a problem occurs (broken zipper); may not ask for help. | Caregiver provides selection assistance same as for 3.6. Provides cues (pre-set alarm) to assist with dressing initiation. Provides other assistance as in 3.6. | Patient will dress self and recognize completion with assistance in selection and donning. Caregiver will provide assistance in selection and donning, will check results and correct errors. Will apply and adjust adaptive equipment. | Same as 3.6. |
| 4.0 | Initiates dressing at customary time of day. Selects items from wardrobe, but may fail to consider time of day, temperature, season, occasion, cleanliness, coordination of colors, or patterns. Dons items slowly in correct sequence. Cannot alter rate of dressing. May ignore or use accessories incorrectly. | Caregiver simplifies selections by reducing number of available garments, or groups garments in ready-to-wear combinations. Suggests changes for inappropriate choices. Corrects hidden errors, assists with arranging desired accessories. Checks and makes adjustments on simple splints. Puts on other adaptive | Patient will initiate and complete dressing at customary time of day with assistance in selection and donning. Caregiver: same as 3.8. | Same as 3.6. Allow ample time for completion of dressing (two to three times average rate). |

| LEVEL | BEHAVIOR | ASSISTANCE | GOAL | WARNINGS |
|---|---|---|---|---|
| | May have difficulty with fasteners requiring fine-motor coordination. May fail to note errors at back (shirt not tucked in, labels sticking out). May be able to put on a simple static splint but may not adjust to fit. | equipment. Stores clothing in visible, easy-to-reach locations. Removes dirty, damaged, poorly fitting garments. | | |
| 4.2 | Initiates dressing at customary time of day. Selects clothing items based on striking features, such as color, one feature at a time. May choose to wear a favorite item (a particular pair of shoes) all the time. May become aware of a feature (such as dirt on shoe) and be unable to shift attention to something else. Fails to see hidden errors as in 4.0. May put on a simple static splint; may recognize a striking error in adjustment and ask for help. | Same as 4.0. Caregiver points out other visible features to correct errors in combinations. | Patient will select clothing based on matching cues and will don common garments independently. Caregiver will provide assistance as necessary with new garments, fasteners, and will monitor and correct dressing errors. Caregiver will apply and monitor complex adaptive equipment. | Same as 4.0. Monitor fit of all adaptive equipment. |
| 4.4 | Finds garments in familiar locations; initiates dressing at usual times. Selects familiar combinations or outfits. May want to wear same outfit over and over or to an event because "I wore it there before". Resists new combinations. May fail to consider weather conditions, season, time of day, occasion, coordination of color, or pattern as factors | Caregiver stores garments in ready-to-wear condition in familiar locations. Groups garments in usual combinations or by type. Points out visible features to be considered in coordinating new items. Monitors results; suggests corrections to hidden or subtle errors. Assists with small or unusual fasteners. Monitors application of simple splints and makes | Patient will initiate and complete dressing using familiar combinations of clothing with assistance with new and difficult fasteners. Patient will apply simple splints or other devices with assistance. Caregiver: same as 4.2. | May be upset if familiar combinations are not available. May argue with suggested corrections of errors. |

| LEVEL | BEHAVIOR | ASSISTANCE | GOAL | WARNINGS |
|---|---|---|---|---|
|  | in selection. May miss hidden errors or subtle problems such as shirts out in back, skirt too short for slip or knee-high hose, missing buttons, tears. Uses accessories in a fixed fashion. May not work fasteners requiring fine-motor adjustments. May be able to learn procedure to put on a dynamic hand splint or a simple preadjusted cuff sling. May be unable to fasten straps or buckles out of view. | needed adjustments. Puts on other adaptive devices. |  |  |
| 4.6 | Searches for desired clothing items in drawers or closet. Changes one item in a familiar outfit to produce a "new" outfit. Does not consider how change affects whole look. May coordinate shoes with outfit. Tries to don tight-fitting items (boots, hosiery) with some success. Fine-motor adjustments (jewelry fasteners, sheer hosiery, small bows, necktie, buckles) may be abandoned. Follows suggested spatial adjustments (location of scarf, tie, strap on splint). | Same as 4.4. Caregiver demonstrates changes in spatial locations that improve results. | Patient will dress self independently and will vary combinations one feature at a time. Will apply simple splints or preadjusted slings. Caregiver: same as 4.2. | Monitor for appropriateness of new combinations. |
| 4.8 | Considers all striking visible features of garments, including color, pattern, condition, general fit. May not attend to less striking qualities (cleanliness, fabric | Caregiver points out consequences of selections, such as being under- or overdressed for the weather or occasion. Demonstrates new sequences of actions | Patient will select garments considering all striking features with caregiver assistance to consider secondary effects. Caregiver: same as 4.6. | Allow additional time for new garments, or for making new combinations. |

| LEVEL | BEHAVIOR | ASSISTANCE | GOAL | WARNINGS |
|---|---|---|---|---|
| | type) or consider social standards or current style in making selections. May don clothing slowly, checking results by examining in mirror from several angles on completion. Learns by rote a sequence of new actions, such as putting on a prosthesis. May recognize predictable problems with fit or function of adaptive equipment. | for donning garments or adaptive equipment. | Caregiver will monitor fit and function of complex adaptive equipment to avoid medical complications. | |
| 5.0 | Varies strength, range of motion, in donning tight-fitting garments or shoes and working clasps, ties, straps. May not consider surface properties (need for ironing, cleanliness) or social standards. | Caregiver provides assistance as in 4.8. | Patient will successfully vary range of motion and strength to don garments. Caregiver will explain secondary effects of selections to avoid undesirable consequences. | May argue with suggestions to change selections. |
| 5.2 | Recognizes and considers all tangible properties of garments (cleanliness, need for ironing, fabric textures) in selections. | Same as 4.8. | Patient will select garments considering surface properties. Caregiver: same as 5.0. | Same as 5.0. |
| 5.4 | Mixes wardrobe items freely. Criteria may be idiosyncratic or "to be different." Results may be odd or socially inappropriate. Effectively manages fine-motor adjustments in hard-to-reach places (unsticks zippers, buttons at back or wrist, buckles on prosthetic devices). Adjusts slings, straps on prostheses for better effects. | Caregiver offers explanations of undesirable secondary effects of selections. Check for proper donning of complex adaptive equipment. | Patient will solve new problems involving spatial properties in dressing. Caregiver: same as 5.0. | May resist suggestions to alter selections based on secondary effects. |

| Level | Behavior | Assistance | Goal | Warnings |
|---|---|---|---|---|
| 5.6 | Uses some esthetic criteria to harmonize or coordinate outfits and accessories. May be aware of current styles. May be aware of proportion and body type as influences in esthetic appearance. Alters donning rate with assistance to conform to time constraint. | Caregiver offers alternative possibilities for selections based on different criteria. Point out time constraints in new situations. | Patient will consider coordination of clothing for pleasing effects with caregiver assistance to identify social consequences. Caregiver: same as 5.0. | Same as 5.4. |
| 5.8 | Selections consider tangible secondary properties (weight of fabric and heat of day) based on previous experience. Varies pace of dressing spontaneously to conform to a new time constraint. | Caregiver offers explanations of consequences of selections in new situations. | Patient will consider tangible secondary effects when selecting garments, and will adjust pace of dressing as needed. Caregiver: same as 5.0. | |
| 6.0 | Speculates and plans for dressing needs, including considering all properties of garments, demands of social situation, donning time, personal resources, for routine, special events. | None needed. | Patient dresses self, including putting on and removing adaptive equipment, independently and in a timely fashion. | |

## 10.2 Self-Awareness Disability: Bathing

Bathing includes using soap, water, towel, and toiletries to clean, rinse, dry, moisturize, and deodorize body and hair. Bathing may be done in bed, or bathroom tub, or shower. Excludes grooming.

| LEVEL | BEHAVIOR | ASSISTANCE | GOAL | WARNINGS |
|---|---|---|---|---|
| 1.0-1.4 | No awareness of need to bathe. May move away from caregiver's touch. | Caregiver gives sponge bath to patient in bed. | Caregiver maintains cleanliness to avoid undesirable medical complications. | Monitor for skin problems due to uncleanliness. |
| 1.6-1.8 | May move arms or legs, or may roll over to assist with bathing with proprioceptive cues. May hold trunk or other body part against gravity with continuous cuing. May resist bathing. | Caregiver gives sponge bath in bed with passive supports. Touches body parts to cue desired movements. | Same as 1.0-1.4. | Monitor for skin problems. Patient may resist bath. |
| 2.0-2.2 | Sits for sponge bath. Moves extremities. Moves trunk to assist or prevent falling to one side. May do a pivot transfer with assistance. Aware of caregiver's efforts to bathe. | Caregiver gives sponge bath in bed or seated in chair. Gives verbal commands to move body parts. | Caregiver will maintain cleanliness of patient to avoid undesirable medical complications. | Watch for discomfort, which may result in striking out. Watch for falls. |
| 2.4-2.6 | May walk to bathroom and step into tub with assistance. Moves body parts on command. May be able to bend at waist to put head under faucet for shampoo. | Caregiver bathes patient (sponge or seated tub bath). Cues to walk to bathroom. Uses bathing chairs, nonskid bath mats. Dries patient in bath to avoid falls. | Patient will cooperate with bathing by moving body parts. Caregiver: same as 2.0. | Baths recommended to avoid falls. May be frightened by risk of fall and refuse to enter tub. |
| 2.8 | Uses grab bars to get in and out of tub. | Same as 2.4. | Patient will cooperate with bathing by using grab bars to stabilize. | Same as 2.4. Grasp of grab bars may be too weak or tight. Moves slowly. |

| LEVEL | BEHAVIOR | ASSISTANCE | GOAL | WARNINGS |
|---|---|---|---|---|
| 3.0 | Grasps washcloth, soap, towel, shampoo, or puts them down when placed in hand. May do back and forth movements for brief periods. | Hands bathing tools to patient while in bath or seated in shower. | Patient will grasp familiar bathing tools when placed in hand. Caregiver will initiate and supervise bathing, providing assistance. | Remove sharp or dangerous objects from reach. Do not leave patient. Watch for falls on wet floors. |
| 3.2 | Spontaneously grasps washcloth, soap, towel, shampoo, and initiates associated movements. Stops and starts actions on command. Does not sequence actions. | Same as 3.0. Starts and stops actions with short commands. | Patient will start and stop actions on command. Caregiver: same as 3.0. | Same as 3.0. If shower is attempted, caregiver will get wet. |
| 3.4 | Picks up washcloth, soap, towel, and wipes easy-to-reach body parts. May wash in one spot, forget to use soap. May forget to rinse or dry off. May not rub hard enough to remove dirt. May quit before complete. May stay in tub or shower a long time if allowed. May initiate bath or shower at odd times. | Reminds patient when to bathe; prohibits too-frequent bathing. Provides essential, safe tools at proper times. Sequences with verbal cues through correct routine. Applies soaps, shampoo, lotions in correct amounts. Reminds patient to wash hidden areas. Washes hard-to-reach areas for patient. Checks water temperatures. | Patient will sustain familiar actions to complete a bath or shower and shampoo with assistance to sequence actions. Caregiver will initiate and supervise bath and shampoo; will sequence through actions. | Do not leave alone. If showers are attempted, watch for flooding and falls. Check water temperatures. Patient may leave tub or shower before done. |
| 3.6 | Actions of washing follow perimeter of body; may try to do back. Imitates caregiver suggestions to rub harder. May wait for water temperature to cool or warm. May forget steps in sequence (rinse or dry). Does not measure amounts of shampoo, lotions, deodorant. May quit before task is completed. | Same as 3.4. Demonstrates simple modifications in actions for more effective results (rubbing harder or less hard). Premeasures amounts of shampoo or lotion. | Patient will imitate modifications in manual actions to complete bathing more effectively. Caregiver will initiate, supervise bathing. Will demonstrate modifications for more effective results. | Same as 3.4. Watch for impulsive actions that may result in falls. |

| LEVEL | BEHAVIOR | ASSISTANCE | GOAL | WARNINGS |
|-------|----------|------------|------|----------|
| 3.8 | Covers all visible body parts with soap and rinses it off. May forget hidden parts or a step. Aware of completion. May stop when a problem is encountered (i.e., no shampoo), but may not ask for help. | Same as 3.6. Caregiver may leave patient for short period. | Patient will follow cues to complete bathing and shampooing routine and will state when he or she is done. Caregiver: same as 3.6. | Restrict access to harmful materials. Expect waste if allowed to measure amounts. Do not leave unsupervised for more than a few minutes. |
| 4.0 | Recognizes need for a bath but may initiate at inappropriate times. When materials are accessible, moves slowly through a familiar sequence until done or exhausted. May not ask for help for a major problem (unusual controls on faucets, no soap, etc.). May not note wet floors. | Caregiver places needed supplies in arm's reach, visible. Provides familiar products. Is available for problem solving. Demonstrates unusual controls on faucets; opens unusual product dispensers. Uses anti-slip bath mats. Checks quality of outcome if desirable. May leave unsupervised with set-up. | Patient will complete bath or shower with set-up to avoid harmful effects. Caregiver will provide familiar, safe set-up, and be available to solve problems, check results. | Store bath supplies in hidden cupboards or lock bathroom door to limit bathing at inconvenient times. Watch for floods, falls. May take 2 to 3 times average to complete task. |
| 4.2 | Recognized need for a bath and may ask if time is appropriate. Collects supplies from visible location. Follows routine. May miss small or hidden places (back of head, ears, fingernails). Recognizes a problem such as lack of soap and asks for help. Attends to one striking feature at a time. | Caregiver stores familiar products in visible locations within 24 inches of tub or shower. Checks quality of results; reminds to wash small or hidden body parts. | Patient will initiate and complete bathing by securing own supplies from visible locations, with assistance to avoid harmful effects. Caregiver: same as 4.0. | Allow ample time for task completion. Remove hazards (electrical appliances) from proximity to bath. |
| 4.4 | Initiates bath, shower, shampoo at customary time and follows typical routine invariantly. May collect supplies from familiar locations. May not vary rate, may not alter amounts (to save | Caregiver purchases familiar bathing supplies and stores in same locations, clearly labeled. Checks for results. Points out missed hidden body parts. Can leave patient alone. | Patient will initiate and complete a familiar bathing routine in own home environment with assistance to avoid harmful effects. Caregiver will provide familiar supplies, | May become upset if routine products are not available. Protect from unseen hazards (slippery floor, electrical appliance near water). |

| Level | Behavior | Assistance | Goal | Warnings |
|---|---|---|---|---|
| | water or materials). May want same products; may not read labels on new products. May use excessive amounts of lotion, shampoo thinking "more is better". May not do fine-motor adjustments to open tight or unusual containers. May resist changing routine to accommodate heat, exercise. Little or no awareness of sharing bathing space and supplies with others; may not hang up towels, clean area of toiletries, etc. | | will correct errors, and will supervise new or potentially harmful procedures. | |
| 4.6 | May alter bathing routine to account for exercise, hot weather, special event. Works at getting dirt from small places with some success. May hunt for supplies in open cupboards. May be willing to try a new product or substitute a product. May follow suggestions that involve changing locations (storing supplies near bathing area, drying off in shower to avoid dripping on floor, hanging up towels after use to clear space). | Caregiver provides needed supplies in open cupboards or shelves. Explains consequences of changes in product use or routine. | Patient will initiate and complete routine bathing with variations in daily schedule, product use, or product storage with assistance to avoid harmful or undesirable effects. Caregiver: same as 4.4. | Remove unseen hazards. May be unable to coordinate bath schedule with others. |
| 4.8 | May coordinate bathing schedule with others. Attends to all striking features of self, and bathing environment. Checks quality of results on completion. May learn a new procedure (bathing to | Caregiver explains secondary effects (i.e., frequency, conservation, social rules of shared space) as needed. | Patient will complete routine bathing independently and will check quality. Patient will understand explanations of secondary effects. Caregiver will explain secondary effects | Same as 4.6. |

| LEVEL | BEHAVIOR | ASSISTANCE | GOAL | WARNINGS |
|-------|----------|-----------|------|----------|
| | conserve water) by rote. Understands secondary effects when these are explained (need to conserve water, drying effects of prolonged or too frequent bathing, scheduling baths to avoid inconvenience to others). Reports low supplies to caregivers. | | that may result in harm or undesirable social consequences. | |
| 5.0 | Initiates and completes routine bathing independently. Varies strength or range of motion to solve a problem (bathing with a physical impairment such as a cast on arm). May fail to anticipate secondary effects or intangible properties of new products (allergies to soaps). | Same as 4.8. | Same as 4.8. | |
| 5.2 | Initiates and completes routine bathing independently. Attends to all surface qualities of skin, nails, hair, and may make bath product selections based on subtle effects produced by these products. Notes all tangible features of bathing environment (wet, slippery floors). | Same as 4.8. | Same as 4.8. | |
| 5.4-5.8 | Independent in all routine bathing. May not read labels of new products; may fail to consider passage of time, alter rate of bathing, or anticipate hazards in a new environment. | Same as 4.8. | Same as 4.8. | |

## 10.3 Self-Awareness Disability: Walking and Exercising

Walking and exercising include awareness of how to move a normal body to different locations in space or through different movement patterns.

| Level | Behavior | Assistance | Goal | Warnings |
|---|---|---|---|---|
| 1.0- 1.6 | Does not ambulate. Does not cooperate with transfer from lying to sitting position. Does not assist with passive ROM exercise. | Bed with side rails. Caregiver turns body to maintain skin integrity. Passive supports to maintain sitting in bed. Passive ROM for joint mobility. | Caregiver will provide safe environment to avoid falls and protect against medical complications due to immobility. | Side rails in proper position. Check for skin integrity. |
| 1.8 | May raise arms to do ROM. May resist passive ROM by pushing away. | Bed with side rails. Caregiver provides continuous cues to do ROM exercise or lift buttocks off bed. | Patient will cooperate with ROM exercise by holding body parts against gravity. Caregiver will assist ROM exercises. | May resist by pushing away. |
| 2.0 | Does not ambulate. Holds body upright while sitting. | Caregiver provides continuous cues to lean to transfer from one seated position to another. | Patient will maintain seated position. Caregiver will assist with seated transfers. | Watch for fatigue or discomfort that may result in striking out. |
| 2.2 | Stands and may take a few steps with assistance. May cooperate with a pivot transfer. Uses "righting reflex" with upper extremities to prevent falling. | Caregiver provides tactile and verbal cues to assist standing, stepping, and making pivot transfers. | Patient will stand and make pivot transfers with assistance. Caregiver will provide cues, assistance in standing, transfers. | Watch for falls. Observe proper body mechanics to avoid back injury. |
| 2.4 | Ambulates slowly and aimlessly through doorways and around furniture. Stands and sits. May pace excessively. | Caregiver confines to safe, level areas. Closes doors to restrict access. Positions chairs before patient sits. | Patient will ambulate in restricted areas without falling. Caregiver will provide safe environment. | May wander or get lost if unrestricted. |
| 2.6 | Walks to a known destination such as bed or bathroom. May push or bang on | Caregiver opens doors to allow access to desired destinations. Assists up stairs or | Patient will walk to known destinations within restricted areas. | Same as 2.4. |

| LEVEL | BEHAVIOR | ASSISTANCE | GOAL | WARNINGS |
|---|---|---|---|---|
| | closed doors. Does not note uneven terrain. Steps up a stair when cued. | steps by cues and physical guidance. Removes area rugs, obstacles. | Caregiver will cue to climb stairs, provide safe walking areas. | May grab unstable objects or people and fall. |
| 2.8 | Grabs railing, bars, or other objects to stabilize position or to sit, stand, or step up. May not note position on chairs before sitting; may grab unstable objects. May cooperate with upper extremity resistive exercises by pushing or pulling with cues. | Caregiver guides to desired locations by walking next to or in front of patient. Points out railings. Positions chairs before patient sits. | Patient will stabilize self when changing body position.<br>Caregiver will provide cues and assistance in climbing stairs, sitting down, and transferring. | |
| 3.0 | Ambulates slowly toward interesting objects or people. Does not notice change in terrain as walks. May briefly increase pace to a faster walk but has trouble stopping or may lose balance or trip. May walk short distances for exercise accompanied by one other. Briefly imitates ROM exercise. | Caregiver confines to safe, level areas. Supervises stair climbing. Reduces distraction from interesting objects by removing them from view. Checks positions of chairs before patient sits. Escorts to new locations. | Patient will ambulate in restricted areas.<br>Caregiver: same as 2.8.<br>Caregiver will escort to new locations. | Same as 2.6. |
| 3.2 | Ambulates slowly within a restricted area toward objects that elicit familiar actions (picking up telephone). Does not seek out objects that are not visible. May wander away from a group or guide if distracted. Alters pace on command but does not sustain and reverts back to slower than normal pace. Climbs stairs slowly but independently. Walks with a | Caregiver restricts access to undesirable locations or objects by closing doors or removing objects from view. Escorts to all new locations. Checks position of chairs before patient sits. Stops perseverative movements with verbal commands. | Patient will ambulate in restricted areas.<br>Caregiver: same as 2.8. | Wanders and may get lost outside restricted areas. |

| LEVEL | BEHAVIOR | ASSISTANCE | GOAL | WARNINGS |
|---|---|---|---|---|
| | group short distances for exercise. ROM exercises may be repeated in a perseverative fashion. | | | |
| 3.4 | Ambulates within two to three familiar, contiguous rooms to access desirable activities (toilet, food, coffee) without assistance. Follows a guide to new locations without awareness of destination. Can alter ambulation pace on command but is easily distracted and reverts to previous pace. May be impulsive when changing body position from sitting to standing, and lose balance. May walk into others; does not note changes in terrain, traffic lights. Walks and talks at the same time with difficulty. Starts, stops, counts repetitive ROM or strengthening exercises with direct supervision. | Caregiver restricts access to new or undesirable locations. Cues patient to alter pace. Reminds patient to change position of body slowly. Can be escorted in community with a small group. Supervises directly all ROM and strengthening exercises. | Patient will ambulate and transfer from sitting to standing positions with caregiver assistance.<br><br>Patient will ambulate in community with caregiver escort.<br>Caregiver will escort patient to new locations. | Wanders and may get lost, especially if allowed to move unsupervised in community. Impulsive actions may result in falls. |
| 3.6 | Ambulates within several familiar living areas separated by closed doors. Aware of inside and outside of premises. May wander to a new location to access a desired activity, get lost, and be unable to retrace steps. May imitate modification in ambulation pace for short periods. May run for a short distance. | Caregiver restricts access to new or undesirable areas by locking doors to outside. Escorts to all new locations outside living areas. Provides cues to modify pace as needed. Provides direct supervision of all graded exercise programs with appropriate cues to ensure proper duration, force of actions. | Patient will modify pace of ambulation in familiar environment.<br>Caregiver will escort to new locations.<br>Caregiver will supervise graded exercise to ensure proper performance of repetitive actions. | Same as 3.4. |

| LEVEL | BEHAVIOR | ASSISTANCE | GOAL | WARNINGS |
|---|---|---|---|---|
| 3.8 | May imitate change in duration or amount in a graded ROM or strengthening exercise but needs cues to maintain. | | | |
| | Ambulates within familiar living areas or areas separated by short distances (such as next-door neighbor, backyard). Aware of destination after arrival and may express surprise. May be unable to retrace steps if lost. May run until tired or stopped. May recognize completion of a program of ROM and strengthening exercises. | Caregiver restricts access to new or undesirable areas. Escorts to all new locations outside immediate neighborhood. | Patient will ambulate and transfer safely within a familiar setting with assistance to avoid getting lost or fatigued from overexertion. Caregiver will escort to new locations in community. | Same as 3.4. |
| 4.0 | Walks or runs within fitness capacity to reach a predetermined familiar destination located a short distance away (mail box, or neighborhood store). May be easily confused by unexpected changes such as removal of landmark/need to detour. May ask to be led in new environment; may resist going to new environments and prefer familiar premises. Transfers from standing to sitting are generally safe though slow. May not note changes in terrain, a stair, an object on ground, and may trip. | Caregiver accompanies to all new locations and environments that are highly stimulus laden or hazardous. | Patient will ambulate and perform transfers independently within a familiar environment to reach a desired location. Caregiver will provide assistance in new or hazardous environments. | May become very anxious in highly stimulus-laden environments such as airports, malls, amusement parks, casinos. May resist going to such places. |

| LEVEL | BEHAVIOR | ASSISTANCE | GOAL | WARNINGS |
|-------|----------|------------|------|----------|
| 4.2 | Ambulates or runs within fitness capacity to familiar destinations within 1/2 to 1 mile. May not vary route. Aware of changes in familiar landmarks. May fail to attend to activity or noises outside of visual field in front as he or she walks but attends to one or two striking landmarks or cues. May ask for help if gets lost. May alter pace in response to perceived problem, such as bumpy terrain. May be able to learn a simple graded exercise program. | Caregiver escorts to all new locations. Points out landmarks to be used as cues to guide direction in new environments. Points out visible hazards requiring adjustments in pace or routes. Checks performance of all graded exercise. | Patient will ambulate and perform transfers independently using one to two visible cues to navigate to reach a desired destination.<br>Patient will ask for assistance if lost.<br>Caregiver will provide assistance to avoid falls, hazards, getting lost. | Same as 4.0.<br>Fails to attend to potential hazards. |
| 4.4 | Ambulates or runs within fitness capacity within fitness capacity within neighbor-hood to reach familiar destinations within a mile or more depending on routine. Chooses to go by familiar routes. Notes striking visible cues at eye level; may fail to attend to signs (except as landmarks), most activity or noise outside visual field, terrain changes. May not alter pace in response to a time constraint. May use a limited number of striking cues to find way in a new environment. May ask for assistance if lost. May follow suggested routes given for safety reasons but does not understand reason behind suggestions. Needs new routes identified | Caregiver provides assistance same as for 4.2.<br>Checks frequently travelled routes for hazards (such as crossing train tracks) and assists patient in identifying safest routes. Accompanies on new routes until well-learned. Monitors all graded exercises until well-learned. | Patient will ambulate to familiar locations with assistance to identify safest routes.<br>Patient will learn new route or exercise program after several days to weeks of practice.<br>Caregiver will provide assistance to avoid hazards or getting lost. | Same as 4.0. |

| LEVEL | BEHAVIOR | ASSISTANCE | GOAL | WARNINGS |
|---|---|---|---|---|
| | by others and learns these after several days to weeks of practice. May be trained to follow an exercise program after doing the program several times. Does not anticipate hazards or secondary effects of incorrect practice of program. May get bored and abandon a repetitive exercise routine. Can count up to 20 repetitions of exercises. | | | |
| 4.6 | Varies routes taken within familiar neighborhood to reach destinations associated with routine activities. Scans visible environment to search for a desired cue, such as a landmark, to guide direction. Follows a verbal explanation of a safety hazard when effects are immediate and visible (railroad crossing). May not understand less visible hazards (a "bad" neighborhood). May attempt to alter pace in response to a time constraint but this is not maintained. Needs new routes identified by others and learns them after several days to weeks of practice. May attempt to alter amount, duration, speed of graded exercise without awareness of potential complications. May shift to next exercise in a program. | Provides assistance same as for 4.4. | Patient will vary routes to familiar locations with caregiver assistance to identify hazards.<br>Caregiver: same as 4.4. | Variations in usual routes do not anticipate hazards or influence of time of day on landmarks or safety of the route. May get lost. "Pleasure hikes" in remote areas should be supervised. Variations in exercise programs should be checked for safety. |

| LEVEL | BEHAVIOR | ASSISTANCE | GOAL | WARNINGS |
|---|---|---|---|---|
| 4.8 | Ambulates or runs to new destinations when routes are pointed out. Learns new routes by rote over several days. Scans environment and notes all striking visible cues. Reads street signs and attempts to use this information in guiding route but still may be unable to find way home if lost. Understands explanations of safety hazards that are visible but secondary (walking alone at night). Learns an exercise program by rote and does it invariantly. | Caregiver accompanies patient to new locations until sequence is learned. Identifies safety hazards. | The patient will ambulate to desired new locations with assistance and will scan environment for safety hazards. Caregiver will provide assistance to ensure safety in walking in community. | |
| 5.0 | May ambulate to new locations by trial and error; may forget newly discovered routes and have to rediscover them. Effectively varies strength and ROM in graded exercise program or program to increase coordination or motor control. May refuse to comply with prescribed exercise programs. | Caregiver identifies potential hazards of walking in unfamiliar areas or from deviating from or refusing to comply with prescribed exercise protocols. | Patient will walk to desired new locations with assistance to identify safety hazards. Caregiver will provide warnings regarding safety hazards. | May refuse to comply with exercise protocols. |
| 5.2 | Notes all visible, tangible features of surrounding environment and uses these to guide walking. | Caregiver provides assistance as for 5.0. | Patient: same as 5.0. Caregiver: same as 5.0. | |
| 5.4 | Ambulates or runs to familiar and new locations independently. Notes spatial arrangements of buildings and streets as | Caregiver identifies safety hazards that are secondary, not visible, including need to plan for water, food, proper clothing, | Patient will ambulate to new locations of desirable activities and will follow an exercise program with assistance to avoid | Same as 5.0. |

| LEVEL | BEHAVIOR | ASSISTANCE | GOAL | WARNINGS |
|---|---|---|---|---|
|  | walks. Discovers new routes and remembers them. May refer to a map for guidance but may not be able to use it effectively. May choose to perform certain exercise activities and refuse others. Understands secondary effects such as conditioning when these are explained. | first aid, emergency plan for hikes in remote areas. Points out secondary complications of altering exercise programs (injury, exhaustion) and precautions for exercise (hot or cold weather, polluted air, etc.). | injury. Caregiver: same as 5.0. |  |
| 5.6 | Compares known routes with suggested routes and may alter. Varies pace of ambulation or exercise in response to a time constraint or other factor (heat, air pollution, state of health). May consider and follow recommended exercise programs, substituting methods when indicated. | Caregiver provides information to assist comparisons or selections in exercise programs or activities. | Patient will compare methods of exercise and follow suggested protocols to avoid harmful effects. Caregiver will provide information as needed to avoid harmful effects. |  |
| 5.8 | Varies pace according to clock and all tangible properties of a traversed route. Follows verbal explanations of secondary or intangible effects to avoid injury or accidents in an exercise program. | Same as 5.6. | Same as 5.6. |  |
| 6.0 | Ambulates to new location considering route with assistance from maps. Understands secondary effects and factors to be considered in pursuing a conditioning program or other exercise program. | None needed. | Patient participates in program of conditioning aware of risks, benefits, and consequences of deviations from prescribed activity. |  |

## 10.4 Self-Awareness Disability: Eating

Eating includes sitting at the table; putting food in the mouth; cutting food into bite-sized pieces; chewing and swallowing without letting food escape; removing food that soils from face, hands, clothes, or eating area; adjusting pace and sequence according to food temperature; adjusting seasonings, and opening packages.

| Level | Behavior | Assistance | Goal | Warnings |
|---|---|---|---|---|
| 1.0-1.2 | Licks lips, salivates, or sniffs in response to food smells. Does not open mouth or swallow on command. Must be tube fed. | Caregiver positions tubes and feeds patient. Monitor intake to ensure adequate nutrition. | Caregiver will provide for nutritional needs of patient with regular tube feedings. | Check weights to ensure adequate intake. |
| 1.4-1.6 | Turns head, opens mouth, or swallows on command. May sit in bed with support to hold body against gravity. May cooperate with hand-over-hand feeding of soft foods. May express food preferences with grunts or smiles. | Same as 1.0 or positions patient with passive supports in bed. Places soft food in spoon and feeds patient with verbal commands to open, swallow. Places spoon in patient's hand, and guides hand to mouth. | Caregiver will provide for nutritional needs of patient with either tube feeding or will feed a soft diet with commands or hand-over-hand methods. | Watch weights. Watch for choking. |
| 1.8 | May pick up soft finger food and place it in mouth. May drink from a cup placed in hand. Does not use utensils such as spoon or fork. May spill food or liquid without awareness. May push caregiver away. | Caregiver places soft finger food in front of patient. Places cup with liquid in hand. Cuts food into bite-sized pieces and places on spoon or fork; guides utensil to mouth with hand-over-hand method or feeds patient. | Caregiver will provide for nutritional needs of patient by providing soft finger foods, liquids in cups, and assistance with other foods. Patient will feed self soft finger foods. | Watch for choking. Precut solid foods and avoid stringy, hard-to-chew food. Check temperature of foods. Watch for spills with liquids. |
| 2.0-2.2 | Sits while eating. Spontaneously picks up food with fingers and places in mouth. May pick up a spoon or cup to eat or drink. Does not note temperature of food, or cut food into bite-sized pieces. May be unable to get | Caregiver assists to transfer to chair or serves on tray in bed or wheelchair. Precuts food. Soft or easy-to-chew food preferred. Remove nonedible objects from view. Fills cups half full to prevent spills; checks food temperatures. Cues to continue eating. | Caregiver will meet nutritional needs of patient by precutting foods and assisting with self-feeding as needed. Patient will feed self with spoon or with fingers with assistance from caregiver. | Same as 1.8. |

| LEVEL | BEHAVIOR | ASSISTANCE | GOAL | WARNINGS |
|---|---|---|---|---|
| | food on spoon. May eat very slowly. May need reminders to keep eating. May place nonedible objects in mouth. Does not note spills. | | | |
| 2.4 | May walk to table and sit when told or may follow guide to table. May pick up spoon or cup and begin to eat or drink without being cued. May start eating as soon as food is seen or served. May eat slowly or not finish meal. May be unable to get food on utensil and may use fingers. May show no awareness of others at the table. May ignore spills, dribbling food on face. Is unaware of temperature of food, sequence of dishes. | Caregiver reminds patient of mealtimes and escorts to table. Precuts food into bite-sized pieces. Checks food temperatures. Assists with opening containers. Cues to wipe face with napkin. | Caregiver: same as 2.0. Patient: same as 2.0. | Same as 2.0. |
| 2.8 | May walk to familiar eating area without an escort when told. May pick up utensils or cup and eat/drink without being cued. May have difficulty keeping small food (peas) or liquids on utensil. Does not cut with knife; eats food as is on plate. May eat until plate is empty or may refuse certain foods. Cannot alter rate of eating, which may be very slow. No awareness of others at table, spills, temperature of foods, table manners. | Caregiver provides assistance same as for 2.4. Takes into account food preferences, increases intake. | Caregiver: same as 2.0. Patient will feed self with conventional utensils with assistance from caregiver to cut food, open containers. | Same as 2.0. Consider food preferences. |

| Level | Behavior | Assistance | Goal | Warnings |
|---|---|---|---|---|
| 3.0-3.2 | May ask for food at any time of the day when hungry. May eat any visible food. May not be able to keep track of mealtimes. May use all utensils except knife; may try to cut food items with spoon/fork edge. No awareness of others at the same table; does not talk, pass dishes, observe usual manners. May be able to open a simple container (milk carton or transparent diet kit) to reach a highly valued item. Leaves opened containers where they drop. May eat excessive amounts of a favorite food (candy). Unaware of spilled food on table, self, floor. May chew noisily or with open mouth. | Caregiver reminds patient of mealtimes. Serves appropriate serving sizes or restricts access to undesirable food items to prevent overconsumption. Cuts meat or other difficult items. Pours liquids. Reminds patient to dispose of trash in proper containers. Plans and supervises all special dietary needs. | Caregiver will provide for nutritional needs with appropriate food portions, restricting access to undesirable foods, assisting with cutting and containers. Patient will feed self with conventional utensils with assistance in cutting foods, opening containers. | May overeat if given free access to preferred food items. Cannot follow dietary restrictions. |
| 3.4 | May anticipate meal times based on familiar signs (kitchen activity/smells). Uses all utensils except knife; cuts with side of spoon or fork. Eating is self-absorbed; rate may be rushed with patient not stopping to swallow between bites or chewing inadequately. May eat strongly preferred food items only; may not understand need to eat balanced diet, follow dietary restrictions, or alter amounts. | Caregiver provides assistance same as for 3.0. Cues patient to chew longer or slow down as necessary. | Caregiver: same as 3.0. Patient: same as 3.0. | Same as 3.0. Failure to observe manners may alienate others. Check food and beverage temperatures. |

| LEVEL | BEHAVIOR | ASSISTANCE | GOAL | WARNINGS |
|---|---|---|---|---|
| 3.6 | May wait for others to sit before eating when requested. May be able to wait short periods for food to be prepared (fast food restaurant). May be able to imitate a modification of a classic eating action (cutting, opening container, chewing with mouth shut). May be able to alter rate of eating for short periods. | Caregiver demonstrates modifications of classic actions for better effects, including conforming to standard table manners. Cues patient when to wait for food to cool or be prepared or served. | Caregiver will provide for patient's nutritional needs and will demonstrate modifications of classic eating actions to increase effectiveness. Patient will feed self, using conventional utensils, with assistance, to comply with special dietary needs. Patient will imitate modifications of classic eating actions. | Same as 3.4. |
| 3.8 | May be trained to present self at dining area at regular mealtimes, or to follow a routine such as waiting for others before eating, passing dishes, sitting until all are finished, checking surrounding areas for spilled food, wiping mouth with napkin. Does not engage in social conversation at the table. | Caregiver trains patient in highly desirable social manners one at a time, over several weeks. Provides assistance with new containers or difficult cutting requiring neuromuscular adjustments. Plans and supervises special dietary needs. | Caregiver will provide for patient's nutritional needs and will train in highly desirable social manners as needed. Patient will feed self, using conventional eating utensils, with assistance, to comply with special dietary needs. Patient will be trained to follow highly valued social routines | Same as 3.4. |
| 4.0 | Initiates coming to table at routine times of day. Uses common utensils in customary fashion. May not attend to spillage or crumbs. Use of knife and fork to cut may be clumsy. May be unable to talk and eat at the same time but indicates awareness of others at table. Needs assistance to cut resistive foods. May be trained to follow specific social manners as in 3.8. May refuse to try unfamiliar foods. Overfills liquid | Regular mealtime routine with familiar menus are preferred by patient. Trains in highly desired social manners as in 3.8. Reminds patient to check temperatures of hot foods. Assists with cutting of difficult items. Cautions patient not to overfill glasses and mugs. Plans for special dietary needs; reinforces understanding of specific foods to avoid. | Patient will feed self with conventional utensils, with assistance, to comply with special dietary needs. Will learn to follow highly desired social routines, one step at a time. Caregiver: same as 3.8. | Assist with handling/consuming hot liquids and foods. Monitor compliance with special diets. |

| Level | Behavior | Assistance | Goal | Warnings |
|---|---|---|---|---|
|  | containers. May not check food temperatures. May remember a specific food restriction (i.e., walnuts) but does not understand or apply a dietary restriction principle (i.e., sugar free, low cholesterol). Needs help to open unusual containers. |  |  |  |
| 4.2 | Initiates coming to table at routine times of day. Uses common utensils in customary fashion. Recognizes visible error (spillage from overfilled cup) and asks for help. Attempts to replicate a visible example to comply with a social standard (i.e., cutting bite-sized pieces, filling glass up to 1 inch from rim, dishing appropriate serving sizes) one feature at a time. Asks for help to determine acceptability of new food items to restricted diets. May have trouble waiting for others, for food to cool or be served, but understands explanations for delays. | Same as 4.0. Caregiver provides visible demonstrations of desired social behaviors. | Patient: same as 4.0. Caregiver: same as 4.0. | Same as 4.0. |
| 4.4 | Initiates coming to table at routine times of day. Uses common utensils in customary fashion. May see and clean up highly visible spills or dropped food items, but doesn't anticipate these errors (pouring liquids too fast, filling dishes | Caregiver monitors compliance with special diets. Assists with unusual containers. Reminds patient of standard social manners when problems occur. Warns patient to take precautions when passing hot, heavy, or liquid dishes. | Patient will feed self with conventional utensils, and will comply with reminders of standard table manners and dietary restrictions. Caregiver will remind patient of standard table manners and will monitor compliance with dietary restrictions. | Watch for handling of hot, heavy, or liquid dishes. May resist changes in diet or new restrictions. |

| LEVEL | BEHAVIOR | ASSISTANCE | GOAL | WARNINGS |
|---|---|---|---|---|
| | being passed, picking up hot plate without hot pad). Attempts to comply with standard social behavior for table manners when reminded. May not be able to eat and converse at the same time. May not be able to alter pace or rate of eating on request. May have trouble waiting as in 4.2 and with opening unusual packages. Recognizes well-learned special diets. May resist changes in diet and menu. | | | |
| 4.6 | May alter rate of eating on request, but may not sustain. Attempts to vary actions to open an unusual container or to cut food more effectively but may not succeed. May be willing to alter food selections or accept diet changes without resistance. Looks across table to converse with others or locate needed food item. | Caregiver provides assistance as for 4.4. | Patient: same as 4.4. Caregiver: same as 4.4. | Same as 4.4. |
| 4.8 | Attends to all striking visible features of food and social situation. Eats and attends to social conversation though may not talk and eat at same time. Manages all utensil use. Follows a schedule prepared by others of mealtimes or special dietary needs. May need to be | Caregiver assists with identifying intangible properties of food to comply with dietary restrictions. Demonstrates use of unfamiliar utensils or procedures. | Patient will feed self independently and will learn use of new utensils or procedures. Caregiver will identify applications of dietary restrictions in new foods. | Monitor new food for compatibility with dietary restrictions. |

| Level | Behavior | Assistance | Goal | Warnings |
|---|---|---|---|---|
| | reminded to check for less tangible food properties (temperature, spiciness) and may not be able to apply principles of dietary restrictions. Learns use of new utensils or procedures of eating new foods by rote. | | | |
| 5.0 | Varies strength or range of motion to use new utensils, open containers. Eats and talks with others. May not see crumbs or other small spills but cleans up when cued. Needs help identifying intangible properties to comply with dietary restrictions. | Caregiver assists with identifying all properties of food to comply with dietary restrictions. | Patient will feed self independently and will learn use of new utensils by varying actions. Patient will comply with dietary restrictions with assistance from caregivers. Caregiver: same as 4.8. | Same as 4.8. |
| 5.2 | Notes crumbs, spills in immediate eating area. Disposes of trash without being told. May use socially acceptable table manners. Needs help with identifying less tangible properties of new foods as in 5.0. May attend to manner of food preparation from outer appearance (baked versus fried). | Caregiver provides assistance as for 5.0. | Patient: same as 5.0. Caregiver: same as 5.0. | Same as 4.8. |
| 5.4 | May be aware of socially acceptable table manners but may choose not to alter behavior. May seek variety in diet. May express strongly held food preferences. May understand explanations of food | Caregiver provides assistance as for 5.0. | Patient: same as 5.0. Caregiver: same as 5.0. | May not comply with dietary restrictions. |

| LEVEL | BEHAVIOR | ASSISTANCE | GOAL | WARNINGS |
|---|---|---|---|---|
| | groups and dietary restrictions but choose to not alter diet. | | | |
| 5.6 | May attempt to discern table etiquette in order to comply with social standards in a new situation. May vary use of seasonings to suit palate. May compare various diets. | Caregiver provides assistance as for 5.0. | Patient: same as 5.0. Caregiver: same as 5.0. | |
| 5.8 | Seeks information about tangible secondary properties of food (i.e., may read a labeled product to determine ingredients or ask about ingredients before eating to comply with special diets). | Caregiver provides information about properties of new foods to avoid harmful effects. | Patient will follow dietary restrictions with assistance from others. Caregiver: same as 5.0. | |

## 10.5 Self-Awareness Disability: Toileting

Toileting includes recognizing the need to void, going to the bathroom, closing the door, adjusting garments, sitting down, voiding, wiping the body clean, readjusting garments, flushing the toilet, washing and drying hands, and leaving the bathroom.

| Level | Behavior | Assistance | Goal | Warnings |
|---|---|---|---|---|
| 1.0-1.4 | No awareness of need to defecate or urinate. Does not assist caregiver in toileting activities. | Caregiver places diapers on patient, checks and changes regularly. | Caregiver will control bowel and bladder accidents and prevent medical complications of incontinence. | Watch for skin problems (rash, breakdown). |
| 1.6-1.8 | No awareness of need or no communication of need to defecate or urinate. May cooperate by rolling onto side to ease placement of bedpan or assist with cleaning when cued. | Same as 1.0, or caregiver positions bedpan at regular intervals. | Same as 1.0. | Same as 1.0. |
| 2.0 | Sits on toilet when so placed by caregiver. May lean to assist wiping when cued. | Caregiver positions patient on toilet or bedpan at regular intervals. Wipes and arranges clothing. | Patient will sit on toilet and cooperate with assistance. Caregiver: same as 1.0. | Do not leave unattended on toilet. |
| 2.2 | May cooperate with a pivot transfer to toilet. Sits or stands on command while being wiped and garments are adjusted. | Caregiver takes patient to bathroom at regular intervals. Gives assistance with tactile, verbal cues to do pivot transfer. Wipes; arranges garments. | Patient will stand/sit on command and cooperate with pivot transfers. Caregiver: same as 1.0. | Watch for falls. Observe proper body mechanics to avoid injury. |
| 2.4 | Follows caregiver through open doorway to bathroom. Sits and stands spontaneously. May not wait to be wiped or have garments adjusted. May put hands under wash water when cued. | Caregiver leads to bathroom at regular intervals. Assists with garments, wiping. Flushes toilet. Cues to put hands under water and applies soap, rinses. | Patient will follow caregiver to bathroom and cooperate with assistance to complete toileting. | Watch for falls. |

| LEVEL | BEHAVIOR | ASSISTANCE | GOAL | WARNINGS |
|---|---|---|---|---|
| 2.6 | May communicate need to use toilet immediately before. May walk to bathroom but not get there in time. May put hands under water when cued. | Caregiver leads to bathroom on request or at regular intervals. Assists with garments; wipes patient, readjusts garments, cues and assists with hand washing. Easy-to-remove garments reduce accidents. | Patient will communicate need to use toilet and cooperate with caregiver assistance. Caregiver will ask patient about need to use toilet at regular intervals and will provide assistance to complete activities. | Same as 2.4. |
| 2.8 | Slowly walks to familiar bathroom. Grabs bars or other objects (toilet paper dispenser) to stabilize self when sitting down or standing up. May grip toilet paper or pants but needs assistance in wiping, adjusting garments. | Caregiver provides assistance as in 2.6. Installs grab bars for stability. | Patient will use grab bars when standing and sitting and will cooperate with caregiver assistance. Caregiver: same as 2.6. | May pull on bathroom hardware. May fall. |
| 3.0 | Recognizes need to use toilet and walked toward bathroom but may get distracted on the way and not arrive in time. May pull down loose-fitting pants or be unable to remove. May take toilet paper in hand but wipes ineffectively or only when cued. May flush when cued if handle offers little resistance. Does washing motions if cued. Men may miss toilet if urinating while standing. | Caregiver leads to bathroom, or checks to make certain patient arrives at bathroom. Assists to remove garments. Places toilet paper in patient's hand, checks results. Assists with fasteners. Cues to flush, washes hands. Assists males with hitting toilet when urinating while standing. | Patient will initiate and complete toileting with appropriate assistance from caregiver. Caregiver will provide appropriate cues to sequence patient through toileting activities and will check results to ensure safe and hygienic outcomes. | Do not leave alone in bathroom. Check results. |
| 3.2 | May communicate need to use bathroom. Grasps and tears toilet paper and wipes back and forth without noting results. | Caregiver provides assistance as in 3.0. | Same as 3.0. | Same as 3.0. |

| Level | Behavior | Assistance | Goal | Warnings |
|---|---|---|---|---|
| | Stops and starts actions on command. May successfully doff and don loose-fitting pants but fails to adjust, tuck in shirt. May be unable to do fasteners. Needs to be sequenced through actions as in 3.0. Men can usually urinate standing up but may miss toilet. | | | |
| 3.4 | Recognizes need to void and goes to familiar bathroom. Operates ordinary door handles but may not close door while in bathroom. Doffs and dons most clothing items slowly; may need help with new or unusual fasteners, sticky zippers. Wipes but does not check results and may wipe over and over, using excessive amounts of toilet paper. May forget to flush, wash hands. May not adjust garments, may leave shirt untucked, or zipper open. | Caregiver checks quality of results. Is available to assist with fasteners. Pretears toilet paper to prevent excessive use. | Patient will initiate and complete toileting in familiar environment with caregiver assistance to avoid ineffective results. Caregiver will check results and correct errors to avoid undesirable medical, social consequences. | Failure to check results may produce skin problems, plumbing problems, undesirable social problems (appearance). |
| 3.6 | May be able to imitate a modification of wiping (i.e., wiping longer, harder, using less paper) for more effective results. Effects are still not noted. | Caregiver provides assistance as in 3.4. | Patient will imitate modifications of actions for better results. Caregiver will demonstrate modified actions, check results, correct errors as needed. | Same as 3.4. |
| 3.8 | May complete sequence of toileting actions with one or two steps left out (door left open, forgets to wash, zip pants up). Can recognize completion and | Caregiver provides assistance as in 3.4. | Patient: same as 3.6. Caregiver: same as 3.6. | Same as 3.6. |

| LEVEL | BEHAVIOR | ASSISTANCE | GOAL | WARNINGS |
|---|---|---|---|---|
| | can inform caregiver when through. May not ask for assistance with fasteners. | | | |
| 4.0 | Initiates toileting activities at customary time of day. Follows usual routine slowly; does not alter rate. Has trouble with some fasteners requiring fine adjustments. Checks results of wiping. May not adjust garments in back. May use excessive toilet paper. Needs to be escorted to a public restroom. | Provides needed supplies in visible locations for customary toileting routine (toilet paper, soap, towel). Checks for errors in adjusting garments and assists with fasteners. Monitors amount of toilet paper used; provides precut amounts if necessary. Escorts to public restrooms. | Patient will initiate and complete usual toileting routine when all supplies are available with caregiver assistance to solve problems and avoid undesirable effects. Caregiver will provide appropriate set-up and assistance with solving problems to avoid undesirable effects. | May take much longer than average to complete toileting. |
| 4.2 | Recognizes difficulties that interfere with completion of toileting and asks for help (no paper, door latch that won't close, inability to operate flush). May be able to report change in bowel or bladder habits. | Provides assistance as in 4.0. | Patient: same as 4.0. Caregiver: same as 4.0. | Same as 4.0. |
| 4.4 | Follows a routine of toileting without variation in a familiar environment. Does not anticipate need to use toilet before going to an event or location with limited access to toileting facilities. Needs to have public restrooms pointed out. May be unable to operate an unfamiliar or stiff flush control. May fail to note errors in clothing adjustment at back. May use too much paper, thinking "more is | Reminds patient to use bathroom before trips, other conditions with limited access to restrooms. Checks for errors in clothing adjustment. Points out locations of public facilities. Demonstrates use of unfamiliar controls. Provides all supplies for toileting in visible locations. | Same as 4.0. | Same as 4.0. |

| LEVEL | BEHAVIOR | ASSISTANCE | GOAL | WARNINGS |
|---|---|---|---|---|
| | better." Does not consider needs of others (limiting time in bathroom, lowering seat, etc.). | | | Same as 4.0. |
| 4.6 | Scans visible environment for a needed supply (toilet paper, paper towel, soap dispenser, sign for a public restroom) but may not find it unless at or near eye level. May be able to alter amount of toilet paper or towels used when effects are explained. | Same as 4.4. | Same as 4.0. | |
| 4.8 | Independently performs usual toileting routine. Notes all striking cues in a new environment to locate a public restroom. May not anticipate need to use bathroom before trips, etc., but can learn to take this precaution for regularly occurring events. May learn bathroom etiquette (amount of time, conservation of paper, putting lid down after use) by rote. | Caregiver identifies social conventions related to toileting when patient must share facilities with others. Reminds to use bathroom before trips, etc. | Patient will independently perform toileting routine with assistance from caregiver to follow social rules. Caregiver will identify desirable behaviors for patient to maintain social and hygienic standards. | |
| 5.0-5.8 | Independently performs all toileting. Can explore a new environment to locate a bathroom without assistance. Can figure out use of stiff or new flush controls and learn use of assistive devices by varying neuromuscular effects (5.0). May not anticipate need for toileting in new | Caregiver identifies sanitary considerations when conventional means for toileting do not exist. | Patient: same as 4.8. Caregiver: same as 4.8. | |

| LEVEL | BEHAVIOR | ASSISTANCE | GOAL | WARNINGS |
|---|---|---|---|---|
| | situations (5.0 to 5.8) or consider sanitary requirements in unusual circumstances (i.e., in absence of conventional toileting facilities) (5.0 to 5.8). | | | |

## 10.6 Self-Awareness Disability: Taking Medication

Taking medication includes recognizing the reason for taking medication, knowing when and how much to take, remembering to take, opening and closing containers, obtaining the correct amount, swallowing, renewing prescriptions, and reporting adverse effects to the physician.

| LEVEL | BEHAVIOR | ASSISTANCE | GOAL | WARNINGS |
|---|---|---|---|---|
| 1.0-1.8 | No awareness of need for medication. May swallow when medication is put in mouth. May hold up head on command. | Caregiver places medication in patient's mouth at proper times of day with verbal cue to swallow. Crushing pills or using liquid forms preferred. Monitors for adverse reactions, side effects. | Caregiver will dispense all required medications in correct amounts at the appropriate time of day to avoid medical complications. | May not be able to swallow pills. |
| 2.0-2.8 | No awareness of need for medication. May place a pill in mouth when it is put in hand or may drink liquid from cup on command. May grasp cup or may refuse to hold cup or to swallow medication. | Caregiver hands pill or premeasured liquid to patient with command to swallow. Crushing pills or liquid forms preferred. | Caregiver: same as 1.0. Patient will swallow medications when given by caregivers. | May not be able to swallow medication in pill form. May refuse to take. |
| 3.0 | No awareness of need for medication. May grasp a pill placed in front of him or her or refuse to pick it up. May place in mouth spontaneously. | Caregiver places pills or premeasured liquid in front of patient. Checks for swallowing or gives verbal cues to swallow. Depot forms may ease compliance. | Caregiver: same as 1.0. Patient: same as 2.0. | Same as 2.0. Do not leave medications in accessible locations. |
| 3.2 | No awareness of need for medication. May pick up pills and place in mouth (repeatedly up to four times). Actions can be stopped or started with commands. | Same as 3.0. | Caregiver: same as 1.0. Patient: same as 2.0. | Same as 3.0. |

| LEVEL | BEHAVIOR | ASSISTANCE | GOAL | WARNINGS |
|---|---|---|---|---|
| 3.4 | May recognize medication by color or shape when it is given daily, but does not note amounts, time of day. Does not understand purpose of medication, side effects, adverse reactions. May attempt to open a container to get pills thinking they are candy. Cannot open child-proof containers. May refuse to take for idiosyncratic reasons. | Caregiver will open containers, premeasure liquids, and give to patient at appropriate time of day. Checks for swallowing. Checks for side effects, adverse reactions. | Caregiver will provide medications in correct amounts at appropriate times of day and will check for compliance, adverse reactions, or side effects. Patient will take medications with assistance from caregiver to avoid harmful effects. | Store all medication in secure locations away from patient in child-proof containers. |
| 3.6 | May initiate taking medication based on a familiar association (breakfast). May recognize color/shape of pills; may note amount. Cannot open child-proof containers. Can wait for medication when asked. Does not understand side effects, and may refuse to take. | Provides assistance same as 3.4. | Caregiver: same as 3.4. Patient: same as 3.4. | Same as 3.4. |
| 3.8 | May be trained to initiate taking medication at a particular time of day. May recognize pills (color or shape) and tell when medication has been altered. May not note amounts; may take all pills offered. | Provides assistance as in 3.4. Trains patient to request medication or go to bathroom to retrieve pills at specific time of day (i.e., after breakfast). Dispenses in correct amounts. Checks compliance/ adverse effects. | Caregiver: same as 3.4. Patient: same as 3.4. | Same as 3.4. |
| 4.0 | Initiates taking a familiar dose of medication at a regular time of day. Recognizes color, shape, and amount of a simple prescription (less than three | Opens containers; dispenses or premeasures and leaves in visible locations to assist with remembering. Checks on compliance, and monitors for | Patient will take simple dosages as prescribed with assistance from caregiver to avoid harmful effects. Caregiver will monitor compliance, watch | Patient may not seek assistance for problems encountered. Changes in routine activity will confuse patient and disrupt compliance. |

| LEVEL | BEHAVIOR | ASSISTANCE | GOAL | WARNINGS |
|---|---|---|---|---|
|  | different pills). May recognize a problem (not the right pill) but may not seek assistance. May know name of medication. May not understand purpose or need for medication. May confuse side effects with desired effects. Cannot measure liquid amounts accurately. | side effects or adverse effects. Renews prescriptions as needed. Measures liquid medications. Caregiver does injections. Assists with compliance when routine schedule is disrupted (time change, vacations, medication changes). Pill sorters recommended. | for undesirable effects, and renew prescriptions. |  |
| 4.2 | Initiates taking a familiar dose of medication at a regular time of day. May recognize deviation from color, shape, amount of a typical prescription and ask for help. Approximates a liquid measure. May not understand effects, side effects, adverse effects as 4.0. May have erroneous ideas of effects that lead to noncompliance. May not be able to open containers. | Same as in 4.0. | Patient: same as 4.0. Caregiver: same as 4.0. | Same as 4.0. |
| 4.4 | Initiates taking a familiar dose of medication at a regular time of day. May follow routine rigidly and may resist changes in prescriptions. May match correct amounts of several different pills with a sample. Measures a liquid amount with a clearly marked measure. May be trained to inject medications over several weeks. Does not note adverse or side effects, or a visible problem (skin | Caregiver monitors medication compliance. Assists with new containers, changes in prescriptions, or schedules, which are departures from routine. Supervises injections or does injections for patient. Monitors for unwanted effects, or side effects. Reorders prescriptions. Stores medication in visible locations. | Patient will take routine medications with assistance from caregiver to avoid harmful effects. Caregiver will monitor compliance and check for adverse reactions, side effects. | Patient may resist changes in routine prescriptions. May refuse to take medications based on erroneous beliefs about effects. |

| LEVEL | BEHAVIOR | ASSISTANCE | GOAL | WARNINGS |
|---|---|---|---|---|
| 4.6 | rash, or infected injection site) unless strikingly visible. Does not anticipate need to renew prescriptions. May be able to open a child-proof container. May attempt to open new containers; may not be successful. May purposefully alter amounts or types of pills for a better effect, but is unaware of potential hazards. May stop medications because feels "well". Visually scans environment to locate medication that is not in usual location. | Caregiver explains problems of deviating from prescriptions. | Patient: same as 4.4. Caregiver: same as 4.4. | Same as 4.4. |
| 4.8 | Follows new prescriptions slowly. Considers three or more variables (time of day, intervals, amounts, type of medication) at one time with difficulty. Learns a new procedure (injecting medication) slowly by rote. Notes all striking features that may indicate adverse reactions or side effects. Follows verbal explanations of secondary effects to be avoided (mixing medications, altering dosages). May follow a schedule set up by others for renewing and securing prescriptions. | Caregiver describes side effects to assist self-monitoring. Monitors new prescriptions until well-learned. Assists with setting up schedule for prescription renewal or when usual procedures are disrupted. | Patient will secure and administer own medication in proper amounts at appropriate time of day with assistance to avoid harmful effects. Caregiver will monitor compliance until new procedures are learned and will check for adverse effects. | Patient may be confused by changes or interruptions in routine of securing and taking medication. |

| Level | Behavior | Assistance | Goal | Warnings |
|---|---|---|---|---|
| 5.0 | Opens new containers. May understand medication schedules but has trouble taking medications on time. May choose to discontinue medications. May recognize side effects that affect ability to do neuromuscular adjustments (tremors, stiffness, sedation). | Caregiver explains effects, side effects, with examples from patient's experience to assist understanding and accuracy of self-reported effects. Assists with identification of benefits including functional improvements. Assists with timely compliance. | Patient will secure and take medications as prescribed and will monitor and report adverse effects to physician. Caregiver will assist compliance by reminding to take and renew prescriptions, and explain effects as necessary. | May choose to not take medications |
| 5.2 | May note tangible changes in skin (subtle bumpy rash or color changes) suggesting medication reaction or injection-site problems and report to physician. May have a vague understanding of the presence of a mental disorder, but confuse symptoms with drug effects or side effects. | Caregiver provides assistance as in 5.0. Assists with understanding mental disorders and role of biological treatments for mental disorders. | Patient: same as 5.0. Caregiver: same as 4.8. | Same as 5.0. |
| 5.4 | May recognize the presence of a mental disorder and consider the effects that medications might have on reducing functional difficulties. May elect to not comply with medical advice, or may choose to alter dosages to fit a personal understanding of what needs. May be able to apply a criteria for altering dosage in response to a particular symptom. May confuse various concepts (side effects, drug synergies, prophylaxis, tolerance, etc.). Can usually report | Caregiver monitors for compliance with criteria for altering dosages. Points out potential harmful results of indiscriminate altering of doses or of noncompliance. | Patient will secure and administer medications accurately and report effects to physician with assistance from caregiver to clarify effects. Caregiver will assist in identifying functional improvements and will clarify effects of medication to enhance compliance. | Same as 5.0. |

| LEVEL | BEHAVIOR | ASSISTANCE | GOAL | WARNINGS |
|---|---|---|---|---|
| 5.6 | effects with some accuracy. Compares prescriptions in effects, cost, convenience or suitability to personal situation. May read *Physician's Desk Reference* or seek advice of others on same medications. May be concerned about social stigma of dependence of medication for chronic conditions. May not understand discussions about potential secondary effects. | Caregiver provides or refers patient to information to assist comparison. | Patient: same as 5.4. Caregiver: same as 5.4. | |
| 5.8 | May understand explanations of inevitable secondary effects to be avoided for safety reasons (forbidden foods, photosensitivity) but may need to have potential secondary effects pointed out (risks of treatment). May consider future needs of up to a week and plan to secure medications. | Caregiver provides assistance as in 5.6. | Patient: same as 5.4. Caregiver: same as 5.4. | |
| 6.0 | May be able to take medication as prescribed. May be able to monitor effects, side effects, check for adverse effects pointed out by physician. May understand relevant concepts and hazards, including situations or activities to avoid, and can state a reasonable plan | No assistance needed. | Patient independently complies with taking medication. | |

| Level | Behavior | Assistance | Goal | Warnings |
|-------|----------|------------|------|----------|
| | to follow in case of emergency related to taking medication (severe allergic reaction). Plans ahead to secure medication supplies. | | | |

## 10.7 Self-Awareness Disability: Using Adaptive Equipment

Using adaptive equipment includes recognizing a physical disability, recognizing an object as a substitute for normal ability, accepting the equipment, and learning to use the equipment.

| LEVEL | BEHAVIOR | ASSISTANCE | GOAL | WARNINGS |
|-------|----------|------------|------|----------|
| 1.0-1.8 | No awareness of physical disability. No understanding of purpose of equipment. With tactile cues may hold up arms, legs, or trunk while splint or straps are applied (1.8). | Caregiver applies equipment (bed rails, safety straps, anti-pressure cushions) and monitors for correct fit. Caregiver selects and maintains all equipment. | Caregiver will apply and monitor use of all adaptive equipment to avoid undesirable medical complications. Patient will cooperate by holding body parts against gravity (1.8). | Check for improper fit or positioning of equipment that may restrict blood flow or cause discomfort. |
| 2.0-2.8 | No awareness of physical disability. No understanding of purpose of equipment. Sits in wheelchair but is unable to propel or propels for a short distance without awareness of destination. Uses grab bars when cued and may assist with use of transfer board (2.4). May push or pull with upper extremities to shift body position in wheelchair when cued (2.8). May attempt to sit, stand, walk, use arms in normal manner requiring restraint to prevent falls, etc. may remove or refuse to wear uncomfortable equipment. | Caregiver applies equipment as in 1.0. Caregiver selects and maintains all equipment. Pushes wheelchairs and locks to prevent aimless wandering. Security locks, gates, extra locks on wheelchairs may prevent getting lost. Slip-proof mats and treads prevent falls in bathroom. Bathing seats, raised toilet seats, assist positioning. | Caregiver: same as 1.0. Patient will cooperate with transfers, positioning, by grabbing bars or pushing/pulling when cued by caregiver. | Watch for falls in transfers, or in ambulation with a new physical disability. May wander and get lost. Watch for discomfort that may result in striking out. Uncomfortable positioning devices may be refused or removed. |
| 3.0 | May recognize the loss of gross motor capability (walking) or limb. Grasps a piece of equipment offered at eye level or may put/throw it down. Does not use walkers, canes, or crutches. | Same as 2.0. Wheelchairs are preferred for ambulation difficulties. Built-up utensils may be offered at eye level. | Caregiver: same as 2.0. Patient will grasp and feed self with built-up spoons; will use wheelchair. | Same as 2.0. |

| LEVEL | BEHAVIOR | ASSISTANCE | GOAL | WARNINGS |
|---|---|---|---|---|
| 3.2 | May recognize the loss of a gross motor capability, limb, or grasp. Spontaneously grasps piece of equipment and begins associated action based on appearance of equipment. Does not sequence actions or note effects. Starts and stops on command. | Same as 3.0. Caregiver washes mitts, built-up utensils whose physical appearance is same as unadapted object will elicit associated actions. | Caregiver: same as 2.0. Patient will do associated actions with equipment that resembles familiar objects. | Remove potentially harmful adaptive equipment. |
| 3.4 | May recognize the loss of gross motor capability, limb, or grasp. May not note loss of strength, coordination, or ROM. May accept adaptations that allow dominant hand to be used in a normal manner (built-up spoon). Does not imitate a modification of a normal action, but repeats habitual actions over and over, or until distracted. May be able to propel wheelchair forward or back but cannot get around furniture, through small doorways; forgets to set brakes and may get lost if allowed outside. May attribute loss of abilities to nonmedical cause ("I'm weak because you don't feed me enough"). | Caregiver applies and supervises use of all adaptive equipment. Wheelchairs preferred for ambulation difficulties; extra locks may prevent wandering. Clears space to increase mobility and avoid damage to furniture. Splints, slings, other passive positioning devices must be regularly checked. Stops repetitive actions. Restrains when lack of awareness of disability may result in falls, etc. | Caregiver will apply and supervise use of all appropriate adaptive equipment to avoid undesirable medical complications. Patient will perform familiar actions with aid of appropriate adaptive equipment with assistance to avoid harmful effects. | Same as 3.2. |
| 3.6 | Imitates a modification of a familiar action to use a piece of equipment (cleaning nails with suction hand brush). May be able to learn to use familiar | Caregiver provides assistance same as in 3.4. | Caregiver: same as 3.4. Patient: same as 3.4. | Same as 3.4. |

| LEVEL | BEHAVIOR | ASSISTANCE | GOAL | WARNINGS |
|---|---|---|---|---|
| 3.8 | object or adaptive device using a normal action with nondominant hand after much repetitive drilling. May recognize the visible effects of a physical disability when this is pointed out, but may not understand medical causes. Awareness of task completion with equipment in place may increase acceptance of equipment. | Caregiver points out visible effects of enhanced performance with equipment use or visible effects of disability to assist with acceptance of equipment and compliance with safety precautions. | Caregiver: same as 3.4. Patient: same as 3.4. | Same as 3.4. |
| 4.0 | May recognize the loss of gross motor capability, marked loss of strength, ROM, coordination, or balance as restricting ability to complete a sequence of actions. May accept adaptive equipment that uses familiar action sequences (velcro button fasteners) to do highly valued tasks. Understands purpose of the equipment when effect is immediate; does not understand secondary effects (prevention of contractures, energy conservation). If equipment requires neuromuscular adjustments in positioning or use, may abandon use, or use in an unsafe way (leaning on crutches or walkers). | Caregiver supervises application or applies adaptive devices for patient. Points out visible cues to assist patient in correct application. Stores equipment in visible locations to assist in remembering to use equipment. Caregiver takes care of all maintenance on equipment. Wheelchairs may be preferred for ambulation disabilities, as patient may not be able to safely use crutches (avoiding brachial plexus injury) or walkers (attending to environment while executing new sequence of actions). | Patient will use adaptive equipment using familiar movement patterns to complete routine tasks with assistance from caregiver to avoid harmful effects. Caregiver will supervise application and use of adaptive equipment, and maintain equipment to avoid undesirable medical complications. | Monitor for correct positioning. Patient may forget to use equipment. |
| 4.2 | Same as 4.0 in recognition of physical disability. May put on a simple splint by | Caregiver provides assistance as in 4.0. | Patient: same as 4.0. Caregiver: same as 4.0. | Same as 4.0. |

| Level | Behavior | Assistance | Goal | Warnings |
|---|---|---|---|---|
| | matching one visible feature at a time. Needs help with more complex equipment requiring adjustment and/or fine-motor fasteners (i.e., prostheses). May be trained to don equipment as part of routine dressing. Uses equipment that requires usual action patterns only. May combine familiar actions into sequences with difficulty (lifting place-step sequence of using a walker). Does not understand potential hazards of incorrect use. | | | |
| 4.4 | Recognition of physical disability same as 4.0. May be trained to use adaptive equipment that requires a sequence of familiar actions (walker) slowly, one step at a time. Notes striking features of equipment (two straps) but not less visible features (relative position or tension of straps). Does not anticipate hazards (failure to lock wheelchair brakes before transfer). Does not generalize use of one piece of equipment to a similar piece; once learned, may resist changes in equipment. | Caregiver supervises donning complex equipment and checks adjustment of all equipment. Takes care of maintenance; stores equipment in easy-to-access locations. Monitors use until well-learned. Checks environment to remove safety hazards (rugs or slippery floors that impede wheelchair, walker use). | Patient: same as 4.0. Caregiver: same as 4.0. | Same as 4.0. |
| 4.6 | Recognition of physical disability same as 4.0. May be able to make a spontaneous | Caregiver provides assistance as in 4.4. | Patient will use adaptive equipment by using familiar movement patterns and will make simple spontaneous | Monitor for undesirable effects of patient's adjustments. |

| LEVEL | BEHAVIOR | ASSISTANCE | GOAL | WARNINGS |
|---|---|---|---|---|
|  | adjustment in position, duration, or strength for better effect (reducing downward pressure on walker with wheels for better mobility). Such adjustments may not be sustained. Scans visible environment for equipment. May attempt to adjust one feature (location of strap, foot rest) without awareness of secondary effects (edema, posture). May understand a verbal explanation of visible safety hazard to be avoided (one-handed cutting board with nail). |  | adjustments for better effects with caregiver assistance to avoid harmful effects. Caregiver will supervise application and use of adaptive equipment, and will maintain equipment to avoid undesirable medical consequences. | Allow enough time for adapted activity performance. |
| 4.8 | Recognizes the loss of gross motor capability, marked loss of strength, ROM, coordination, sensation, or balance and can name several visible effects of loss during the process of doing an activity. May not anticipate effects of loss in new activity. May learn a series of new actions slowly by rote, attending to all striking visible effects on objects. May learn use of walker with wheels, electric self-feeder, swivel eating utensils. May don arm slings and prostheses, checking for correct positioning by close examination. Does not do spontaneous | Caregiver monitors application and use of equipment until well learned. Caregiver provides explanations of secondary effects or hazards to be avoided. Caregiver solves problems requiring neuromuscular adjustments and monitors and provides for maintenance of equipment. | Patient will learn use of new equipment that does not require continuous neuromuscular adjustments with caregiver assistance to avoid harmful effects. Caregiver will supervise use of appropriate adaptive equipment until well-learned and will identify secondary effects to be avoided for safety reasons. Caregiver will provide appropriate maintenance. |  |

| Level | Behavior | Assistance | Goal | Warnings |
|---|---|---|---|---|
| | neuromuscular adjustments or anticipate secondary effects. | | | |
| 5.0 | Recognizes physical disability and potential of adaptive equipment to vary functional capacity. May learn use of new equipment by varying strength and ROM and noting best effects. May forget solutions to problems (varying pressure on a walker with wheels). Does not consider spatial or surface properties before acting (slowing gait for uneven terrain, maneuvering wheelchair in small space). May use adapted jar openers, key holder, walker seats that require neuromuscular adjustments. May choose not to use equipment. | Caregiver monitors application and use of new equipment until well-learned. Points out secondary effects to be considered for safety reasons. Assists with identifying simple principles of judging distance and space (checking door width in public restroom for wheelchair access). Monitors and provides for maintenance of equipment. | Patient will learn use of equipment requiring neuromuscular adjustments with caregiver assistance to avoid harmful effects. Caregiver: same as 4.8. | Watch for impulsive behavior that may be unsafe (doing wheelies in wheelchair). |
| 5.2 | Recognizes physical disability as in 5.0. Attends to all tangible properties of objects and environment including changes in the condition of skin surfaces, cleanliness of equipment, qualities of floor or terrain that affect ambulation, correct positioning of equipment. Uses walkers safely on uneven surfaces. May have trouble varying spatial properties, such as required by maneuvering | Caregiver provides assistance as in 5.0. Assists with problem solving for spatial properties. Provides explanations of hidden properties or secondary effects to be avoided for safety reasons. | Patient will learn use of equipment requiring neuromuscular adjustments and will solve problems requiring attention to all tangible features with caregiver assistance to avoid harmful effects. Caregiver: same as 4.8. | Same as 5.0. |

| LEVEL | BEHAVIOR | ASSISTANCE | GOAL | WARNINGS |
|---|---|---|---|---|
| | wheelchairs in small spaces, or using reachers or dressing sticks. | | | |
| 5.4 | Recognizes physical disability as in 5.0. Varies spatial properties (posture, position or objects in space) in learning use of equipment. Maneuvers wheelchair in tight space, uses extension aids, adjustable rotating razors, one-handed can openers. Varies use to discover better methods. May resist following recommended use until a problem is encountered. May not attend to hidden or secondary properties (energy expenditure, load on a reacher). May not anticipate routine maintenance of equipment. May choose to not use equipment when it requires too much energy or it so time consuming or for little-valued tasks. | Caregiver provides explanations of potential secondary effects to be avoided for safety or other reasons. Reminds patient to perform routine maintenance or checks needs for patient. Equipment may be stored away from view. Demonstrations of undesirable outcomes may increase understanding and compliance with suggested precautions. | Patient will learn use of equipment requiring neuromuscular adjustments and will solve problems requiring attention to all tangible features with caregiver assistance to avoid harmful effects. Caregiver: same as 4.8. | Same as 5.0. |
| 5.6 | Discusses/compares methods of equipment use (primary and secondary effects) to select best approach. Makes estimates of volume in space (judging whether a wheelchair will fit in a bathroom stall). May be concerned with social implications of equipment use (pros and cons of prosthetic hand versus hook). | Caregiver provides assistance as in 5.4. | Patient will compare methods to solve problems in equipment use. Caregiver will identify potential secondary effects to avoid undesirable consequences. | Same as 5.4. |

| Level | Behavior | Assistance | Goal | Warnings |
|---|---|---|---|---|
| | Potential secondary effects may not be understood (energy expenditures). | | | |
| 5.8 | Generates new plan of action in presence of adaptive equipment. May anticipate inevitable secondary effects (equipment maintenance). Needs potential secondary effects explained (brachial plexus injury from leaning on crutches, damage to joints from not observing joint protection principles). | Caregiver provides explanations of potential secondary effects to avoid injury or damage to equipment. | Patient will plan out actions with assistance to identify potential harmful effects.<br>Caregiver: same as 5.6. | |
| 6.0 | Speculates about adaptive equipment use in new situations by imagining problems and most effective solutions. Considers known relevant sensorimotor models and potential secondary effects. Can understand verbal or written information about use of new equipment, including precautions, complications, and preventive maintenance. | Caregiver provides information to assist patient in considering alterative solutions to problems as needed. | Patient will use adaptive equipment effectively and safely, providing for regular maintenance to ensure optimal function. | |

## 11.0 Situational Awareness Disability: Housekeeping

Housekeeping includes recognizing the accumulation of dust, dirt, and clutter; getting cleaning supplies; sweeping, mopping, or vacuuming floors; washing, dusting, and polishing furniture, windows, mirrors, utilities, and bric-a-brac; cleaning toilet, bathtub, shower, sinks, and counters; keeping drawers, closets, and cupboards tidy; picking things up and putting them away; deciding when things need to be repaired, replaced, or discarded; and emptying the trash. This category excludes preparing food, sharing in family activities.

| LEVEL | BEHAVIOR | ASSISTANCE | GOAL | WARNINGS |
|---|---|---|---|---|
| 1.0-2.8 | Does not participate in housekeeping activities. | Caregiver does all housekeeping activities. | Caregiver will do all housekeeping tasks. | Store all household cleaners and tools away from view. |
| 3.0-3.2 | No awareness of need for housekeeping. May pick up cloth and initiate back and forth movements to clean but does not note effects. | Caregiver provides assistance same as for 1.0. | Same as 1.0-2.8. | Same as 1.0-2.8. |
| 3.4 | No awareness of need for housekeeping. May pick up common cleaning tool such as cloth or broom and begin actions of cleaning. Does not note results. Quits when distracted. May initiate tasks when objects are in visible locations (pick up clothes or empty a trash can). | Caregiver hands patient drying or dust cloth and points out locations to dry/dust. Does not expect good results. Redirects attention as needed. Sequences through actions. Stores tools away from view to prevent undesired use. | Caregiver will provide common cleaning tools that use repetitive action; will supervise use to avoid harmful effects. Patient will sustain repetitive actions and cooperate with assistance. | Do not expect effective results. |
| 3.6 | No awareness of need for housekeeping. May follow the perimeter of an object as he or she cleans or wipes it and may imitate a demonstrated change in the duration or location of an action (may dry a dish longer, or sweep under a table when shown). Sees striking effects | Same as 3.4. | Caregiver will do all housekeeping tasks. Will supervise use of common tools using repetitive actions to avoid harmful effects. Patient will follow demonstrated changes in location or duration of action demonstrated by caregiver. | Same as 3.4. |

| Level | Behavior | Assistance | Goal | Warnings |
|---|---|---|---|---|
| | (clothing picked up from floor) but not subtle effects (clean or polished surface, tidy drawer). | | | |
| 3.8 | No awareness of need for housekeeping. May follow directed sequence of actions (put away dishes, sweep and empty trash cans). May sense completion of task when all objects or supplies are used (dishes put away). May wipe entire surface of an object (tabletop) but neglect sides, back, or other parts (table legs). | Caregiver provides common tools (broom, dust pan, dust rags, drying towel) and sequences through with verbal cues. Preferred tasks involve striking changes (such as moving objects around) and tools that are extensions of the hand. Caregiver does other tasks, checks for quality, and makes corrections. | Caregiver will supervise selected housekeeping tasks by providing tools, monitoring use, checking results. Caregiver will sequence patient through actions. Patient will follow demonstrated and verbal cues to complete selected housekeeping tasks. | Same as 3.4. |
| 4.0 | Initiates a well-learned housekeeping routine when supplies are accessible; sequences own actions to completion. Incorrect sequences are not self-corrected, but a correction may be imitated. Does not vary actions or tool use for better effects. Attends to striking effects (visible mold on toilet) but may not note dust, untidy clutter, broken objects, disorganization in drawers). Asks for the next step in an unfamiliar task. Works until done, out of time, or exhausted. | Caregiver stores supplies for well-learned tasks (dusting, sweeping) in accessible locations. Stores harmful or dangerous materials away from view. Checks sequence of actions and corrects errors. Checks quality of cleaning for hygienic results. Caregiver plans and prioritizes housekeeping activities including securing supplies, organizing cupboards and drawers, doing repairs, solving new problems. Supervises use of potentially harmful substances. | Patient will complete selected routine housekeeping tasks with supervision to follow correct sequences and avoid harmful effects. Caregiver will supervise selected housekeeping tasks, monitoring use of potentially harmful tools, and checking effects. | Restrict access to unfamiliar tools or materials with potential harmful effects. Supervise use of cleaning supplies for safety. Check quality of cleaning results. |
| 4.2 | Initiates and completes a routine of housekeeping activities. May be able to set a priority for tasks important to him or | Caregiver provides assistance as in 4.0. Points out relevant cues, one at a time, to solve problems. | Patient will complete selected routine housekeeping tasks with supervision to note visible cues and avoid harmful | Same as 4.0. |

| LEVEL | BEHAVIOR | ASSISTANCE | GOAL | WARNINGS |
|---|---|---|---|---|
| | her, may become fixated on the priority and be difficult to shift attention to other important tasks. Cleans, polishes, sweeps, arranges objects, attending to striking visible features, one feature at a time. | | effects. Caregiver will supervise selected housekeeping tasks, assisting patient to solve problems and avoid harmful effects. | |
| 4.4 | Initiates and completes a routine of housekeeping activities at the usual time of day. Sweeps, cleans, polishes, puts objects away to match a previous performance, a demonstrated sample, or a visible cue. Fails to see dirt or dust in the corners, or hidden surfaces. May change posture but not move objects, while cleaning or dusting. Modifications in strength or fine-motor movements to produce desired results may be attempted but abandoned. May use excessive amounts of cleaner, polish, or water, thinking more is better. Fails to take into account secondary properties of cleaning agents (soap film, irritating fumes, combustion potential). May resist changes in routine or products. May imitate step-by-step demonstrations of new procedures or products. Remembers to recycle waste by appearance (newspaper, soft drink can) and may be | Caregiver provides familiar housekeeping tools and supplies in accessible locations. Supervises use of new or potentially harmful cleaning products. Checks quality of cleaning for hygienic results. Assists with securing supplies, organizing cupboards and drawers, doing repairs, solving new problems. Caregiver does cleaning or polishing involving awareness of surface properties or uses tools requiring neuromuscular adjustments. | Patient: same as 4.2. Caregiver: same as 4.2. | Watch for excessive use of cleaning or polishing agents. Check for hygienic results of cleaning especially in hard-to-see or hard-to-reach locations. May organize objects by visible cues. May fail to differentiate between similar products (wood and ceramic cleaning agents). |

| LEVEL | BEHAVIOR | ASSISTANCE | GOAL | WARNINGS |
|---|---|---|---|---|
| | confused by new products with similar appearance (glossy paper with printing). May throw away repairable objects. | | | |
| 4.6 | Scans environment for needed supplies, dirt, clutter, when cleaning, polishing, putting things away. May attempt to vary strength and coordination (rubbing harder) for better results, without success. May choose to vary tool or supply use with no awareness of potential harmful consequences. May imitate demonstrated alterations in spatial arrangements of objects, as in organizing closets or cupboards, or putting away objects. | Caregiver provides assistance as for 4.4. Demonstrates more effective storage arrangements for household materials. Monitors use of potentially harmful products for safe use and checks variations in tool or product use for undesirable consequences. | Patient: same as 4.4. Caregiver: same as 4.4. | Watch for variations in typical tool or product use that may have undesirable consequences. |
| 4.8 | Initiates and completes a routine of housekeeping activities in a fixed manner. Learns new procedures slowly by rote. Notes all striking visible effects of cleaning, dusting, mopping, polishing, and checks quality of results by close examination when done. Moves objects around without assistance to put them away. Corrects visible errors one at a time, without awareness of secondary effects. May follow verbal explanations of visible secondary effects to avoid for | Caregiver assists rote learning of new products or procedures by adding one step at a time and verifies memorized sequences. Points out secondary effects to be considered for safety reasons (adequate ventilation with toxic cleaning agents, combustible potential of chemical combinations, storing toxins away from food items). Assists with securing needed supplies based on typical monthly use. Assists with organizing cupboards and drawers for most efficient object retrieval. | Patient will complete housekeeping activities and will learn by rote new procedures with assistance to avoid harmful effects and to check problem-solving methods. Caregiver will provide assistance with rote learning for new procedures or products and will verify new learning. Will identify potential secondary effects to avoid for safety reasons. | Identify household hazards posed by electrical, gas, appliances; toxins; poisons; improper trash disposal; storage of sharp objects. |

| LEVEL | BEHAVIOR | ASSISTANCE | GOAL | WARNINGS |
|---|---|---|---|---|
|  | safety reasons (cleaning with gloves to avoid skin rash). May not anticipate housekeeping supply needs but reports low supplies to caregiver. May not anticipate typical use of housekeeping supplies when arranging in cupboards. May follow recycling procedures or safety precautions by rote. |  |  |  |
| 5.0 | Effectively varies range of motion and strength while sweeping , mopping, polishing, cleaning to produce better results without assistance. Learns a new sequence of actions (how to use a new product) demonstrated several steps at a time. Does not change pace while working or consider surface, spatial, intangible properties of objects. May set and follow a weekly schedule of housekeeping activities but has trouble adhering to it. | Caregiver identifies relevant surface or spatial properties for solving problems (streaks on glass; crumbs or dust on surfaces). Identifies undesirable secondary effects or intangible properties to consider (potential damage to walls, countertops from tape or sharp instruments, electrical load tolerances for household outlets, contamination of food from improper storage of toxic cleaning products, plumbing problems related to putting too much or improper food in garbage disposal, or too much paper in toilet). Reminds patient of essential housekeeping tasks as needed. | Patient will initiate and complete routine housekeeping with assistance to solve problems involving surface or spatial properties. Caregiver will identify secondary effects, tangible and spatial properties to be considered to avoid harmful effects. | Same as 4.8. |
| 5.2 | Solves problems in housekeeping activities that require awareness of all tangible properties (stains; streaks; shine on polished wood or metal; grain on | Caregiver identifies relevant spatial properties to assist with problem solving and verifies new solutions using surface properties. Identifies secondary effects | Patient will initiate and complete routine housekeeping activities with assistance to solve problems involving spatial properties and will follow verbal | Same as 4.8. |

| Level | Behavior | Assistance | Goal | Warnings |
|---|---|---|---|---|
| | wood surfaces; tarnish on metal surfaces; surface dirt) by altering amounts of cleaners and making neuromuscular adjustments. Does not anticipate potential effects or problems. May forget solutions. Follows a weekly schedule of housekeeping activities but has trouble altering pace. May appear impulsive. Discriminates between special tools, cleaning supplies (glass versus metal cleaners). | and intangible properties to avoid harmful effects as in 5.0. Assists with supply acquisition based on identified priorities. | explanations of secondary effects to avoid for safety reasons. Caregiver will identify secondary effects and spatial properties to be considered to avoid harmful effects. | |
| 5.4 | Solves problems in housekeeping activities that require awareness of spatial properties: searches in drawers, cupboards, closets for needed supplies (may leave a mess); moves objects flexibly when cleaning or putting things away; cleans between objects and considers walls, ceilings. Remembers new solutions to problems. May abandon tedious tasks (polishing silver). Sets own standard for cleanliness or household organization or arrangement that may not be efficient, orderly, or esthetically pleasing. May argue with explanations offered to enhance function or esthetic appearance. | Caregiver verifies new solutions using spatial properties. Identifies intangible or secondary effects as in 5.0. Provides verbal explanations of ways to enhance function (storage of supplies) or esthetic appearance. | Patient will initiate and complete routine housekeeping with assistance in noting all tangible properties to solve problems. Caregiver will identify secondary effects to avoid undesirable effects. | Same as 4.8. |

| LEVEL | BEHAVIOR | ASSISTANCE | GOAL | WARNINGS |
|---|---|---|---|---|
| 5.6 | Moves household objects flexibly in space to clean and organize a more functional or esthetic appearance. May attempt to coordinate overall household decor or consider current style in selections. May seek information from household publications or others to improve methods. Social convention may alter routines (more cleaning for a house guest). Long-term effects (of decorating or remodeling on property value) may not be considered. | Caregiver provides information to assist in comparing methods, including social standards and potential secondary effects. | Patient will compare methods to vary and improve housekeeping with assistance to avoid undesirable effects. Caregiver: same as 5.4. | Same as 4.8. |
| 5.8 | Plans new methods in presence of household objects. Reads instructions to use new products. Varies pace to accommodate clock and tangible properties of objects. May not consider the needs of others. Asks for clarification of potential secondary effects. | Caregiver provides explanations of potential secondary effects. | Patient will plan out new methods of solutions to housekeeping problems when objects are present. Caregiver: same as 5.4. | |
| 6.0 | Plans out solutions to new problems with no objects present. Considers potential secondary effects including hazards posed by chemical, electrical, or toxic hazards posed by chemical, electrical, or toxic properties; expense; environmental impact; social considerations; long-term effects for persons and property. | No assistance is needed. | Patient will plan and complete a safe, effective housekeeping routine including planning for long-term needs. | |

## 11.1 Situational Awareness Disability: Preparing/Obtaining Food

Preparing/obtaining food includes taking an inventory of foodstuffs on hand, planning a balanced diet, preparing a grocery list, obtaining food, storing food, following a recipe, timing dishes, setting table, serving food, cleaning food preparation area and utensils, washing the dishes and the table, and discarding spoiled or uneaten food. This category excludes eating and sharing in family activities.

| Level | Behavior | Assistance | Goal | Warnings |
|---|---|---|---|---|
| 1.0–3.2 | Does not plan, prepare, or place food on the table. Does not assist with clean-up after meals. Does not pass dishes at the table. May serve self excessive amounts of food. May eat from refrigerator when hungry. Does not observe dietary restrictions. | Caregiver plans, obtains, prepares, and serves all food. Caregiver does all clean-up and food storage. | Caregiver will provide healthful diet for patient, taking into account dietary restrictions, food preferences of patient. | Remove all sharp or hot objects or materials from view. Monitor when patient is near hot stove. |
| 3.4 | **A. Planning** Does not plan for food. **B. Obtaining** May eat from refrigerator. Cannot wait for service at restaurant. Does not shop. **C. Preparing** May be able to do repetitive manual actions in food preparation (snapping beans, washing vegetables, hulling strawberries). Does not note effects; may be slow and or little real help or may be impulsive, or need frequent redirection. **D. Serving** When directed and handed objects, may | Caregiver plans, obtains, prepares, and serves all food. Hands necessary objects for patient to set table, checks results and corrects errors. Provides repetitive action tasks as possible in food preparation, and checks results. Stops repetitive actions or changes to new actions when needed. Redirects attention back to task. Restricts access to sharp tools and appliances; handles hot, heavy, liquid dishes. Monitors servings for amounts, and compliance to dietary restrictions. | Caregiver will provide healthful diet for patient, taking into account dietary restrictions and food preferences. Patient will sustain repetitive actions to assist with food preparation or clean-up as directed by caregiver. | Restrict access to sharp tools; dangerous appliances; hot objects or surfaces; heavy or liquid dishes. Watch for impulsive or repetitive actions that may be dangerous. Watch for distractibility. |

| LEVEL | BEHAVIOR | ASSISTANCE | GOAL | WARNINGS |
|---|---|---|---|---|
| | be able to set table. Correct location of objects may be ignored. If allowed to serve self portions, may take inappropriate quantities and does not alter amounts when cued. Does not observe dietary restrictions. Does not pass hot, heavy, or liquid dishes safely. <br> E. Cleaning Up <br> Does not note or clean up spills. When directed, may clear table, may be able to rinse or dry dishes or silverware. <br> F. Storage <br> Does not recognize need to properly store food, discard spoiled food. | | | |
| 3.6 | A. Planning <br> Does not plan for food. <br> B. Obtaining <br> May eat from refrigerator. May be able to sit and wait for short period to be served at table or in fast food restaurant when told. Does not shop. <br> C. Preparing <br> May be able to modify a repetitive action such as peeling a missed spot on a carrot, snipping parsley into smaller bits, washing lettuce longer, though the reason for the modification is not | Caregiver plans, obtains, and serves all food. Demonstrates locations for repetitive actions in food preparation or clean-up tasks, and checks results. Sequences actions for patient to ensure outcomes, redirecting attention as necessary. Avoids tasks requiring use of sharp tools, appliances, hot surfaces, handling of liquids, or tasks requiring precise outcomes. | Caregiver: same as 3.4. Patient will modify repetitive actions to assist with food preparation or clean-up as directed by caregiver. | Same as 3.4. |

| Level | Behavior | Assistance | Goal | Warnings |
|---|---|---|---|---|
|  | understood. Assistance may be of little real help.<br>D. Serving<br>May be able to set table with correct placement of plates and other utensils with demonstration. May be able to alter food serving size when cued. Serves cold or room temperature dishes safely.<br>E. Cleaning Up<br>May be able to clear table or dry and put away clean dishes in correct locations when directed.<br>F. Storage<br>May not recognize need for proper food storage. |  |  |  |
| 3.8 | A. Planning<br>Does not plan for food.<br>B. Obtaining<br>May be trained not to eat food from refrigerator, or to present self in a dining area for a meal, or to go through a cafeteria line and select a limited number of dishes.<br>C. Preparing<br>May be trained to make a simple sandwich with one or two ingredients (peanut butter and jelly). Persists doing actions until all supplies are used or a | Caregiver plans and shops for all food. Provides safe activities using repetitive actions to help in food preparation (peeler, scrub brush, spoons) and checks effects. Sequences actions of patient to ensure functional outcomes. Avoids tasks requiring handling hot, heavy, or liquid dishes. Avoids exposure to dangerous kitchen appliances. Verifies results, pointing out a visible outcome. Checks that stored food is properly covered. | Caregiver; same as 3.6.<br>Patient will persist at doing repetitive actions and will recognize a completed task. | Same as 3.4. |

| LEVEL | BEHAVIOR | ASSISTANCE | GOAL | WARNINGS |
|---|---|---|---|---|
| | surface is covered (shells all peas; covers bread with jelly; covers cookie sheet with presliced cookies) and stops. Recognizes a highly visible effect when this is pointed out (potato skin left unpeeled). Recognizes completion of task.<br>D. Serving<br>Places all visible plates and utensils on table or covers surface. May be trained to select certain foods or serving size after much repetition. May be trained to follow a valued social procedure related to serving, such as waiting for others to sit before starting to eat or pass dishes.<br>E. Cleaning Up<br>When directed, removes all dirty dishes from table; rinses or dries all utensils, and recognizes completion. Washes dishes but does not check results. May remove spills or crumbs from immediate eating area when cued by caregivers.<br>F. Storage<br>May be trained to place left-over food in refrigerator; may not place in proper containers. | | | |
| 4.0 | A. Planning<br>Does not plan for food. May make unreasonable or unhealthful requests for | Caregiver plans for food needs of patient. Restricts access to unhealthful or undesirable foods. Regular mealtime | Patient will prepare a well-learned simple meal with assistance from caregiver to provide necessary ingredients and to | Restrict access or supervise use of all electrical or gas appliances, sharp tools. Store all undesirable foodstuffs or |

| LEVEL | BEHAVIOR | ASSISTANCE | GOAL | WARNINGS |
|---|---|---|---|---|
| | food and not understand explanations.<br><br>B. Obtaining<br>May initiate coming to the table or dining room at routine times of day. May depend on an environmental cue (lunch whistle, arrival of food carts) to recognize mealtimes. May follow an inflexible routine for obtaining food (eating at or only one restaurant) and go hungry if anything out of the ordinary restricts access to food. May order same items from a menu or purchase same food items at store day after day. May not follow dietary restrictions or understand balanced diet.<br><br>C. Preparing<br>May prepare a simple cold or room temperature meal that has a few ingredients (sandwich, salad) and that is well-learned. Does not vary method of preparation. May use well-known amounts; may not measure, time procedures, or follow a recipe. If usual ingredients are missing, may abandon task. May cut or burn self when using sharp or hot equipment. May forget to turn off stove, leave water running, or fail to prevent a fire or electrical accident. | routine and familiar menus are preferred by patient. Provides safe tools and familiar cold or room-temperature ingredients in visible locations for snacks. Prepares all hot meals or dishes requiring use of appliances or sharp knives. Cautions patient when passing hot or heavy serving dishes. Pours liquids. Checks results of clean-up for missed dirt or soap on plates and utensils, or for correct stacking in dishwasher. Checks storage of leftovers and for spoilage. | avoid harmful effects. Patient will order a familiar meal in familiar restaurant with assistance from caregiver to adjust to unexpected changes.<br>Caregiver will plan for nutritional needs of patient taking into account food preferences and dietary restrictions. Caregiver will provide safe tools and ingredients in visible locations for preparation of familiar cold meals. Caregiver will remind patient of dietary restrictions and solve all new problems. | equipment away from view. Check for availability of usual offerings if patient dines out alone. |

| LEVEL | BEHAVIOR | ASSISTANCE | GOAL | WARNINGS |
|---|---|---|---|---|
| | D. Serving<br>Initiates picking up a tray or dish and serving self at meals. Aware of others at table and passes dishes. May not check temperatures or weight of serving dishes before picking them up.<br>E. Cleaning Up<br>Initiates clearing table, or following a well-learned clean-up routine. Washes or rinses visible dirt from dirty plates; may miss less visible dirt, soap residue. Cannot vary methods of washing to produce better results. Puts away dishes in familiar locations.<br>F. Storage<br>May put leftovers in refrigerator but may not cover; does not distinguish between foods that will keep and those that should be discarded or consider potential future use. Does not check stored food for spoilage. | | | |
| 4.2 | A. Planning<br>Does not plan for long-term food needs. May go to the store repeatedly, whenever food is desired, and buy for immediate needs only. May not check inventories before shopping. May set a priority (getting a particular ingredient for | Caregiver plans for long-term food needs, taking into account nutritional needs, food preferences, dietary restriction. Reinforces compliance with dietary restrictions by identifying forbidden foods by sight, clarifying new food items, and demonstrating proper food portions. | Patient will prepare a well-learned simple meal; will recognize visible errors and ask for help.<br>Caregiver will plan for long-term food needs. Caregiver will provide safe tools and ingredients in visible locations for preparation of familiar cold meals and | Same as 4.0.<br>Do not leave in kitchen alone when using dangerous tools or equipment. |

| Level | Behavior | Assistance | Goal | Warnings |
|---|---|---|---|---|
|  | a meal). May become fixated on the priority and find it difficult to shift attention to other important tasks. May select prepackaged, complete dinners or eat from cans.<br>**B. Obtaining**<br>Follows a standard routine for obtaining food at usual time of day (goes to dining room or familiar restaurant or grocery store). May search immediate area for a particular food item (pantry, grocery shelf). May ask for help when items are not found.<br>**C. Preparing**<br>Prepares a well-learned simple meal. Recognizes visible deviation from an external sample or stored model (runny pancake batter) but may not identify reason for problem. May attempt to solve a problem by matching one visible feature at a time or by asking for help. May prefer preparation with immediate results, such as heating up canned or frozen food. May cut or burn self or fail to observe precautions with gas and electrical appliances. May be unable to open unusual or hard-to-open containers. May not read directions for preparation on new products, or follow a new recipe. | Provides safe, familiar ingredients and tools for simple meal preparation, and monitors use of hot, sharp tools and appliances as in 4.0. Checks quality of clean-up and storage of food as in 4.0. | supervise use of appliances and sharp tools. Caregiver will be available for problem solving. |  |

| LEVEL | BEHAVIOR | ASSISTANCE | GOAL | WARNINGS |
|---|---|---|---|---|
| | D. Serving<br>May alter size of portions served by matching sample.<br><u>E. Cleaning Up</u><br>Recognize visible dirt or a problem (no detergent, washer is full) and asks for help.<br><u>F. Storage</u><br>May recognize spoilage (bad smell/visible mold) and asks if food should be discarded. | | | Check patient's awareness of proper use of appliances. Supervise use of all tools or substances with potential harmful effects. Solve problems involving neuromuscular adjustments (cutting meat off bones, opening new containers). |
| 4.4 | <u>A. Planning</u><br>Does not plan for long-term food needs. May go to store repeatedly, whenever food is desired, and buy for immediate needs only. May follow a fixed diet and go hungry if usual food items are unavailable. May not check food inventories and may run out of essentials frequently. May choose to use canned, frozen, prepackaged meals exclusively. Does not consider nutritional needs or special dietary restrictions unless these are well-learned.<br><u>B. Obtaining</u><br>Follows an established routine for obtaining food. Goes to familiar restaurants, grocery stores, missions, | Caregiver plans for long-term food needs and monitors inventory of essential food items, or reminds patient to check for needed items before shopping. Reinforces compliance with dietary restrictions as in 4.2. Monitors use of all hazardous tools and appliances and new procedures, assisting with avoiding undesirable effects. Solves all new problems. Checks quality of clean-up and food storage or points out dirt, improper storage procedures, and demonstrates solutions. Monitors stored food for spoilage. Stores food and sage tools in familiar, visible locations for easy access. | Patient will prepare well-learned dishes with assistance from caregiver to avoid harmful effects and solve new problems related to food preparation, storage, and clean-up.<br>Caregiver will plan or assist patient in planning for long-term food needs and will supervise preparation and storage of food to avoid harmful effects. Caregiver will monitor clean-up for hygienic results. | |

| Level | Behavior | Assistance | Goal | Warnings |
|---|---|---|---|---|
| | family eating area. May not eat if something prevents usual access (closure of restaurant). Searches area within 3 to 4 feet for needed food items in a grocery store or pantry and recognizes by size, shape, or general appearance. Does not read labels to check compliance with dietary restrictions but recognizes a familiar special diet.<br><br>C. Preparing<br>Prepares simple, well-learned dishes that may be hot or cold. Uses food and equipment in familiar locations, or within 3 to 4 feet. Uses amounts that are standard and may not deviate from these. May read a new recipe but does not follow it or follows with difficulty, one step at a time. Can use a clearly marked measuring device. Attends to the visible, primary effects related to food preparation and of tools; fails to note secondary, or intangible properties (heat, burning at bottom of a pan, combustibles near flame, electrical hazards, contamination of work surfaces or tools from nonvisible materials. Imitates demonstrated solutions. May burn or cut self, fail to turn off gas or stove, not note a hazardous situation. | | | |

| LEVEL | BEHAVIOR | ASSISTANCE | GOAL | WARNINGS |
|---|---|---|---|---|
| | D. Serving<br>Sets table to match a familiar outcome. Attempts to conform with standard social practices of waiting for others, passing food, when requested. May not consider need to share a limited quantity of food. May not check for temperature or weight before picking up.<br>E. Cleaning Up<br>May recognize and clean up a highly visible spill or dropped food items; does not note crumbs or less striking dirt. May not think to remove waste from work area during food preparation. Initiates clearing the table and follows an established clean-up routine. Needs cuing to clean in corners, hidden locations (inside refrigerator), and does not make neuromuscular adjustments in strength to remove sticky, greasy, or baked-on food from pots and pans.<br>F. Storage<br>May follow established routine for storage of new and left-over food. May not anticipate spoilage or check stored items on regular basis. May recognize visible signs of spoilage (mold) or a bad smell. May not recognize infestations of small bugs (rice, flour). May not think to | | | |

| Level | Behavior | Assistance | Goal | Warnings |
|-------|----------|------------|------|----------|
| | cover foods; may not separate foods to reduce contamination from smells in refrigerator. | | | |
| 4.6 | A. Planning<br>Same as 4.4.<br>B. Obtaining<br>Follows established routine for obtaining food. Scans visible counters, shelves, for needed items in pantry or grocery store. May be willing to substitute for a missing familiar item.<br>C. Preparing<br>May attempt to individualize a dish by changing, adding, or eliminating an ingredient, without awareness of the effects on the outcome. May ask for supplies used in the past that are not visible. May attempt to vary amount of strength or fine-motor coordination used in cutting, peeling, mixing, for better effects without success. Maintains awareness of the passage of time for about 15 minutes or when cued.<br>D. Serving<br>Scans visible counters and tables for items needed to set table in usual fashion. May ask for previously used items. May enjoy changing table cloth, | Caregiver provides assistance as 4.4 except demonstrates changes in spatial locations (location of cutting, placement of appliances), and explains functional reasons. Explains undesirable consequences of variations when needed (adding more/less leavening agents, or spices). Monitors use of appliances, equipment, and explains or demonstrates hazards to avoid (no metal in microwave oven, no plastics near heat, unplugging electrical appliances, etc.). | Patient will prepare well-learned dishes with assistance from caregiver to avoid harmful effects and solve new problems. Patient will scan environment for needed items and will vary actions from a standard.<br>Caregiver will plan or assist patient to plan for long-term food needs and will supervise preparation and storage of food to avoid harmful effects. Caregiver will monitor clean-up for hygienic results. | Same as 4.4.<br>Watch for variations in actions, typical tool use, or food combinations that may have harmful effects. |

| LEVEL | BEHAVIOR | ASSISTANCE | GOAL | WARNINGS |
|---|---|---|---|---|
| | plates, or other feature of table. May not understand need to limit serving sizes.<br>E. Cleaning Up<br>May attempt to alter strength, use of tools in order to clean difficult-to-clean pots and pans.<br>F. Storage<br>May adjust clear plastic coverings over open containers so that they are air-tight, or open and close plastic storage containers by varying actions. May scan all visible items in refrigerator for signs of spoilage when asked. | | | |
| 4.8 | A. Planning<br>Does not plan for long-term food needs. May learn to follow by rote a plan for purchasing food items that include a balanced diet or special dietary needs. Takes inventory of food on hand by careful examination of all visible objects.<br>B. Obtaining<br>May follow a weekly schedule for purchasing food at grocery store. May locate a new restaurant, mission, or eating area by noting all visible cues or by following directions pointed out by others. Scans all shelves above and below eye level to locate needed items in | Caregiver assists with making lists of essential food items, which consider balanced diet, dietary restrictions, and food preferences to do weekly shopping. Demonstrates new tasks one step at a time and validates discovered new solutions to facilitate rote learning. Explains hazardous secondary effects to avoid for safety reasons. Checks periodically for compliance with safety procedures and food storage methods. Solves problems requiring variations in strength or range of motion in tool use, opening and closing containers. | Patient will learn new methods of food preparation by rote with caregiver assistance to avoid harmful effects and to solve problems.<br>Patient will note all visible effects in food preparation.<br>Caregiver will assist in planning for long-term food needs, will assist new learning by rote, and will monitor regularly for safety and to check problem-solving methods. | Daily checks for safety when patient lives independently. |

| LEVEL | BEHAVIOR | ASSISTANCE | GOAL | WARNINGS |
|---|---|---|---|---|
| | pantry or store.<br>**C. Preparing**<br>Memorizes a new sequence of actions to prepare a dish, slowly, one step at a time. Attends to all striking features (shape, color, texture, size) as he or she works. Follows a written recipe in a rigid manner, asking for verification of meaning of directions. By rote, may follow a demonstrated safety procedure such as turning pot handles inward, or unplugging appliances after use, or angling cuts away from fingers. May solve problems involving changing a spatial location (moving objects around kitchen) but not requiring continuous neuromuscular adjustments (frosting a soft cake, cutting meat off a bone). Closely watches the clock to time dishes for short periods; needs cues (timers) for longer periods.<br>**D. Serving**<br>Learns proper amounts of serving portions, including not overfilling glasses or bowls.<br>**E. Cleaning Up**<br>Closely checks plates, utensils, after washing for visible dirt. Washes all visible counters and working areas. | | | |

| LEVEL | BEHAVIOR | ASSISTANCE | GOAL | WARNINGS |
|---|---|---|---|---|
| 5.0 | F. Storage<br>Follows a routine by rote for storing new and left-over food. May treat all foods the same (saving all left-overs or throwing everything out on a fixed schedule). May not understand intangible properties that influence disposal (shelf life, humidity, nature of food).<br><br>A. Planning<br>May make reservations for eating out but may fail to remember or arrive late. May make a schedule for grocery shopping but fail to adhere to it.<br>B. Obtaining<br>Same as 4.8.<br>C. Preparing<br>Varies strength and range of motion effectively for better results in food preparation. Opens new or difficult containers; adjusts methods of cutting (slice, chop, mince); mixing (stiff dough). May forget discovered solutions to problems. May abandon tedious tasks.<br>D. Serving<br>Passes heavy serving dishes safely. | Caregiver provides assistance as for 4.8. Validates solutions to problems involving neuromuscular effects. Caregiver solves problems involving awareness of surface and spatial properties. | Patient will solve problems in food preparations that involve variations in neuromuscular effects with caregiver assistance to avoid harmful effects.<br>Caregiver will assist in planning for long-term food needs, will validate discovered solutions to problems, and will monitor regularly for safety and to check problem-solving methods. | Weekly checks for safety when patient lives independently. |

| Level | Behavior | Assistance | Goal | Warnings |
|-------|----------|------------|------|----------|
| | E. Cleaning Up<br>Cleans difficult dirt off pots and pans or work surfaces by varying actions.<br>F. Storage<br>Same as 4.8. | | | |
| 5.2 | A. Planning<br>May make a weekly schedule for shopping or eating out but may impulsively change lists or schedules. May rely on lists to guide shopping.<br>B. Obtaining<br>Discriminates between items based on brands, condition of food, or price.<br>C. Preparing<br>Solves problems in food preparation involving tangible properties (washes and peels vegetables thoroughly, cuts out bad spots, greases pans carefully, notes contaminated surfaces). Notes textures (as in bread), sheen (as in candy, sauces, frostings), and consistency of color or texture. Discriminates between specialized tools. Throws trash away as he or she works.<br>D. Serving<br>Same as 5.0.<br>E. Cleaning Up<br>Notes and cleans up crumbs and spills on | Caregiver identifies consequences of impulsive shopping, or failing to follow special dietary precautions. Validates solutions to problems involving tangible properties and assists with problems requiring awareness of spatial properties. Identifies visible secondary effects to be avoided for safety reasons in use of tools and appliances; monitors for safety in food preparation and storage. | Patient will solve problems in food preparation that involve all tangible properties with caregiver assistance to avoid harmful effects.<br>Caregiver: same as 5.0. | Weekly checks for safety when patient lives independently. |

| LEVEL | BEHAVIOR | ASSISTANCE | GOAL | WARNINGS |
|---|---|---|---|---|
| | table/work area. Notes and cleans grease on pans. May not clean in corners, or may not persist if cleaning task is tedious.<br><br>F. Storage<br>Notes tangible changes indicating spoilage (color, mold, dryness, curdling). May not store food for efficient use; may not take usual care to prevent spoilage or food poisoning. | | | Check new kitchens to identify potential safety hazards. |
| 5.4 | A. Planning<br>May argue with need to maintain a schedule or plan for food needs. May state importance of food budget but not follow it.<br><br>B. Obtaining<br>Searches in closed cupboards, drawers, cabinets, for needed food, tools, or equipment. May ask for a tool or food item to be used in a new context. Finds items in a new market successfully.<br><br>C. Preparing<br>Moves tools and appliances around work space flexibly. Makes fine-motor adjustments with tools (chops, peels, or carves slippery/small items). May freely vary combinations of ingredients and dishes without consideration of social or | Caregiver identifies consequences of failure to follow dietary guidelines, budgetary constraints, or safety procedures in food preparation and storage. Assists with identification of secondary effects when needed for problem solving or safety. Suggests alternate methods of tool use. | Patient will solve problems in food preparation that involve varying spatial properties with assistance from caregiver to avoid harmful effects.<br>Caregiver: same as 5.0. | |

| LEVEL | BEHAVIOR | ASSISTANCE | GOAL | WARNINGS |
|---|---|---|---|---|
| | esthetic consequences. Alters tool use for desired effects.<br>D. Serving<br>Flexibly alters table set-up, serving portions.<br>E. Cleaning Up<br>Cleans interior and exterior spaces (stove, cupboards, pots). Moves dishes around in dishwasher to fit. Cleans in corners and hard-to-reach areas, but may not persist at tedious cleaning.<br>F. Storage<br>May question need to follow storage guidelines of others. | | | |
| 5.6 | A. Planning<br>May consult recipes or ask advice of others for meal planning. May consider coordinating textures, appearance of foods.<br>B. Obtaining<br>Selection of stores/restaurants includes awareness of current trends or recommendations of others.<br>C. Preparing<br>Varies food combinations to achieve an effect pleasing to eye or palate. Adjusts and blends spices or herbs. Can vary pace of working with assistance. May | Caregiver identifies consequences of failure to follow dietary guidelines, budgetary constraints, safety procedures in food preparation and storage. Assists with comparing primary and secondary effects to solve problems. Reminds about the passage of time. | With assistance, patient will compare methods to solve problems in food preparation to avoid harmful effects. Caregiver: same as 5.0. | Same as 5.4. |

| LEVEL | BEHAVIOR | ASSISTANCE | GOAL | WARNINGS |
|---|---|---|---|---|
| | forget about the passage of time when busy. May have trouble coordinating timing of several dishes. | | | |
| | D. Serving | | | |
| | May alter table settings to harmonize with an occasion, style of food. | | | |
| | E. Cleaning Up | | | |
| | Same as 5.4. | | | |
| | F. Storage | | | |
| | Estimates storage area needs and reorganizes. Compares storage methods. | | | |
| 5.8 | A. Planning | Caregiver provides assistance with planning an overall organization. Caregiver points out relevant social considerations in meal planning and preparation. Identifies secondary effects to consider for safety reasons. | Patient will plan in the presence of material objects to accomplish food preparation with assistance from caregivers to avoid harmful effects. Caregiver will assist with planning overall organization and will identify intangible and secondary effects to be avoided for safety reasons. | Same as 5.4. |
| | Plans new dishes, menus when materials are present. May be able to anticipate menu requirements of up to a week. May consider inevitable but not potential secondary effects of plans. | | | |
| | B. Obtaining | | | |
| | May use resources such as newspaper ads or coupons to suggest where to obtain food. | | | |
| | C. Preparing | | | |
| | May follow new recipes. Varies pace and times actions according to the clock, past experience, and tangible properties. | | | |
| | D. Serving | | | |
| | Plans serving sizes so that limited food quantities are equally distributed; may | | | |

| Level | Behavior | Assistance | Goal | Warnings |
|---|---|---|---|---|
| | solicit individual requests and include this in adjusting portions.<br><br>E. Cleaning Up<br>Plans a method of clean-up when all materials are present, which tends to increase efficiency.<br><br>F. Storage<br>May divide, wrap, label, and date bulk items for freezing or storage. May position items in drawers, cupboards for easier access. Seeks explanations of potential secondary effects to avoid. | | | |
| 6.0 | A. Planning<br>Plans for nutritional needs of self and others, including special dietary needs, for periods of a month or longer. Speculates about new problems (menus and preparation for a camping trip in an unfamiliar locale) without materials present.<br><br>B. Obtaining<br>May determine shopping locations and food selections by price comparison done beforehand, or by awareness of quality/variety/other relevant and valued criteria. May use restaurant guides or reviews to determine selections when eating out. | No assistance needed. | Patient will obtain and safely prepare a healthful diet for self and dependents, taking into account dietary restrictions. | |

| LEVEL | BEHAVIOR | ASSISTANCE | GOAL | WARNINGS |
|---|---|---|---|---|
| | C. Preparing<br>Speculates about problems in food preparation, uses cookbooks or other references for information. Considers anticipated problems and secondary effects.<br>D. Serving<br>Considers needed serving sizes for guests and plans for adequate amounts.<br>E. Cleaning Up<br>Anticipates clean-up needs. Plans for required time, materials, space; may clean as he or she prepares to minimize effort after a meal.<br>F. Storage<br>May plan storage of food to minimize spoilage, contamination, and to maximize efficient access. Storage of leftovers considers nature of food and possible future use. Items are checked periodically for spoilage. | | | |

## 11.2 Situational Awareness Disability: Spending Money

Spending money includes understanding the value of local currency; recognizing situations that require payment for goods and services, being aware of current prices; calculating cost, change, and remaining money; accounting for money spent; adjusting to price changes as well as changes in personal income; anticipating future purchases; paying bills; using credit; balancing a checkbook; and planning of financial security.

| Level | Behavior | Assistance | Goal | Warnings |
|---|---|---|---|---|
| 1.0-3.0 | Does not handle money or is given no opportunity to do so. May not recognize that money transactions are occurring. | Caregiver manages all financial matters for patient, including planning, spending, and saving. | Caregiver will manage patient's finances to avoid undesirable consequences. | May lose money if allowed to have it. |
| 3.2 | May recognize local currency and its value. May hand money to another person when cued, but is not aware of amount of transaction, change, or may not recognize that a transaction is occurring. | Same as 1.0-3.0. | Caregiver: same as 1.0. | Same as 1.0. |
| 3.4 | May recognize local currency. In a familiar exchange situation (paying at grocery store) may hand money to another person but may not attend to the amount given or received. May not understand that he or she owes money for a service. Usually not aware of amount or source of his or her income. | Same as 1.0. Caregiver gives patient money to hand to others but checks for correct amounts of change. | Caregiver: same as 1.0. | If given money, may give away or lose it. |
| 3.6 | May be able to place coins in slots to buy a soda or to pay fare on the bus when sequenced through steps. | Caregiver manages all financial planning for patient. Sequences patient with verbal cues through simple exchange of money. | Caregiver will plan and manage patient's finances and will sequence patient through simple monetary transactions to avoid harmful effects. | Same as 3.4. |

| LEVEL | BEHAVIOR | ASSISTANCE | GOAL | WARNINGS |
|---|---|---|---|---|
| | | | Patient will follow cues given by caregiver in all money exchanges. | |
| 3.8 | May be trained to do the steps in a simple transaction involving a fixed amount of money (buying a cup of coffee at a coffee shop or a soda from a machine). Recognizes completion of the transaction. May be trained to ask for assistance in all other money transactions. May remember an old price, but be unable to adjust to current prices. | Caregiver manages all financial planning for patient. Trains patient in highly valued and routine exchanges for a direct service or product; sequences through steps of all other exchanges, or does these for patient. | Caregiver will plan and manage patient's finances and will train patient to perform highly valued routine exchanges, supervising to avoid harmful effects. Patients will recognize completion of a routine exchange for direct product or service. | Same as 3.4. |
| 4.0 | Completes a simple monetary transaction for a small purchase without assistance (notes price of article, hands over cash, checks change). May be unusually slow in all actions. May be aware of a few highly valued amounts (monthly disability check, or rent); otherwise does not know prices of most goods or services. May try to manage own funds but over- or underspends. | Caregiver provides daily allowance for small, routine purchases. Plans budget of a monthly income, providing for essential services (rent, medication) to avoid over- or underspending. Manages all unusual or large purchases and plans for ongoing and long-term needs. | Patient will make small routine purchases independently or manage a daily allowance with assistance from caregiver to avoid harmful effects. Caregiver will assist patient with budgeting of a monthly income, providing a daily allowance for routine purchases. Caregiver will manage on-going, long-term, and unusual monetary transactions. | May not recognize need for assistance and resist help. |
| 4.2 | May be able to set a priority for an expense that is highly valued; may become fixated on the item and fail to appropriately make adjustments when necessary. | Caregiver provides assistance as for 4.0. Assists with spending priorities as necessary. | Patient: same as 4.0. Caregiver: same as 4.0. | Same as 4.0. |

| Level | Behavior | Assistance | Goal | Warnings |
|---|---|---|---|---|
| 4.4 | Manages routine purchases for immediate needs. May use paper and pencil, a calculator, or may count cash very slowly. May use credit cards or checks if highly familiar but may not know balance in account and exceed bank or credit limits. May be able to state amounts of very routine or essential purchases correctly. May not be able to make a monthly budget without assistance. May not remember to account for taxes, redemption values, or tips in figuring costs. May not be able to make adjustments to price or income changes. May spend as if he or she has unlimited funds, or far fewer funds than he or she does have. May resist changing usual routine of money management (learning to use an automated teller). | Caregiver assists in identifying monthly expenses and setting priorities for routine expenditures. Assists with making adjustments to changes in routine expenses or income. Monitors all checkbook and credit card use to avoid overdraft or excessive credit use. Plans long-term financial needs. | Patient will manage routine expenditures in cash with assistance from caregiver to make a monthly budget, and to monitor bank and credit card use to avoid harmful effects.<br><br>Caregiver will assist with making monthly budget and will monitor all use of bank or credit accounts. | May overspend if given access to bank or credit card accounts. |
| 4.6 | May be willing to vary usual routine to manage money (using an automated teller to make deposits or get cash). May attempt to vary his or her usual procedures and not anticipate resulting problems. | Caregiver provides assistance as for 4.4. Demonstrates desirable modifications in money management routine. | Patient: same as 4.4.<br>Caregiver: same as 4.4. | Same as 4.4. |
| 4.8 | By rote, slowly follows budget or learns money management procedures | Caregiver assists with making a monthly budget, and demonstrates all procedures | Patient will do routine money management by following a budget and | Daily checks for money-related problems if patient lives independently. |

| LEVEL | BEHAVIOR | ASSISTANCE | GOAL | WARNINGS |
|---|---|---|---|---|
| | identified by others. May need assistance to adjust to changes in income, expense, or usual banking procedures; to prepare for infrequent major expenses; and to manage emergencies such as stolen money or credit cards. | for managing money until well-learned (check writing, depositing money, reading statements). Monitors with daily assistance to solve problems and makes adjustments. Plans for long-term needs. | procedures by rote, with assistance from caregiver to avoid harmful effects. Caregiver will provide assistance with learning rote procedures and will assist with problem-solving and long-term planning. | Weekly checks for money-related problems if patient lives independently. |
| 5.0-5.2 | May be able to identify a monthly budget of routine expenses from past experience without assistance but has trouble adhering to it. May run up bills beyond ability to pay, or may overextend credit. May have trouble balancing checkbook. May not prepare for infrequent major expenses, or account for small, incidental fees. Can learn new banking procedures by following a series of demonstrated steps. Needs to have secondary effects related to money management explained by others (cost difference between a cash and credit purchase, consequences of overdrafts). Does not plan for long-term financial security. Spending may be impulsive. | Caregiver demonstrates all new banking procedures. Identifies consequences of failure to follow budget or proper procedures. Assists with planning for infrequent of hidden expenses. Provides weekly checks to monitor effectiveness of money management and is available to solve new problems. Assists with planning long-term financial security. | Patient will manage routine weekly and monthly income and expenses with assistance from caregiver to solve new problems, avoid harmful effects, and plan for future financial security. Caregiver will demonstrate new banking procedures, identify consequences to avoid undesirable effects, assist with solving new problems, and plan for long-term financial security. | |
| 5.4-5.6 | Generates a monthly budget, usually including routine, incidental fees. Usually aware of current prices for routine and | Caregiver provides assistance same as for 5.0-5.2. | Patient: same as 5.0. Caregiver: same as 5.0. | May resist following recommended procedures and alter actions only after undesirable consequences have occurred. |

| Level | Behavior | Assistance | Goal | Warnings |
|---|---|---|---|---|
| | highly valued commodities. May purposefully vary methods of banking, or depart from budget without awareness of consequences. May argue with requests to adhere to budget or proper banking procedures. Problems (such as overdrafts) may be excused or minimized. Priorities set for expenditures may not consider the needs of others. Can remember solutions to problems and can understand explanations of secondary effects but is apt to change behavior only after an undesirable effect has occurred. Does not anticipate predictable changes in expenses (i.e., cost of living) but adjusts after they occur. | | | |
| 5.8 | May be able to plan out a new budget when all needed information (i.e., specific figures and expenses) is present. May need assistance to plan on overall organization. Asks for explanations of secondary effects to be avoided; does not anticipate but can include the needs of others when these are identified. May not consider long-term financial planning (retirement accounts, wills, etc.). | Caregiver assists with planning new budget by identifying all salient expenses, including needs of others. Assists with identifying secondary effects, priorities, long-term needs to consider in planning | Patient will manage routine income and expenses and will plan out a new budget when all needed items are identified. Caregiver will assist in planning a new budget by identifying all salient considerations and will assist with long-term financial planning. | |

| Level | Behavior | Assistance | Goal | Warnings |
|-------|----------|------------|------|----------|
| 6.0 | Plans use of money by considering income and expenses, including infrequent expenses. Plans for long-term financial security for self and dependents. Uses written materials or consults others to learn about relevant resources (bank or savings accounts, investment opportunities, retirement accounts, tax considerations). | No assistance needed. | Patient will plan for and manage routine and long-term financial activities. | |

## 11.3  Situational Awareness Disability: Shopping

Shopping includes deciding on items needed, visiting stores and malls to examine goods, checking mail order catalogues and advertised sales or specials, remembering intent to purchase, locating goods within a store, comparing goods and prices, recognizing budget and adjusting purchases according to what one can afford, deciding on method of payment, and protecting currency, checks, and credit cards from theft. This category excludes spending of money.

| Level | Behavior | Assistance | Goal | Warnings |
|---|---|---|---|---|
| 1.0-3.2 | Does not have an opportunity to go shopping or walks aimlessly around shopping area without noting merchandise. | Caregiver does all shopping for patient, including deciding on needed items, locating, and purchasing items. | Caregiver will manage all shopping for patient. | Stimuli at shopping malls may overwhelm patient; patient may wander and get lost. |
| 3.4-3.8 | Follows a guide to a shopping area; looks in windows or at displays. May not have any intent to purchase; may take items without paying; or may want to buy an item but fail to note price or whether he or she has money. May pick up and handle familiar items. | Caregiver does all shopping for patient as in 1.0-3.2. Monitors patient whereabouts to prevent wandering or taking things when in shopping areas. | Caregiver: same as 1.0-1.3. Caregiver will monitor patient's actions and whereabouts on shopping outings to prevent undesirable consequences. | Do not leave patient alone in shopping areas. Patient may pick up, drop, take merchandise. Patient tolerates short trips only (thirty minutes). |
| 4.0 | May walk a short distance to a familiar shop to purchase a familiar item or items. May be immobilized by changes in shops, price, or appearance of merchandise. Completes a simple monetary transaction but may do so very slowly. May know the price of a few highly valued items but generally does not note or anticipate cost, compare prices, or adhere to a budget. Does not take precautions to | Caregiver accompanies to all new shopping locations or environments that are highly stimulus laden or hazardous. Assists patient in identifying shopping needs, amount of money required, and provides cash for purchases consistent with budgetary restrictions for small and routine purchases. Manages purchases for costly or unusual merchandise. Does necessary price comparison. | Patient will shop for familiar items in familiar shops and with assistance from caregiver for other purchases to avoid harmful effects.<br>Caregiver will assist patient with identifying shopping needs, will provide adequate cash for simple purchases, and will accompany to new shopping locations. | May resist assistance with shopping. May resist going to new shopping areas. May become highly anxious in shopping malls. May be able to tolerate short (1 hour) shopping trips only. |

| LEVEL | BEHAVIOR | ASSISTANCE | GOAL | WARNINGS |
|---|---|---|---|---|
| 4.2 | protect self from theft; may resist going to new shopping areas. If items are not in usual locations may not ask for help.

May go to familiar shops repeatedly to purchase immediate needs with cash. Does not make a list, or compare prices or anticipate cost as in 4.0. May become fixated on purchasing a particular item without considering whether he or she needs or can afford the item. Looks in familiar locations for items, matching one striking cue at a time (color or shape of box). May ask for help if item is not in usual location or appearance of item has changed. | Caregiver provides assistance as for 4.0. | Patient: same as 4.0. Caregiver: same as 4.0. | Same as 4.0. Patient may insist on purchasing an item that is unrealistic or impractical. |
| 4.4 | Goes to familiar stores to shop for routine items. May go without needed items if something prevents usual access, including changes in price or appearance. Matches visible features two at a time with stored models for the item, or with an exact representation (such as a picture from an advertisement). Does not compare products in terms of price, quality; does not read labels to determine ingredients, nature of materials, operating instructions, hazards, or other features. | Caregiver accompanies patient to all new shopping areas. Assists in making lists to reduce number of trips. Identifies substitutions or alternative products when usual items are unavailable. Suggests where familiar items can be purchased most reasonably based on price comparisons, when maximizing use of patient's funds is desirable. Monitors all checkbook or credit card use (see "Spending Money"). Limits cash given to patient to immediate purchase needs. | Patient will do routine shopping in familiar locations with assistance from caregiver to avoid undesirable effects. Caregiver will assist with shopping requiring price or product comparison, use of unfamiliar stores or purchase of unfamiliar items, or taking into account budgetary constraints. | May overspend if given access to credit cards or checking accounts. |

| Level | Behavior | Assistance | Goal | Warnings |
|---|---|---|---|---|
|  | May not consider cost of items in relation to overall budget. May search and note objects within 3 to 4 feet in front of him or her when shopping. May not note other surroundings, including signs, special advertisements, aisle labels, or unsafe conditions. May not take precautions to protect against theft of goods or money. | Suggests ways for patient to protect self from theft of goods or money while shopping. |  |  |
| 4.6 | May vary usual shopping routine, including visiting a new store or substituting a different brand for an unavailable product. Searches open cupboards and shelves in stores, moves stacked clothing to see items underneath. Scans visible environment for a desired cue (such as an aisle number or sign). | Caregiver provides assistance as for 4.4. | Patient will do routine shopping in familiar locations, and will scan environment for cues to locate desired items. Will accept caregiver assistance to avoid undesirable effects. Caregiver: same as for 4.4. | Same as for 4.4. Watch for unexpected problems resulting from variations in shopping routines. |
| 4.8 | Shops for routine items at familiar locations. Learns directions to new shopping areas by rote. May learn to use a shopping list, or to compare label prices in store, or to use money-saving procedures (use of coupons, etc.), from others by rote. Such procedures are followed rigidly. May be able to learn safety precautions to protect against theft. Turns items over to locate a price | Caregiver assists with rote learning of shopping tricks to reduce costs (cutting coupons, making lists) and identifies stores for new of infrequently purchased items. Assists with price and product comparison for best use of limited funds. Identifies visible secondary effects to consider (space for furniture, whether a garment goes with other wardrobe items, care instructions). Explains secondary | Patient will, by rote, shop for routine items and will learn new ways to shop more efficiently. Caregiver will assist with rote learning of desired methods and will identify undesirable secondary effects to avoid. | Daily checks for shopping-related difficulties if patient lives independently. |

| LEVEL | BEHAVIOR | ASSISTANCE | GOAL | WARNINGS |
|---|---|---|---|---|
| | tag and size. May not read or consider care labels (clothing), ingredients (foodstuffs) or other secondary effects including whether item is practical or affordable. | effects (effects of purchase on budget, warranties, qualitative differences in products). | | |
| 5.0-5.2 | May make a daily or weekly schedule for shopping needs, to which he or she has trouble adhering. Turns objects over to examine all tangible properties including care labels, fiber content, color-fast quality, quality of construction. May not consider potential secondary effects of purchase; shrinkage in size selection, appropriateness to budget, or event. May be impulsive in spending. May discriminate between specialty department stores, labels, brand names versus generic. | Caregiver assists with learning of desired shopping tricks to reduce costs by demonstrating methods several steps at a time. Assists with product and price comparisons, identifies intangible properties of objects and secondary effects of purchases on budget. Identifies special bargains or sales that are out of the ordinary. Points out consequences of impulsive spending. | Patient will do routine daily/weekly shopping with caregiver assistance to consider intangible properties and secondary effects. Caregiver will identify secondary effects of purchases to avoid harmful effects and will assist with unusual purchases. | May follow an inflexible shopping routine or may have trouble getting to stores when they are open. Weekly checks for shopping-related problems if patient lives independently. Watch for impulsive spending. |
| 5.4 | Does routine shopping for daily/weekly purchases. May investigate new stores or purchase new products to see what they are like. Searches in stores to locate desired items. May compare prices but not consider secondary effects of purchasing, such as the distance traveled, warranty, or qualitative differences of products. May have to return purchases | Identifies intangible properties and secondary effects of purchases to assist with problems solving and to avoid harmful effects. Points out consequences of over-spending. | Patient: same as 5.0. Caregiver: same as 5.0. | Same as 5.0. |

| Level | Behavior | Assistance | Goal | Warnings |
|---|---|---|---|---|
| | frequently. May overspend and alter behavior only after undesirable consequences have occurred. | | | |
| 5.6 | Compares pros and cons of stores, products, methods of payment. May use catalogs, newspaper ads, read consumer magazines for help. May need assistance to account for hidden properties or costs such as travel time, time expenditure, seasonal price variations, etc.). | Caregiver assists in planning for new or unusual purchases and for long-term shopping needs. Identifies hidden costs, or other properties to consider, including the needs of others, financial benefits of specific sales, seasonal price variation, buying in bulk quantities. | Patient: same as 5.0. Caregiver: same as 5.0. | |
| 5.8 | Plans for new purchases in the presence of objects (in the store, catalogs). Considers inevitable secondary effects such as washing/storage of items, time spent in shopping. May not anticipate needs of others, or potential effects. Sets own pace. | Caregiver provides assistance as for 5.6. | Patient: same as 5.0. Caregiver: same as 5.0. | |
| 6.0 | Shops within a set of individualized priorities; anticipates and accepts the consequences of big purchases; compares products based on price, quality, and other relevant factors, when objects are not present. Plans for long-term shopping needs, including anticipating needs of others. | No assistance is needed. | Patient will manage all shopping needs, including setting priorities, considering needs of others, considering consequences of purchases for overall budget. Will compare goods and services and make adjustments to availability of commodities as necessary. | Provide visible objects to assist planning. |

## 11.4 Situational Awareness Disability: Doing Laundry

Doing Laundry includes recognizing when clothing is dirty; sorting according to method of cleaning and by color; loading washing machine or sink and washing; sorting for drying; loading dryer, hanging to dry or lying flat to dry; ironing by need and setting for fabric; hanging things up or folding for storage; doing simple mending to replace buttons or torn seams; putting clothing or linen away. This category includes hand laundry, machine laundry, and dry cleaning.

| LEVEL | BEHAVIOR | ASSISTANCE | GOAL | WARNINGS |
|-------|----------|------------|------|----------|
| 1.0-3.2 | Does not do laundry or is given no opportunity to do laundry. Dirty clothes and linens are removed by others and laundered. May be aware of wet clothing only as it affects subjective sense of comfort. Unaware of dirty, wrinkled, torn clothing. | Caregiver does all laundry for patient, including sorting, washing, drying, ironing, and putting away. | Caregiver will manage all laundry needs of patient. | Remove all toxic supplies from view. |
| 3.4 | May not realize that clothing/linen is dirty. May have no awareness of different methods of doing laundry and may not understand explanations. May do repetitive actions of washing articles by hand but does not attend to results or follow a typical sequence of wash/rinse/dry. May be able to remove flat sheets from beds or fold towels haphazardly. May not be aware of need for ironing, mending, or putting away clothing in hamper when directed. | Caregiver does laundry of linen/clothing for patient. Directs patient to place dirty clothing in hamper or remove flat sheets from beds. | Caregiver will manage all laundry needs of patient.<br>Patient will follow directions to remove bedding or place dirty items in hamper. | Watch for ineffective or harmful results if allowed access to laundry supplies. |
| 3.6 | May be able to fold towels or other garments by lining up straight edges. | Caregiver directs patient to place dirty laundry in hamper, demonstrates removal | Caregiver: some as 3.2.<br>Patient will follow demonstrated changes | Restrict access to toxics (bleach, spray-on spot removers) and hot irons. |

| Level | Behavior | Assistance | Goal | Warnings |
|---|---|---|---|---|
| 3.8 | May be able to remove fitted sheets with demonstration. | of fitted sheets from beds, corrects way to fold flat garments. Does all other washing, drying, mending, ironing, and putting away. | in repetitive actions to fold clothing or remove bedding. | |
| | May be able to imitate modifications in actions to fold garments to achieve a particular size or shape. May fold all available items or drape all laundry on clothes line without redirection. | Caregiver sequences patient through actions of folding or hanging laundry or does these tasks for patient. Does all other washing, drying, mending, ironing, and putting away. | Caregiver will sequence patient through actions of folding or hanging laundry and will manage all other laundry needs. Patient will follow directions to complete folding or hanging of laundry. | Same as 3.6. |
| 4.0 | Initiates a request for clean clothing, or places dirty clothes in hamper. May be unreliable in recognizing need for laundry. Sequences self to complete hand or machine washing but may not distinguish between hand or machine, or dry cleaning fabrics. May not sort or measure soap. May use a dryer or hang garments on line but may not note heat settings; may hang up garments that should be dried flat. Folds and places clean linen/clothing in usual locations. May burn fabrics or self with iron. If a problem occurs, may abandon task. | Caregiver monitors all laundry tasks for incorrect sequences, methods of washing and drying, amounts of water or soap, failure to sort. Reminds patient to initiate laundry if unreliable or does laundry for patient. If patient is allowed to use machines, caregiver checks heat and time settings (washing machines, dryers). | Patient will initiate a familiar routine of laundry with assistance from caregiver to follow correct sequences and to avoid harmful effects. Caregiver will assist patient with following correct sequences to complete a routine laundry task or will do laundry for patient. | May resist suggested change in routine. Watch for harmful effects of not following correct sequence of actions. Use of machines or irons without supervision not recommended. |
| 4.2 | May sort laundry by color or other single striking cue (towels). May view doing laundry as a priority and initiate it | Provides assistance same as for 4.0. Assists with solving problems resulting from changes in tools supplies, or from | Patient will initiate and complete routine laundry activities with caregiver assistance to solve problems resulting | Same as 4.0. |

| LEVEL | BEHAVIOR | ASSISTANCE | GOAL | WARNINGS |
|---|---|---|---|---|
| | regularly, or even when unnecessary. Recognizes errors that fail to match previous experience (heavy soiling, bleeding colors, torn garments, too much soap, new machine at the laundromat) but cannot suggest solutions; asks for help. | failure to sort, use correct washing or drying methods, temperatures of water or heat, amounts of soap or bleach, etc. Provides matching cues, one at a time, to assist with washing, folding, hanging out clothes (i.e., marks correct temperature settings on dryer or washer with tape; stores needed items in visible, easily accessible locations). | from changes in the environment or failure to consider all relevant properties. Caregiver will provide visible matching cues to assist patient to complete routine laundry tasks, and will solve problems and remove hazards. | |
| 4.4 | Initiates and completes routine laundry activities at usual time (uses a familiar machine or washes by hand; goes to familiar laundromat). May sort items by two visible properties at a time (color, type of garment, or by temperature of water listed on care label) or may group laundry by idiosyncratic criteria. May not distinguish between fabric types, delicates, or dry cleaning fabrics. May not check for stains, temperature settings for dryer or water, or for mending needs. May follow a schedule rigidly, or a procedure (such as always adding bleach or a certain amount of soap) rigidly. May not anticipate or be able to adjust to special laundry needs. May forget to clean lint traps. May not wait for iron to heat up before using; may not check water | Provides assistance same as for 4.2. Stores all needed laundry supplies in familiar, visible locations. Reminds patient to check lint traps regularly, pick up dry cleaning, and assists in anticipating special needs (trips, special occasions). Monitors use of hazardous tools and supplies (turning off irons, use of bleach). | Patient: same as 4.2. Caregiver: same as 4.2. | Check irons after use. Check for overloading machines. Check sorting criteria. Do laundry of special or fragile garments. |

| Level | Behavior | Assistance | Goal | Warnings |
|---|---|---|---|---|
|  | level, temperature settings before starting to iron. May forget to turn off iron. |  |  |  |
| 4.6 | May scan immediate environment for needed supplies. May choose to vary from usual routine (wash on a different day, or alter groupings when sorting). | Provides assistance same as for 4.4. Needed objects may be stored within scanning distance of work area. | Patient: same as 4.4. Caregiver: same as 4.4. | Same as 4.4. |
| 4.8 | Initiates and completes routine laundry activities in a fixed manner. Memorizes new procedures (learning use of a new machine, laundromat, or new schedule) slowly by rote, one step at a time. Examines clothing carefully for stains or needed mending. May try to read new care labels but needs assistance to comprehend them. May note and try to correct a visible error (such as a missing button or a stubborn stain) but may not understand cause if due to hidden properties (overloaded machine, unlabeled fabric properties). May not anticipate special needs, including amount of time needed to complete laundry before an event. | Demonstrates new procedures or methods for doing laundry by adding one step at a time and be available to verify results. Provides explanations of intangible properties and secondary effects to consider in sorting, determining wash methods, temperature settings for water, heat, irons. | Patient will learn new methods of doing laundry by rote with caregiver assistance to avoid harmful or undesirable effects. Caregiver will provide assistance with rote learning for new procedures and will identify intangible properties and secondary effects to be considered to avoid harmful effects. | Daily checks for problems related to laundry if patient lives independently. |
| 5.0 | May set and follow a weekly schedule but has trouble adhering to it. Effectively | Caregiver reminds patient of essential laundry tasks as needed; demonstrates | Patient will vary range of motion and strength to solve new problems in laundry | Weekly checks to solve problems in laundry activities if patient lives independently. |

| LEVEL | BEHAVIOR | ASSISTANCE | GOAL | WARNINGS |
|-------|----------|-----------|------|----------|
| | varies range of motion and strength to rub stains or hard to remove dirt from garments. Learns a new sequence of actions (how to use a new washing machine or laundry product) demonstrated several steps at a time. Uses iron effectively. | new product use or clarifies written instructions to ensure proper use. Identifies hidden properties and hidden properties and secondary effects to assist with problem solving, selecting proper washing methods or temperature settings, and care of unusual, new, unlabeled articles. Identifies proper storage and handling of toxic cleaning agents. | activities with assistance from caregiver to avoid harmful effects. Caregiver will identify secondary effects to avoid undesirable consequences. | |
| 5.2 | Notes all tangible features of garments (stains and less obvious dirt on garments, effects of steam versus dry ironing on wrinkles, etc.). Discriminates between fabrics types (color-fast, shrink potential, water or chemical wash). Notes water temperature, appropriate detergent. May be impulsive. | Provides assistance as for 5.0. | Patient will solve problems involving tangible properties in laundry activities with assistance from caregiver to avoid harmful effects. Caregiver: same as 5.0. | Same as 5.0. |
| 5.4 | Varies from usual routine or methods to explore better effects. May question need to do less obvious or tedious steps (pretreating spots, or rearranges to fit. Aware of spatial capacity of washing machines and adjusts load sizes. May not anticipate secondary effects (leaving dyes or bleaches in the laundry area, failing to remove clothes from the dryer | Provides assistance as for 5.0. | Patient will solve problems involving spatial properties with assistance to avoid harmful effects. Caregiver: same as 5.0. | Same as 5.0. |

| Level | Behavior | Assistance | Goal | Warnings |
|---|---|---|---|---|
| | to prevent wrinkling). May not allow enough time to do laundry before an event. | | | |
| 5.6 | Compares laundry methods, substitutes products/methods based on consideration of primary and known secondary effects. May fail to consider potential secondary effects. | Caregiver points our potential secondary effects to avoid. | Patient will compare methods to solve problems in laundry with assistance to avoid harmful effects. Caregiver: same as 5.0. | |
| 5.8 | Plans out new solutions with objects present. May not consider the needs of others (sharing apartment laundry facilities). May not consider potential secondary effects. | Caregiver assists with organizing new laundry routines that consider the needs of others. Verifies new solutions. Identifies potential effects to avoid damage to garments, machines, persons. | Patient will plan solutions to problems when objects are present. Caregiver: same as 5.0. | |
| 6.0 | Plans out solutions to new laundry problems with no objects present. Considers hazards of improper use, storage, combining of cleaning agents; potential ways to damage garments or linens; the needs of others in scheduling or purchasing supplies. Allows adequate time for laundry completion for routine and special events. | No assistance required. | Patient will plan and complete laundry activities for self and others in a safe, effective, flexible manner. | |

## 11.5 Situational Awareness Disability: Traveling

Traveling includes using a vehicle as a means of conveyance for the self or objects, inside buildings and around the community. Vehicles include carts, wagons, wheelchairs, bicycles, cars, buses, trains, and airplanes. Traveling may consist of selecting a destination; deciding on means of transportation, route, time to go and return; collecting objects for the trip; and finding one's way there and back. This category excludes walking, major role disability.

| LEVEL | BEHAVIOR | ASSISTANCE | GOAL | WARNINGS |
|---|---|---|---|---|
| 1.0-1.6 | Lies on bed with wheels or gurney while pushed by caregiver to destination. No awareness of traveling. | Bed with side rails. Checks that restraints are tied securely. | Caregiver will arrange for transportation of patient in gurney or bed. | Check restraints. |
| 1.8 | May sit up in a wheelchair when tied in while being pushed to destination. | Caregiver restrains to prevent sliding out of chair. | Caregiver will arrange for transportation of patient in gurney or wheelchair to essential destinations. | Check restraints. Essential travel only is recommended. |
| 2.0-2.2 | Sits in wheelchair to be pushed by caregivers. Rights self if starts to fall (2.2). May seem to enjoy riding in chair or may try to get out. | Positions wheelchair and provides cues to provides cues to perform transfers into chair; restrains to prevent patient standing up (2.2). | Caregiver will arrange and provide assistance for transportation of patient in wheelchair for short distances. Patient will sit in wheelchair for short trips. | Travel for short distances only is recommended. Discomfort may resist in striking out or attempts to leave chair. |
| 2.4 | May follow a guide to a car or other vehicle. May need assistance to step up into car. May enjoy riding in a vehicle, looking at the scenery for short trips. No awareness of destination. | Caregiver makes travel arrangements for short trips. Guides patient to vehicle. Gives verbal and physical guidance to step into vehicle. | Caregiver will arrange and provide assistance for travel in vehicles for short distances, or will push wheelchair to desired destinations. Patient will sit in vehicles/wheelchair to reach destinations determined by others. | Patient may leave vehicle or chair if left alone and wander off. Lock car doors. |
| 2.6 | Walks toward vehicles when told, steps in. May push on closed doors to get in or out. | Caregiver directs patient to car. Makes arrangements for short trips. | Caregiver: same as 2.4. Patient: same as 2.4. | Same as 2.4. |

| Level | Behavior | Assistance | Goal | Warnings |
|-------|----------|-----------|------|----------|
| 2.8 | May grab door handle or back of seat to assist with getting in and out. May push and pull on wheelchair to propel self for a short distance. | Caregiver provides assistance as for 2.4. Cues to grab handles or bars on vehicles to assist with getting in and out. | Caregiver: same as 2.4. Patient will sit in vehicles or wheelchairs to reach destinations determined by others. Will grab handles to assist entering and leaving vehicles. | May propel wheelchair into walls or furniture. |
| 3.0 | May grab door handles when entering/leaving vehicles. May propel wheelchair in circles. | Makes all arrangements and accompanies on short trips (private car or taxi). | Patient: same as 2.8. Caregiver: same as 2.4. | Same as 2.8. |
| 3.2 | May attempt to open doors of vehicles or may accidentally open while vehicles are moving. | Caregiver provides assistance as for 3.0. Locks doors on inside. | Patient: same as 2.8. Caregiver: same as 2.4. | Lock doors on inside. |
| 3.4 | May sit for periods up to 30 minutes in a private car or taxi driven by others. May not be aware of destinations, but may recognize some features of a highly familiar route. May need breaks for trips longer that 30 minutes. May propel wheelchair forward or backward for short distances but may not get around furniture, through small doorways; forgets to set brakes and may get lost if allowed outside. May attempt to get on a bike or skateboard if familiar, but may fall. May attempt to enter or leave vehicles before they are stopped. | Caregiver makes all travel arrangements including determining destinations, mode of transport, departure time, packing. Stops for breaks as needed. Provides manual activity (eating), music, conversation, to capture attention and reduce restlessness. Clears space to increase mobility and limit damage to walls and furniture when patient is in wheelchair. Restricts access to bicycles, skateboards, and public transportation. | Patient will sit in vehicles to reach destinations determined by caregiver. Caregiver will arrange accompanied trips with assistance to avoid discomfort due to restlessness or distractibility. | Restrict access to community or public transportation if patient wanders. Do not leave alone on trips. |

| LEVEL | BEHAVIOR | ASSISTANCE | GOAL | WARNINGS |
|---|---|---|---|---|
| 3.6 | May wait for vehicles to stop before leaving when cued. May get into any available car, bus, train, or elevator without consideration of destination or cost. | Caregiver provides assistance as for 3.4. | Patient: same as 3.4. Caregiver: same as 3.4. | Watch for impulsive actions such as getting on a bus or waiting elevator. |
| 3.8 | Sits for periods of up to an hour in a private car or taxi, and expresses awareness of destination after arrival. May be able to ride on bus or train with caregiver for short trips. | Caregiver determines destinations, arranges means, and pays for short trips. Accompanies on bus or other form of public transportation. May sequence through actions of paying fare or ticket. | Patient will sit in vehicles driven by others for up to an hour. Caregiver will arrange transportation for short trips; will accompany on public transportation. | Accompany on all trips using public transportation. |
| 4.0 | May initiate traveling to a familiar destination a short distance away by a highly familiar means (bus, bicycle). May become easily confused by unexpected environmental changes. Aware of destination throughout trip. May resist going to unfamiliar locations or altering a familiar mode of transportation. May not tolerate travel more than 1 hour. May forget critical items or steps (taking bus fare) and does not consider travel time or other secondary effects (hazards of route). Attends only to a few striking visible cues in environment in immediate vicinity with possible hazardous results (may not be aware of cars, traffic signals, or uneven terrain). | Caregiver makes travel arrangements for all but highly routine and local excursions. Accompanies patient to all new locations. Checks that patient has essentials for short, unaccompanied trips, including telephone numbers, money to call if lost or stranded. Discourages use of bicycles on busy streets. Shows alternate routes and accompanies patient until well-learned. | Patient will initiate and complete short trips to familiar destinations by familiar means with caregiver assistance to avoid harmful effects. Caregiver will plan and accompany patient to all new or distant locations and will monitor local trips to avoid harmful effects. | May become very anxious in new or stimulus-laden environments (bus or airport terminals). |

| Level | Behavior | Assistance | Goal | Warnings |
|---|---|---|---|---|
| 4.2 | Initiates travel to a familiar destination by familiar means. May become fixated on one feature/step and have trouble completing the activity (such as calling a cab) or may go through the actions slowly, irritating or inconveniencing others. Can sit unaccompanied for periods of up to an hour on bus, train, taxi, or subway and uses familiar landmarks, one at a time, to guide getting on or off. Asks for assistance if lost or if landmarks change. Does not alter familiar routes or travel to new locations without assistance. | Caregiver monitors familiar travel arrangements made by patient and makes all new travel arrangements. Provides telephone numbers, money for emergencies, and specifies what to do if lost. Accompanies on new or distant travels. | Patient: same as 4.0. Caregiver: same as 4.0. | Same as 4.0. |
| 4.4 | Initiates travel to familiar destinations at routine times in vehicles driven by others. Needs new routes or travel procedures identified by others. Learns these by noting visible cues after days to weeks of practice. May be able to use a limited number of striking cues to find his or her way in a new environment. May express interest in driving a car or motorcycle but fails to attend to all necessary cues in environment to do so safely. May not allow adequate time for travel or fail to consult other schedules before starting out. May fail to consider travel needs for | Caregiver provides assistance as in 4.2. Assists with planning travel needs, longer trips. Identifies ways to safeguard property and money. Discourages use of motor vehicles or motorcycles. Discourages use of skates or skateboards without protection of helmet, knee pads. | Patient will initiate and complete routine travel in vehicles operated by others and will accept assistance for new or distant travel. | May be upset by changes in usual travel routines. Advise against operating motor vehicles. |

| LEVEL | BEHAVIOR | ASSISTANCE | GOAL | WARNINGS |
|---|---|---|---|---|
| | longer trips: expenses; medication supply; clothing needs based on anticipated weather, activities, length of trip. May insist on driving a car or traveling alone to new locations with negative consequences. | | | |
| 4.6 | May vary familiar routes traveled without awareness of consequences. May impulsively take a trip to a new location and get lost. May scan environment for information to guide travel (posted schedule, gate numbers). Does not anticipate problems or travel needs in new situations, as in 4.4. | Caregiver provides assistance as in 4.4. | Patient: same as 4.4. Caregiver: same as 4.4. | Watch for problems resulting from variations in usual travel routes or "spontaneous" travel. |
| 4.8 | Learns new routes or travel procedures (reading a bus schedule) slowly by rote. May follow safety precautions pointed out by others related to travel. Does not anticipate hazards. May learn use of a wheelchair slowly but has difficulty maneuvering in tight locations or in estimating space requirements. If allowed to operate a motor vehicle, may do so slowly, or dangerously, unable to anticipate or react quickly to the movements of others. | Caregiver assists with rote learning of new travel routes or procedures by adding new steps one at a time. Identifies safety precautions (guarding money, labeling luggage, carrying emergency telephone numbers), and assists with anticipating travel needs for lengthy trips. Encourages use of public transportation as alternative to operating motor-driven vehicles. | Patient will travel to new locations and learn new travel procedures by rote with assistance to avoid harmful effects. Caregiver will assist rote learning of travel routes/procedures. | Operation of motor vehicles may be dangerous. |

| Level | Behavior | Assistance | Goal | Warnings |
|---|---|---|---|---|
| 5.0 | Varies range of motion and strength to learn use of wheelchair, bicycle, skateboard, skates, or to pull a cart or shift gears in a car. Can make a schedule for traveling to new locations but has trouble adhering to it; may miss bus, train, or other scheduled transport frequently. May need assistance to read and understand an unfamiliar schedule for bus/train. | Caregiver assists with planning departure times to ensure making travel connections. Identifies safety hazards that are secondary or hidden. Assists with planning for essential travel needs, including emergency money and telephone numbers. | Patient will travel to new locations using new methods of transport with caregiver assistance to avoid harmful effects. Caregiver will identify relevant secondary effects and safety precautions to consider in traveling. | Patient may miss scheduled transportation. |
| 5.2 | May be able to read and understand bus/train schedules on grids. May be able to adhere to travel schedules by relying on alarms, calendars. May impulsively leave on a trip without planning for money, clothing, medication needs or without notifying others. | Caregiver explains consequences of unplanned excursions to unfamiliar locations. | Patient: same as 5.0. Caregiver: same as 5.0. | Impulsive travel may occur. |
| 5.4 | Travels to new locations independently. Considers spatial arrangements of streets, buildings, and is generally aware of distances travelled. Has trouble estimating time requirements and may miss scheduled connections. May get lost frequently. May try to use a map, but without success. Discovers new routes and remembers them. May be able to operate a motor vehicle but with | Caregiver identifies safety hazards in traveling to new locations, and assists in planning travel needs including response to emergencies. Points out consequences of failure to consider schedules, needs of others. Encourages use of helmets with motorcycle or bicycle operation. | Patient will travel to new destinations with caregiver assistance to avoid harmful effects. Caregiver: same as 5.0. | Operating motorcycles or cars may be hazardous. Patient may resist assistance. |

| Level | Behavior | Assistance | Goal | Warnings |
|---|---|---|---|---|
| | increased incidence of problems (accident, running out of gas, parking tickets) due to failure to anticipate and consider the movements of other motorists and pedestrians and to plan own actions. May not recognize his or her behavior as hazardous. May question need to plan out schedules or identify travel needs. | | | Patient may ignore needs of others in traveling and may appear self-centered. |
| 5.6 | Compares travel routes and methods to a destination. May consult travel brochures, maps, others. Estimates volume of objects in space and moves accordingly (moves wheelchair in and around new environments effectively, parks a car in tight space). Keeps track of travel times. May fail to consider the needs of others, hazards, travel needs in new settings. | Caregiver provides assistance as for 5.4. | Patient will compare travel routes and methods with caregiver assistance to avoid harmful effects. Caregiver: same as 5.0. | |
| 5.8 | Plans new travel arrangements in the presence of material objects (schedules, calendar, lists of needed items). May need assistance to plan overall organization. May be able to collaborate with others in making decisions. New secondary considerations and effects may need to be identified (need for insurance, | Caregiver assists with making new travel arrangements by providing material objects and suggesting overall organization. Identifies essential safety considerations, and new secondary and intangible effects. | Patient will plan new travel arrangements in the presence of material objects with caregiver assistance. Caregiver: same as 5.0. | |

| LEVEL | BEHAVIOR | ASSISTANCE | GOAL | WARNINGS |
|-------|----------|------------|------|----------|
| | money conversion, inoculations for overseas travel, jet lag, time-zone changes, need to conform to local customs when traveling, etc.). | | | |
| 6.0 | Plans out travel methods and routes by considering several possible courses of action. Factors considered include needs of others, limitations of time and expense, implications for job or family life, travel needs for duration of trip. Considers safety and plans to avoid known or potential harm to self and others. Operates motor vehicles with appropriate level of care. | No assistance is needed. | Patient will plan and complete travel by selected means to routine and new destinations safely. | |

## 11.6 Situational Awareness Disability: Telephoning

Telephoning includes understanding how to use the telephone; deciding to make a call; obtaining and dialing the numbers; leaving messages; answering the telephone; relaying messages; accounting for time-zone changes; recognizing an emergency and using emergency numbers; and paying the telephone bill.

| LEVEL | BEHAVIOR | ASSISTANCE | GOAL | WARNINGS |
|---|---|---|---|---|
| 1.0-3.0 | Does not use the telephone or does not have opportunity to use telephone. | All telephoning is done for patient. | Caregiver will handle all telephone calls for patient. | Locate telephone cords away from pathways to prevent tripping. |
| 3.2 | May pick up telephone within reach and place on ear; telephone may not have rung. May not converse, or may converse when no one is on the line. May leave receiver off hook. Is unable to make call or relay message. | Caregiver locates telephones away from view and reach. All telephoning is done for patient. | Caregiver: same as 1.0. | Locate telephones away from view and reach. |
| 3.4 | Picks up telephone when it rings and says "Hello." May be able to call for another person or may hang up the telephone if call is not for them. May not relay a message or understand message given. May be able to dial one or two well-known numbers over and over. May call for no reason. May forget to hang up the receiver. Cannot locate numbers in the telephone book or though information. | Caregiver makes all telephone calls for patient or supervises dialing from private telephones. Restricts access to public phones to avoid loss of money. Sequences patient through actions of dialing for social calls. Answers telephone or instructs patient to ask caregiver to come to the telephone for messages. | Patient will use telephone with supervision to call familiar numbers. Caregiver will sequence patient through steps to complete telephone calls. | May call familiar or emergency numbers over and over. |
| 3.6 | May be able to imitate a modification in an action such as waiting for caregiver or answering machine to answer the | Caregiver demonstrates modifications in actions that increase effective use of telephone. | Patient will use telephone with supervision to call a few familiar numbers and will imitate desired modifications in | Same as 3.4. |

| Level | Behavior | Assistance | Goal | Warnings |
|---|---|---|---|---|
| | telephone when it rings or pushing telephone into cradle to ensure that it is hung up properly. The reasons for such modifications are not understood. May be trained to dial 911 but cannot judge when to properly use emergency numbers. | | actions. Caregiver will supervise or make telephone calls for patient to ensure outcome, and will demonstrate modifications in action. | |
| 3.8 | May be trained to complete a simple telephone call involving a new number and procedure (i.e., caregiver work number or 911). Does not generalize procedure to new situation and may be unable to determine when to call. | Caregiver provides assistance, same as for 3.6. Trains patient to learn highly valued number and related actions. | Patient will use telephone with supervision to dial a few familiar numbers and will be trained to dial highly valued numbers. Caregiver will supervise or make telephone calls or ensure outcome, and will train patient to make highly valued calls. | Does not judge when an emergency exists. May dial 911 at inappropriate times. |
| 4.0 | Initiates and completes a call to a familiar number (picks up receiver, dials number, waits for response, converses or leaves message, and hangs up). May be able to use a public telephone if familiar to call a known number; may attempt to use and forget to bring money or put in the wrong amount. May be able to repeat a simple message for another. If problem occurs so that call is not completed, may abandon the task. May not ask for help. Does not consider best | Caregiver looks up new numbers and makes unfamiliar calls (operator assisted, pay telephones, out-of-area direct dialing). Is available to take messages and solve problems with call completion. Informs of appropriate times of day for calling; restricts access to telephone if used excessively or inappropriately. Does not expect patient to learn to operate unfamiliar and complex equipment (answering or fax machines, calling cards). | Patient will initiate and complete calls to familiar numbers and will complete calls to new numbers with caregiver assistance to avoid harmful effects. Caregiver will monitor telephoning to solve problems, make new calls, and avoid harmful effects. | May call emergency or other numbers excessively. May ignore time of day when calling. |

| LEVEL | BEHAVIOR | ASSISTANCE | GOAL | WARNINGS |
|---|---|---|---|---|
| | time of day for calling or changes in time zones or costs of calls. May forget reason for call. | | | Same as 4.0. |
| 4.2 | Dials a new number written down by checking it one digit at a time. May be able to call information for a new number but writes it down very slowly; may have to call back to hear it again. May not use the telephone directory or yellow pages. May not be able to locate infrequently used numbers in an address book. Remembers reason for calls, but may call the same person each time he or she has a reason, making several calls instead of one. Does not consider the other person's schedule, the time of day, the costs of calls, changes in time zones. Needs assistance to make calls on unfamiliar telephones, with lengthy numbers or complex procedures. Recognizes problems and requests assistance. | Caregiver provides assistance same as for 4.0. Posts regularly used numbers, including emergency numbers, at eye level next to telephone. Places paper and pencil in visible location next to telephone for messages or for making lists for future calls. | Patient will complete calls by matching written numbers and will request caregiver assistance for locating new numbers or solving problems in telephoning. Caregiver will provide written numbers, will monitor telephoning to solve problems and avoid harmful effects. | |
| 4.4 | Initiates and completes routine telephone calls to familiar numbers from private and pay telephones. May prefer to call the operator for new numbers. Writes down new numbers or messages slowly. May | Caregiver provides lists of frequently used and emergency numbers at eye level or within 3 to 4 feet of telephone. Highlights important numbers for easy recognition in address books or | Patient will complete routine telephone calls with assistance from visible cues and will accept caregiver assistance to avoid harmful effects. Caregiver: same as 4.2. | May make calls at inappropriate times of day or may run up big telephone bills. |

| Level | Behavior | Assistance | Goal | Warnings |
|---|---|---|---|---|
|  | attempt to use address book or directory by looking for a striking cue (a picture advertisement in yellow pages, bold-face type, page number). May make calls at odd hours or in the middle of the night, or talk at length without regard for other person's schedule. Cannot alter rate of speech to fit a time limit. Does not consider costs of calls, time-zone changes in long-distance calling. | directories. Assists with making calls requiring unfamiliar procedures or to different time zones. Specifies conditions for using 911. Trains, step by step, in use of unfamiliar equipment such as answering machines, if desirable. |  |  |
| 4.6 | May be able to alter rate of speech to fit a time limit (3-minute call). May vary usual procedure of making/receiving a call without anticipating resulting problems. May find a number in an address book or telephone directory by searching a page for a particular word or name. May not locate items in yellow pages by using classifications and sub-classifications. | Caregiver provides assistance as 4.4. Provides step-by-step demonstration of variations in telephone routine. | Patient will complete routine telephoning. Will scan visible environment for cues to make calls, and will accept assistance to solve problems. Caregiver: same as 4.4. | Watch for problems resulting from varying telephone routine. |
| 4.8 | Learns use of new telephone, answering machine, or pay telephone by rote, noting all striking features of objects. Applies new learning rigidly, and does not vary actions; adjusts to changes in procedures or numbers with difficulty. Follows emergency guidelines rigidly and | Assists patient with rote learning of new telephone technology or procedures by adding steps one at a time using patient's own telephone/equipment. Identifies emergency telephone procedures and verifies comprehension. Assists with identifying socially | Patient will learn use of new telephone technology or telephone etiquette by rote with assistance from caregiver to avoid harmful effects. Caregiver will assist patient in rote learning of new telephone procedures and will identify harmful secondary effects. |  |

| LEVEL | BEHAVIOR | ASSISTANCE | GOAL | WARNINGS |
|---|---|---|---|---|
| 5.0-5.4 | may be slow to act. May memorize correct times to call others. May limit calls to a predetermined amount of time. May need assistance to adjust to changes in telephone procedures, to learn use of new technologies, to find subclasses in the telephone directory, and to identify telephone etiquette.<br><br>Learns new telephone procedures by imitating several steps at a time. May look up new numbers in directory or address books independently. May not use yellow pages, or may fail to use subclasses (government agencies listed under city). May become confused by new options and ignore them (answering machines, call waiting, FAX machines, television telephone order-recording options) or may learn to use by trial and error. May confuse three-digit special services (411 and 911). Use of telephone appears to be self-centered (may make collect calls, may not consider time of day, others' schedules, may not limit number or length of calls). May run up large telephone bills. May not distinguish between various types of long distance calls and make expensive | appropriate calling times and other guidelines. Assists with finding numbers using subclasses in yellow pages. Identifies secondary effects of excessive telephoning.<br><br>Caregiver identifies consequences of failing to consider cost, length, types of calls. Demonstrates use of new equipment serially and check comprehension. Handles complex optional equipment. Assists with planning telephone use to stay within limited budgets. Assists with use of the yellow pages. | Patient will manage telephoning needs with caregiver assistance to anticipate and avoid harmful effects. Caregiver will identify secondary effects of telephoning to avoid. | Patient may appear self-centered in telephone use. May run up expensive bills. |

| LEVEL | BEHAVIOR | ASSISTANCE | GOAL | WARNINGS |
|---|---|---|---|---|
| | person-to-person calls. Has trouble adjusting rate of speech to a time limit. May try to talk on the telephone and do other things at the same time with resulting errors in other tasks. | | | |
| 5.6 | Compares well-learned procedures with other methods and alters, (makes a call in a few different ways, depending on circumstances). Varies rate of speech to adjust to a timed call but may lose track of time as converses. May consider telephone etiquette, including use of special services (911). May use directories successfully. Seeks explanations of secondary effects before places a call (cost, convenience to others, time-zone changes). May not anticipate telephone needs in special situations (travel). | Caregiver provides assistance same as 5.0. | Patient compares and substitutes telephone procedures with assistance to consider secondary effects to avoid. | Same as 5.0. |
| 5.8 | Plans out new telephone calls requiring novel procedures when options and secondary effects are identified by others | Caregiver points out options and secondary effects (cost, schedules of others, time-zone considerations) to assist in planning for new calls. | Patient will plan new telephone calls with assistance to identify secondary effects. Caregiver will assist with planning by identifying secondary effects. | |
| 6.0 | Plans out new telephone calls independently, considering secondary effects such as cost, availability of other | No assistance is needed. | Patient will plan and execute telephoning by considering various options and their consequences. | |

| LEVEL | BEHAVIOR | ASSISTANCE | GOAL | WARNINGS |
|-------|----------|------------|------|----------|
|  | person, time-zone changes. Considers and selects best method (private, pay, car, or company telephone) in light of consequences. Conducts conversation with awareness of other's situation and time. Plans use of directories and special telephone services. |  |  |  |

# Chapter 8

# Teaching the Physically Disabled

## Tina Blue, OTR

**T**his chapter adds physical problems to a part of the body and describes how teaching a person how to adapt to physical limitations is affected by cognitive disabilities. The physical impairments include sensation, range of motion, strength, abnormal reflexes/tone, gross upper-extremity coordination/motor control, and fine-motor coordination. The overall roles of the occupational therapist, patient, and caregiver are described. Considerations for arriving at effective treatment goals are specified.

The second part of this chapter adds environmental compensations for physical impairments to body parts: architectural barriers/safety, wheelchairs, orthotics, and prosthetics. This chapter provides a general approach to environmental compensations. More specific approaches to adaptive equipment are discussed in Chapter 9.

The third part addresses training techniques used to teach new ways of doing functional activities with physical disabilities. The greater specificity of the decimal system is used in this section to clarify training procedures specific to occupational therapy. The topics covered include dressing, transfers, joint protection, and energy conservation techniques. These topics are addressed from the perspective of teaching that does not necessarily involve adaptive equipment.

## Occupational Therapist, Patient, and Caregiver Roles

Occupational therapists are mandated by definition to facilitate the adaptive process to help patients master their highest level of potential function in selected meaningful activities. Included are the ability to recognize their disability and direct a caregiver to do things not physically possible for the patients. When a cognitive disability is present the patient may not recognize his or her disability or be able to corroborate with the therapist to identify realistic treatment outcomes. A reliable caregiver will need to be included in the treatment planning at the beginning to identify goals (Allen, 1989). The caregiver should also be present during the treatment process to learn how to apply treatment methods and the necessary physical and cognitive assistance required to ensure maximum performance capability and safety of the patient. The patient and caregiver are also given information about the expected natural course of healing with regard to when performance typically begins to plateau and minimal improvements in performance are expected (Finger, 1988). With the cognitively disabled, the therapist plays a key role in the integration of these relationships.

## Treatment Considerations

Effective treatment goals and methods are arrived at during an initial evaluation that accomplishes the following:

- Obtains a premorbid history of functional performance.

- Describes a patient's current functional status: type of disability (e.g., personal care disability, body disposition disability, dexterity disability, etc.); level of cognitive assistance; and level of physical assistance.

- Identifies expected changes in life style in terms of physical independence and occupational disability; patient/caregiver awareness of the consequences of potential disability.

- Identifies the nature of the social support system currently available to the patient, especially the availability of an acceptable caregiver.

- Measures the impairment status as it relates to the disability (e.g., impaired range of motion and strength that causes a body disposition and/or dexterity disability).

- Identifies activities that are important to the patient/caregiver and will be used to establish treatment goals.

- Predicts the rehabilitation potential, the targeted functional outcomes, and the significance in the reduction of the disability within the context of the patient's life (Allen, Foto, Spering, & Wilson, 1989).

Most current protocols for teaching the physically disabled tend to assume a normal ability to learn. Do not assume all patients operate at level 6. Administer the Allen Cognitive Level (ACL) task evaluation to screen for cognitive ability (Allen, 1985). If it is not possible for the patient to do the ACL, observe performance in another activity the patient can do before selecting treatment goals and methods. This may be especially challenging for assessing the patients at the lower cognitive levels of 2 and 3, who are either not physically able to, or refuse to, manipulate the leather lacing. Activities commonly found in rehabilitation settings, like the Minnesota Rate of Manipulation Test (MRMT) or form boards can be used to assess ability to imitate and sustain repetitive actions, check effects of actions with objects (e.g., turning discs over to expose a different color), and use shape and/or color to guide actions.

Verbal information from the patient cannot in and of itself be used as a valid determination of cognitive ability. Patients can be quite disabled despite undisturbed language function. There is often a discrepancy between verbal and motor abilities, which is often more pronounced with patients who have had central nervous system damage (Kaplan & Smith, 1986). For example, a patient with right hemispheric damage may talk like someone at level 5 but perform motor actions at level 3.

When treatment involves teaching information to the patient, cognitive ability overrides the physical disability when selecting treatment goals and methods. A good example would be teaching joint protection and energy conservation techniques, expecting the patient to generalize methods to everyday living. In all of these types of self-administered programs, expected functional outcomes depend on the patient's ability to learn and carry over information. Therefore, the cognitive ability to learn is more important than the physical problem.

When the cognitive level cannot be validated because the physical impairment is so severe that it prevents the patient from being able to manipulate material objects, the physical impairment will override the cognitive level. Select initial treatment goals and methods that address the physical impairments and observe for opportunities to evaluate cognitive abilities.

When severe physical limitations are present that do not necessarily affect cognitive functioning, do not assume level 6 and observe for cognitive ability. These patients can be observed in task performance situations involving directing a caregiver. Is the patient directing the caregiver in a goal-directed manner? Is he or she able to plan the caregiver's actions in new learning situations considering his or her own level of physical disability in relation to safety and efficiency factors? Computers may also be helpful in evaluating cognitive ability by analyzing programs for level of task demand (i.e., solving problems involving sequencing actions and arranging spatial properties).

Experienced therapists realize that level 6 patients may perform very safely and efficiently in their community. These people learn to use environmental alterations, adaptive equipment, and housekeeper/chore person to function despite severe physical handicap.

## Functional Outcomes, Treatment Methods, and Cognitive Assistance

The next two sections will describe treatment methods and the amount of cognitive assistance required to achieve functional outcomes by the 6 cognitive levels.

Physical impairments can be improved with therapeutic intervention in the postacute phase of treatment. Residual impairments cause or contribute to the disability and may be either improved or compensated for in the rehabilitation phase to reduce disability. There are no hard and fast rules here since most patients are still in the postacute phase of recovery when they come to rehabilitation. Therefore, guidelines for treatment will include both the postacute and rehabilitation phases.

The choice of treatment is infinite and should be determined by professional judgment. However, specific treatment techniques will be included to be used as comparative guidelines to modify treatment approaches for patients with varying degrees of cognitive impairment. We will start with level 6 where there is no limit on what can be taught, shifting to teaching the caregiver to give standby assistance at level 5, and using visually cued, situation-specific training at level 4. Treatment methods change to drilling patients in repetitive actions at level 3 as the burden of caregiver responsibility increases, to ensure functional outcomes and the safety of the patient. Treatment methods shift to primarily training the caregiver at levels 2 and 1 when maximum to total assistance is required to perform activities and prevent medical complica-

tions. Caregiver assistance codes are included to describe the amount of cognitive assistance required to ensure functional outcomes, and can also be used by therapists to describe the amount of cognitive assistance used during treatment. A description of the codes can be found in chapter 3, page 25.

The primary motivation for presenting the levels in this way is to provide therapists with a means of predicting successful functional outcomes of treatment and ensuring the safety of their patients. It is suggested that, while reading the levels, the reader compare the way treatment information is presented to the patient and the relative importance of caregiver assistance. Precautions are discussed to prevent safety problems and to help therapists adjust treatment methods for the level of cognitive disability.

Physical Impairments: Sensation

| Level | Functional Outcome | Treatment Methods | Caregiver Assistance | Precautions |
|---|---|---|---|---|
| 6 | Improve impaired upper extremity sensation to reduce body disposition and/or dexterity disabilities. Prevent medical complications. | Assess cutaneous, kinesthetic, and stereognostic sensation. Teach patient sensory reeducation or desensitization techniques using verbal, written, and/or diagrammed instruction. Teach methods like Tinel's sign to self-monitor progress of nerve repairs. Teach proper positioning for parts at risk for injury (e.g., flaccid shoulder). Patient will be able to understand conceptual and abstract medical explanations of condition. Teach patient to compensate for asensory areas visually and by planning actions to prevent mechanical injury. | | |
| 5 | Same as level 6. | Demonstrate treatment program based on testing results. Identify potentially hazardous activities that may cause mechanical damage to asensory areas (e.g., smoking, cutting food). Demonstrate visual, biomechanical, and mechanical compensations. Point out visible and tactile cues that demarcate affected areas. Demonstrate methods like Tinel's sign to self-monitor progress of nerve repairs. Point out awkward prehension patterns that result from | Standby: To check treatment compliance; point out potentially hazardous situations. | Avoid abstract medical explanations of condition with patient. Provide concrete examples of consequences of treatment noncompliance (e.g., pictures in books, existing injured areas). Avoid or adapt splinting to affected areas. Provide written, individualized home program. |

Sensation, *continued*

| LEVEL | FUNCTIONAL OUTCOME | TREATMENT METHODS | CAREGIVER ASSISTANCE | PRECAUTIONS |
|---|---|---|---|---|
| | | median/ulnar nerve injuries, and have patient practice making neuromuscular adjustments while doing functional activities. Provide visual and verbal cuing to point out ineffective motions, abnormally positioned parts at risk for injury (e.g., flaccid shoulder), and potentially hazardous situations. Train caregiver in methods to facilitate treatment compliance. | | Caregiver to prevent medical complications. Avoid using abstract medical explanations with patient. Avoid splinting over asensory areas. |
| 4 | Same. | Alert caregiver and patient to areas that are at risk for injury. Train patient to use unaffected parts to check water temperature. Train caregiver to clearly label ambiguous appliance controls. Initiate training patient in sensory reeducation techniques one step and part at a time. Supervise use of abrasive modalities for cuing to adjust pressure and duration of repetitive movements. Set up goal-directed activities for stereognosis, like "treasure hunt" in rice bins, provided patient has samples of items being searched for in intact hand to facilitate comparison. Teach caregiver methods like Tinel's sign to monitor nerve | Minimum: To initiate and follow through with home programs; supervise patient in potentially hazardous activities; cue patient to reposition parts at risk for injury; alter home environment to compensate for disability. | |

Sensation, *continued*

| LEVEL | FUNCTIONAL OUTCOME | TREATMENT METHODS | CAREGIVER ASSISTANCE | PRECAUTIONS |
|---|---|---|---|---|
| | | repair progress. Demonstrate use of simple adaptive equipment to protect asensory areas and compensate for awkward prehension resulting from residual impairments (e.g., built-up handles, extended dispenser handles, velcro fasteners, etc.). Incorporate task-analyzed crafts and/or familiar functional activities that incorporate both upper extremities. Cue patient to reposition flaccid extremities at risk for injury. Train caregiver how to setup and assist with activities at home. | | |
| 3 | Compensate for impaired upper extremity sensation to prevent medical complications. | Grossly assess cutaneous and kinesthetic sensation and alert caregiver to protect areas that are impaired. May train caregiver in sensory stimulation techniques, like massage and passive range of motion. Apply and demonstrate use of simple adaptive equipment that compensates for awkward grasping patterns (e.g., built-up, cuffed utensils) and encourages use of affected hand while doing classic repetitive upper extremity motions. Supervise caregiver performance with patient. | Moderate: To supervise patient in potentially hazardous situations; reposition parts that are abnormally positioned and at risk for injury (e.g., flaccid upper extremities). Apply stimulation techniques and monitor patient's response. | Caregiver to prevent medical complications. Avoid splinting over asensory areas. Keep verbal directions simple with patient (i.e., noun and verb). |

Sensation, *continued*

| LEVEL | FUNCTIONAL OUTCOME | TREATMENT METHODS | CAREGIVER ASSISTANCE | PRECAUTIONS |
|---|---|---|---|---|
| 2 | Same as level 3. | Grossly assess cutaneous sensation and alert caregiver. May train caregiver in sensory stimulation techniques, if not noxious to patient. Supervise caregiver performance while monitoring patient's response. If splinting is necessary, opt for comparable positioning with less resistive materials (e.g., foam, tubing, etc.). Train caregiver to check frequently for correct fit to prevent chaffing. | Maximum: To apply stimulation techniques; check splint fit and body positioning. | Caregiver to prevent medical complications. Avoid or adapt splinting over asensory areas. Avoid restraining over impaired areas. |
| 1 | Same. | Alert caregiver to suspected impaired areas. Train in sensory stimulation techniques. Use alternative splinting to suspected impaired areas. Train caregiver to apply positioners and to check frequently for chaffing/systemic changes. | Total: Same as level 2. | Caregiver to prevent medical complications. Avoid splinting or restraining over suspected impaired areas. |

Physical Impairments: Range of Motion

| Level | Functional Outcome | Treatment Methods | Caregiver Assistance | Precautions |
|---|---|---|---|---|
| 6 | Improve impaired range of motion to reduce body disposition and/or dexterity disabilities; prevent medical complications. Compensate for residual limitations. | Teach patient range of motion exercises and special techniques to prevent undesired movements or damage to weak musculature or surgically repaired joints. Use splints as applicable with instructions for wear and care. No limit on type or amount of information given. Incorporate use of adaptive devices as needed to compensate for residual limitations. | | |
| 5 | Same as level 6. | Demonstrate to patient correct and incorrect movements. Use verbal and visual cues to correct maneuvers. Demonstrate correct and incorrect splint application. Use functional activities like crafts to reinforce generalization to other activities using desired movements. Demonstrate use of adaptive devices as needed to compensate for residual limitations. Train caregiver in methods for standby assistance to facilitate treatment compliance. | Standby: To cue for undesired movements; check for treatment compliance. | Avoid abstract medical explanations or use of diagrams with patient. Opt for slower, safer gains with concrete goals since patient may be impulsively anxious to achieve gains faster than advised. Provide concrete examples of consequences of treatment (e.g., pictures, patient's own worsening deformity). Write out individualized program for exercises and splint wear and care. |

Range of Motion, *continued*

| LEVEL | FUNCTIONAL OUTCOME | TREATMENT METHODS | CAREGIVER ASSISTANCE | PRECAUTIONS |
|-------|--------------------|--------------------|----------------------|-------------|
| 4 | Same. | Train patient in exercises, one part and action at a time. Provide constant tactile, visual, verbal cuing to correct improper positioning, undesired or unsafe motions. Manually support weak joints for safety (e.g., flaccid shoulder). Demonstrate donning and doffing splints, one step at a time; preadjust straps. Supervise task-analyzed crafts or familiar tasks that incorporate desired actions; encourage bilateral upper extremity use to prevent "guarding" affected extremity. Train caregiver in methods and home program for exercises and splint wear. | Minimum: To continue training; cue/correct undesired or unsafe maneuvers; initiate home program for exercises, splint wear and care; readjust splint position and straps as needed. | Caregiver to prevent medical complications. Avoid use of abstract medical explanations or use of diagrams with patient. Patient may need assistance with diagonal maneuvers. Avoid use of unfamiliar adaptive equipment that would require making new neuromuscular adjustments. Do not expect patient to generalize training. |
| 3 | Same. | Initiate drilling patient to imitate repetitive active range of motion exercises. Provide visual and tactile cuing to halt perseveration or unsafe maneuvers. Incorporate simple repetitive activities that reinforce motions (e.g., MRMT, pegs, hygiene, grooming). Train caregiver how to don/doff splints, readjust straps for home wear and care. Also train caregiver regarding home exercise program and supervise performance with patient. | Moderate: To continue drilling in active range of motion exercises; apply passive range of motion exercises for safety; initiate and follow schedule for exercises and splint wear and care. | Caregiver to prevent medical complications. Avoid having patient do self-range of motion exercises to prevent overstretching of weak joints. Keep verbal directions to patient simple (i.e., noun and verb). Use splints with caution; patient may take them off or use them in an unsafe manner. |

Range of Motion, *continued*

| LEVEL | FUNCTIONAL OUTCOME | TREATMENT METHODS | CAREGIVER ASSISTANCE | PRECAUTIONS |
|---|---|---|---|---|
| 2 | Improve impaired range of motion to reduce body disposition disabilities associated with patient care; prevent medical complications associated with joint deformities. | Train caregiver in application of active range of motion exercises; facilitate postural actions by demonstrating repetitive body movements, incorporating actions with familiar objects (e.g., tossing beach ball, using feeding utensils, etc.). Patient may also be set up with reciprocal pulleys for continuous up and down movements if shoulder is not weak or flaccid. Train caregiver in application of splints/positioners. Supervise caregiver performance with patient. | Maximum: To apply active and passive range of motion exercises; follow schedule for exercises, wear and care of splints/positioners. | Caregiver to prevent medical complications. |
| 1 | Same as level 2. | Train caregiver in application of passive range of motion exercises, splints/positioners. Supervise caregiver performance with patient. | Total: To apply exercises; follow schedule for exercises, wear and care of splints/positioners. | Same as level 2. |

Physical Impairments: Upper Extremity Strength

| LEVEL | FUNCTIONAL OUTCOME | TREATMENT METHODS | CAREGIVER ASSISTANCE | PRECAUTIONS |
|-------|--------------------|--------------------|----------------------|-------------|
| 6 | Improve impaired strength to reduce locomotor, body disposition, and/or dexterity disabilities. Compensate for residual limitations. | Teach graded resistive exercises and activities. Include techniques that prevent undesired compensatory movements or damage to weak, subluxed, or surgically repaired joints. Provide information regarding increasing resistance as safely tolerated per protocol. Instruct in use and care of mobile arm supports, suspension slings, and other adaptive devices that compensate for residual limitations. | | |
| 5 | Same as level 6. | Demonstrate resistive exercises; cue to correct unsafe positioning, speed, and duration of motions. Monitor patient's response to program and increase resistance per protocol. Demonstrate use and care of adaptive devices to compensate for residual limitations. Supervise task-analyzed activities to increase strength and reinforce safety principles. Train caregiver in methods to provide standby assistance and ensure treatment compliance at home. | Standby: To cue for positioning, speed, and duration motions; check for treatment compliance; remind patient to monitor vital functions as applicable. | Opt for slower, safer gains with concrete goals since patient may be impulsively anxious to achieve gains faster than advised (e.g., thinking "over-exercising" is better). Provide concrete examples of consequences of treatment noncompliance (e.g., pictures of dislocated joints, patient's own pain and stiffness). Avoid abstract medical explanations to patient. Provide individualized plan for exercises and activities including rest periods. Incorporate need to warm up and check vital functions, as applicable. |

Upper Extremity Strength, *continued*

| LEVEL | FUNCTIONAL OUTCOME | TREATMENT METHODS | CAREGIVER ASSISTANCE | PRECAUTIONS |
|---|---|---|---|---|
| 4 | Same. | Train patient in resistive exercises, one part at a time. Provide constant visual and tactile cuing to correct ineffective or unsafe maneuvers, errors in duration, and speed of movements. Adjunct with familiar or task-analyzed functional activities that incorporate desired motions and resistance using bilateral upper extremities. Increase resistance per protocol. Set up mobile arm supports/suspension slings, position patient's arm, and train in task-specific settings. Train patient in use of simple adaptive devices that compensate for residual weakness (e.g., levered dispenser handles), and/or ones that can be operated with normal movement patterns (e.g., looped scissors). Train caregiver in home program for exercises, activities, and equipment wear and care. Supervise patient's performance to facilitate compliance with methods. | Minimum: To continue training and cue for/correct undesired motions including speed and duration; initiate an individualized program, including setting up new activities and monitoring vital functions. | Caregiver to prevent medical complications. Avoid use of abstract medical explanations, use of written or diagrammed instructions with patient. Patient may need assistance with diagonal maneuvers that target specific muscle groups. Avoid use of unfamiliar adaptive equipment that requires making new neuromuscular adjustments. Do not expect patient to generalize training. |
| 3 | Same. | Initiate drilling patient to imitate repetitive resistive exercises and activities (e.g., dowel with weight, clothespin ladder, theraputty, hand grippers, theraband, wringing wet towel, etc.). | Moderate: To continue drilling; initiate and follow home program, including setting up activities, applying adaptive equipment and monitoring vital functions. | Caregiver to prevent medical complications. Avoid diagonal or fine-motor maneuvers where patient is required to make intentional new neuromuscular |

Upper Extremity Strength, *continued*

| LEVEL | FUNCTIONAL OUTCOME | TREATMENT METHODS | CAREGIVER ASSISTANCE | PRECAUTIONS |
|---|---|---|---|---|
| | | | | adjustments that target specific muscle groups. Avoid activities that would elicit undesired motions. Keep verbal directions to patient simple (i.e., noun and verb). Avoid use of adaptive equipment that would require patient to be goal-directed and/or to learn new neuromuscular adjustments. |
| | | Provide visual and tactile cuing to halt perseverative or unsafe movements. Determine amount of resistance and adjust according to protocol. Monitor vital functions as needed. Provide adaptive equipment that uses characteristic motions to compensate for residual limitations in grasp and pinch (e.g., built-up utensils, extended door knobs, etc.) Train caregiver in home program for exercises, activities, equipment use and care. Supervise performance with patient. | | |
| 2 | Improve impaired strength; preserve active range of motion to reduce personal care disability associated with patient care. | Train caregiver to facilitate postural actions for active and active-assistive exercises; incorporate movements with familiar objects (e.g., built-up feeding utensils, large-handled cups, tossing beach ball). Supervise caregiver performance with patient to ensure compliance with methods. | Maximum: To apply active and active-assistive exercises; apply adaptive equipment, initiate activities; follow individualized schedule including rest periods and monitoring vital functions as applicable. | Caregiver to prevent medical complications. |
| 1 | Preserve active movement when possible; assist weak movements for purposes of patient care (e.g., positioning). | Train caregiver in sensory stimulation techniques to try and elicit active movement from extremities. Supervise caregiver performance with patient. | Total: To apply sensory stimulation techniques; assist active movement. | Goals not applicable for specific strengthening. Caregiver to prevent medical complications. |

Physical Impairments: Abnormal Reflexes/Tone

| Level | Functional Outcome | Treatment Methods | Caregiver Assistance | Precautions |
|-------|--------------------|--------------------|----------------------|-------------|
| 6 | Improve abnormal reflexes/tone to reduce locomotor, body disposition, and/or dexterity disabilities. | Facilitate normal postural reactions, muscle tone, and selective movement through the use of sensorimotor, neurodevelopmental positioning and handling, PNF techniques, Affolter, and/or Brunnstrom's approach, as applicable. Instruct patient in basic neurophysiological principles. Train in specific techniques that will carry over planned methods. Patient should be able to follow instructions and use internal and external feedback systems to plan, organize, and terminate motor actions. After a period of training and practice, patient should be able to understand and carry over principles learned to independently correct or prevent unwanted movements and incorporate them into motor actions performed during ADLs after discharge if residual impairments are not severe. | If patient is moderately to severely physically impaired, he or she may direct caregiver to set up environment and provide external key points of control through tactile cuing. | |
| 5 | Same as level 6. | Demonstrate basic neurophysiological principles while performing treatment. Provide verbal, visual, and tactile cuing to correct position set, timing, and duration of transitional movements. Assist with planning actions; incorporate movements | Standby: To cue patient while he or she performs transitional movements in functional tasks at home. | Avoid abstract medical explanations to patient. May not be as effective with severe kinesthetic and proprioceptive impairments since this limits internal feedback system information. |

Abnormal Reflexes/Tone, *continued*

| LEVEL | FUNCTIONAL OUTCOME | TREATMENT METHODS | CAREGIVER ASSISTANCE | PRECAUTIONS |
|---|---|---|---|---|
| 4 | Same. | into functional tasks and provide opportunities to practice generalization in many different settings. Train caregivers in methods and supervise performance with patient for facilitating carryover to home setting.<br><br>Train patient in situation-specific settings while incorporating positioning and handling techniques. Establish position and demonstrate cause and effects of techniques on patient's own body. Demonstrate desired movements one step at a time. Provide visual and tactile cuing to correct repeated errors in postural adjustments, pattern, speed, and duration of transitional movements. Train caregiver in basic neurophysiological principles and treatment methods. Supervise caregiver performance with patient to facilitate compliance with methods in discharge setting. | Minimum: To continue training; set up activities; establish position set and provide cuing to correct undesired postural adjustments and transitional movements. | Patient will require long-term repetitive training in task-specific situations. Patient may have difficulty making correct neuromuscular adjustments for transitional movements. Patient may need assistance with diagonal maneuvers. Patient will need assistance with planning actions before execution. Techniques will probably not be actively effective with severe sensory impairments. Patient not a candidate for techniques that require *learning* goal-directed actions. |
| 3 | Compensate for abnormal reflexes/tone to reduce personal care, body disposition, and dexterity disabilities associated with patient care. | Incorporate synergistic movements into familiar, repetitive activities to accomplish simple self-care. (*May try sensorimotor/NDT approaches if patient is reliably cooperative and caregiver is willing to | Moderate: To set up activities, continue drilling, and use sequence through actions. *If sensorimotor approaches are being tried, will have to provide external support for position set; give constant | Patient not a candidate for techniques that require learning goal-directed actions. Keep directions to patient simple (e.g., noun and verb). *If patient is very distractible, may |

Abnormal Reflexes/Tone, *continued*

| Level | Functional Outcome | Treatment Methods | Caregiver Assistance | Precautions |
|---|---|---|---|---|
| | | continue drilling and judge effectiveness of methods. Provide visual and tactile cuing to halt perseveration.) Use simple built-up or cuffed utensils to compensate for impaired grasp as needed. Train caregiver in compensations and handling techniques as applicable. Supervise performance with patient to facilitate compliance with methods in discharge setting. | visual and tactile cuing to correct errors while eliciting familiar repetitive actions. | counteract effects of NDT. *Patient will not be able to alter movements, speed, or duration of transitional actions without constant visual and tactile cuing. |
| 2 | Same. | Train caregiver in handling to reduce tone at key points of control for purposes of positioning; use of positioners to stabilize body parts and maintain positioning. Incorporate synergistic movements into drinking with adapted cups as able. Supervise performance with patient to facilitate compliance with methods. | Maximum: To physically guide patient into reflex-inhibiting patterns. Apply positioners and readjust as needed to maintain positioning. Initiate feeding with devices, as indicated. | Patient may actively resist handling if he or she is distressed or in pain. |
| 1 | Compensate for impaired reflexes/tone to prevent deformities and reduce body disposition disability associated with patient care. | Train caregiver in reflex-inhibiting patterns and use of positioning devices. Supervise performance with patient. | Total: To apply techniques and positioners. Making readjustments as needed. | |

Physical Impairments: Gross Upper Extremity Coordination/Motor Control (*See also "Abnormal Reflexes/Tone")

| LEVEL | FUNCTIONAL OUTCOME | TREATMENT METHODS | CAREGIVER ASSISTANCE | PRECAUTIONS |
|---|---|---|---|---|
| 6 | Improve impaired gross motor coordination/motor control to reduce body disposition disability. Compensate for residual limitations. | Teach gross motor coordination exercises. Teach compensatory techniques like weighting body parts, using resistive activities and adaptive equipment. Apply sensorimotor approaches as applicable. Teach muscle reeducation techniques and incorporate into functional tasks. Consult with patient before considering resistive bracing due to its expense and patient's potential concern regarding cosmesis. | | |
| 5 | Same as level 6. | Teach exercises and demonstrate use of compensatory techniques including use of adaptive devices. Apply sensorimotor approaches as applicable, providing verbal, visual, and tactile cuing to correct positioning, timing, and duration of motions. Demonstrate muscle reeducation techniques and cue to guide effective actions. Demonstrate desired and undesired outcomes. Incorporate supervised, task-analyzed activities to reinforce generalization of methods. Consult with patient and caregiver before considering resistive bracing. Train caregiver in methods to facilitate carry over at home. | Standby: To cue for ineffective positioning and motions; check for treatment compliance. | Avoid abstract medical explanations to patient. Provide individualized written program for exercises. |

Gross Upper Extremity Coordination/Motor Control, *continued*

| LEVEL | FUNCTIONAL OUTCOME | TREATMENT METHODS | CAREGIVER ASSISTANCE | PRECAUTIONS |
|---|---|---|---|---|
| 4 | Same. | Demonstrate gross motor exercises, one pattern of movement at a time. Apply sensorimotor approaches as applicable; demonstrate cause and effect of actions; provide visual and tactile cuing to correct ineffective positioning, timing, and duration of motions. Patient will also require step-by-step demonstration in task-specific situations to learn muscle reeducation techniques. Set up task-analyzed or routine activities to learn new neuromuscular adjustments. Provide constant supervision and assistance to identify and correct undesired outcomes. Compensate for residual impairments by weighting body parts and demonstrating use of adaptive equipment that incorporates normal actions. Train caregiver in techniques and supervise performance with patient to facilitate compliance of methods in discharge setting. | Minimum: To continue training; set up new activities; initiate exercise program; cue for/correct undesired positions and motions. | Avoid use of abstract medical explanations, diagrams, or written instructions with patient. Patient will require long-term repetitive training for muscle reeducation and disassociating gross motor patterns caused by CNS damage or functional surgeries. Patient may need assistance with diagonal patterns. Patient may not be a candidate for resistive bracing due to the level of neuromuscular adjustment required to operate device. |
| 3 | Same. | Initiate drilling patient in familiar, repetitive gross motor activities (e.g., brushing hair, wiping tables, tossing beach ball, bean bags, etc.). May try sensorimotor approaches if patient is | Moderate: To continue drilling. Initiate and follow home program, including setting up activities and sequencing through normal actions. If sensorimotor approaches are effective, will have to | Patient not a candidate for activities that would require him or her to be goal directed. Avoid demonstrating diagonal patterns of movement to patient, or give constant cuing |

Gross Upper Extremity Coordination/Motor Control, *continued*

| LEVEL | FUNCTIONAL OUTCOME | TREATMENT METHODS | CAREGIVER ASSISTANCE | PRECAUTIONS |
|-------|--------------------|--------------------|-----------------------|-------------|
| | | cooperative with efforts; provide external support to maintain positioning while eliciting repetitive actions. Compensate for residual limitations by weighting body parts and/or incorporating abnormal compensatory movements into familiar repetitive activities. Train caregiver in treatment methods. | provide external support to maintain positioning while eliciting repetitive motions. | for effective results. Keep verbal directions to patient simple (i.e., noun and verb). Patient is not a candidate for resistive bracing. |
| 2 | Compensate for impaired gross motor coordination/motor control to reduce personal care and disability associated with patient care. | Train caregiver in application of methods to facilitate postural actions. Supervise performance with patient to facilitate compliance with methods. | Maximum: To demonstrate postural actions, weight body parts, incorporating movements with weighted feeding utensils, and adapted cups (see Fine-Motor Coordination). | |
| 1 | Not applicable for specific compensation. Realistic objective would be to train caregiver to preserve movement efforts for purposes of care. | Train caregiver. | Total: To assist AROM when possible. | |

Physical Impairments: Fine-Motor Coordination

| Level | Functional Outcome | Treatment Methods | Caregiver Assistance | Precautions |
|---|---|---|---|---|
| 6 | Improve impaired fine-motor coordination to reduce dexterity disability. Compensate for residual limitations. | Teach fine-motor coordination exercises and activities. Instruct in wear and care of splints that dynamically assist prehension and/or position hand for function. Compensate for residual impairments with adaptive equipment. | | |
| 5 | Same. | Demonstrate specific placement and prehension patterns, desired and undesired outcomes of methods. Provide verbal, visual, and tactile cuing to correct undesired outcomes. Provide opportunities to practice using new movement patterns by having patient do craft activities. Point out comparable functional activities patient can generalize to. Demonstrate use and care of supportive and/or dynamic splints and adaptive equipment to compensate for residual impairments. | Standby: To cue patient during exercise and activities. Check for treatment compliance. | Avoid abstract medical explanations. Provide individualized written program for exercises, splint wear and care. |
| 4 | Same. | Engage patient in task-analyzed clinic activities that reinforce correct positioning, prehension patterns, and bilateral upper extremity use. Provide constant supervision to correct ineffective movement patterns using step-by-step | Minimal: To continue training, set up activities, cue for/correct undesired positions and motions; ensure correct splint fit and do long-term maintenance. Correct ineffective use of adaptive equipment. | Avoid abstract medical explanations to patient. Making fine-motor adjustments will be particularly difficult at this level; compensate with positioning and/or simple adaptive techniques (e.g., velcro |

Fine-Motor Coordination, *continued*

| LEVEL | FUNCTIONAL OUTCOME | TREATMENT METHODS | CAREGIVER ASSISTANCE | PRECAUTIONS |
|---|---|---|---|---|
| | | demonstration and tactile cuing. Provide simple adaptive equipment to compensate for residual impairments (e.g., built-up utensils, adapted writing utensils, static wrist splints, etc.). Demonstrate wear and care of devices to patient and caregiver. Integrate equipment into clinic activities and situation-specific tasks (e.g., writing, grooming, dressing, etc.) Train caregiver in treatment methods and supervise performance with patient. | | fasteners) and equipment when possible. Avoid dynamic splints and complicated devices that may require additional new learning and neuromuscular adjustments. Patient will require long-term repetitive training to learn new fine-motor adjustments. |
| 3 | Same. | Initiate drilling to engage patient in familiar repetitive fine-motor actions that reinforce functional prehension and upper extremity use (e.g., MRMT, pegs, washing hands, writing, folding linen, etc.). May also use task-analyzed craft activities if not too frustrating to patient, with assistance to sequence through steps (e.g., picking up and gluing large tile to trivet). Provide simple adaptive equipment to reinforce classic motions and compensate for residual impairments (e.g., built-up or cuffed utensils). Train caregiver in home program and supervise performance with patient. | Moderate: To continue drilling. Initiate and follow home program, including setting up activities and sequencing patient through normal actions. Apply and maintain equipment and splints. | Patient is not a candidate for activities that would require him or her to be goal directed. Keep verbal directions simple with patient (i.e., noun and verb) Use static splints with caution. Patient may try to take them or use them in an unsafe manner. If impairment is severe, opt for caregiver compensation versus frustrating patient with demands to make neuromuscular adjustments that are beyond his or her capacity to learn. |

Fine-Motor Coordination, *continued*

| LEVEL | FUNCTIONAL OUTCOME | TREATMENT METHODS | CAREGIVER ASSISTANCE | PRECAUTIONS |
|-------|--------------------|--------------------|----------------------|-------------|
| 2 | Compensate for impaired fine-motor coordination to reduce personal care disability associated with patient care. | Provide simple adaptive equipment (e.g., built-up feeding utensils, large-handled cups) to compensate for residual impairments. Train caregiver in application of devices and methods to facilitate postural actions. Supervise performance with patient. | Maximum: To place adaptive equipment in patient's hand and facilitate postural actions for eating and drinking. | |
| 1 | N/A. | N/A. | Total: To compensate for residual impairments. | |

Environmental Compensations: Architectural Barriers/Safety

Environmental compensations are used to reduce disabilities and prevent medical complications associated with residual physical impairments. Following are guidelines consistent with the previous format to analyze treatment methods according to 6 cognitive levels. Note: Levels 1 and 2 patients are not typically cared for at home and usually are discharged to skilled nursing facilities. However, in the event that a family wishes to assume caregiver responsibility, guidelines have been included to protect the patient.

| Level | Functional Outcome | Treatment Methods | Caregiver Assistance | Precautions |
| --- | --- | --- | --- | --- |
| 6 | Compensate for impaired mobility and architectural barriers to reduce personal care, locomotor, and/or body disposition disabilities, and prevent medical complications. | Collaborate with patient to consider home and environmental architectural barriers to plan needs for safety equipment, relevant adaptive equipment, and home/work modifications. Conceptualize environments through use of diagrams and/or models. Facilitate ability to speculate about future needs, research community resources, and make plans as needed for most safe and efficient performance. | Patient to direct others for physical assistance. | |
| 5 | Same as level 6. | Collaborate with patient and caregiver to anticipate home/work and environmental architectural barriers. Identify need for safety equipment and other environmental adaptations by using three-dimensional models and/or generalizing needs from hospital and clinic settings. Plan actions for patient to use relevant assistive/adaptive equipment. Attend home/work environment with patient and caregiver to confirm needs. Anticipate | Standby: To provide cuing to anticipate hazards, point out more efficient actions. | Make final assessment of equipment needs after making a home visit and before ordering equipment. |

Architectural Barriers/Safety, *continued*

| LEVEL | FUNCTIONAL OUTCOME | TREATMENT METHODS | CAREGIVER ASSISTANCE | PRECAUTIONS |
|---|---|---|---|---|
| 4 | Same. | need for extra assistance and provide a plan to direct others. Provide opportunities to role play, asking passersby for assistance. Teach caregiver methods to facilitate carry over.<br><br>Collaborate with caregiver and patient to confirm future needs. Emphasize avoiding potential problems and simplifying task environments. Teach caregiver to identify and remove potential safety hazards in the home and community. Adapt home environment to minimize barriers and avoid potentially hazardous situations (e.g., nonslip mats, rearrangement of furniture, grab bars, bath benches, etc.). Initiate training of patient in standard procedures. Train caregiver in methods and supervise performance with patient to facilitate compliance with safety standards. | Minimum: To continue training patient with environmental aids; removal of safety hazards and assisting with unfamiliar architectural barriers. | Caregiver to prevent medical complications associated with potential safety hazards.<br>Make at least two home visits: one with caregiver to confirm before ordering equipment (arranging for installation if possible), one with caregiver and patient to practice methods in situation-specific settings.<br>Do not expect patient to generalize procedures learned in clinic to home and community environments. |
| 3 | Compensate for impaired mobility and architectural barriers to reduce personal care, locomotor, and/or body disposition disabilities associated with patient care; prevent medical complications and protect environment. | Collaborate with caregiver to confirm future needs. Protect patient by adapting home environment (e.g., nonslip treads, stabilizing rugs, wiping up floor spills, avoiding changing basic familiar pattern of furniture, safety rails, using stove | Moderate: To continue drilling; complete sequencing of standard procedures; protect patient and environment. | Same as level 4.<br>Patient and environment will need to be protected due to non-goal-directed behavior.<br>Simplify verbal instructions with patient (i.e., noun and verb). |

Architectural Barriers/Safety, *continued*

| LEVEL | FUNCTIONAL OUTCOME | TREATMENT METHODS | CAREGIVER ASSISTANCE | PRECAUTIONS |
|---|---|---|---|---|
| | | burner and electrical outlet covers, etc.). Begin drilling patient in standard procedures with environmental aids. Protect environment by using toilet seat cover locks and removing valuables that might be knocked over, etc. Train caregiver in methods and supervise performance with patient. | | |
| 2 | Same as level 3. | Collaborate with caregiver to anticipate future needs, including environmental adaptations and safety equipment. Initiate facilitating postural actions to use grab bars and bath seats. Provide environmental adaptations to ensure patient safety (e.g., padding guardrails, use of joint pads, restraints, positioners, etc.). Adapt home environment to facilitate wheelchair/bed maneuverability. Train caregiver in methods and supervise performance with patient. | Maximum: To facilitate postural actions to use environmental aids; protect patient and environment. | Caregiver to prevent medical complications. Protect the environment in the event patient is independently mobile. Make at least two home visits: one to confirm needs with caregiver before ordering equipment, one with caregiver to practice methods. |
| 1 | Compensate for impaired mobility and architectural barriers to reduce body disposition disability associated with total patient care; prevent medical complications. | Collaborate with caregiver to anticipate future needs. Provide environmental adaptations to ensure patient's safety, such as padding guardrails, applying joint pads and positioning devices. Train caregiver in proper restraining techniques | Total: To position and protect patient. | Caregiver to prevent medical complications. Make at least one home visit to adapt home environment with caregiver and assess for additional safety and patient care needs. |

Architectural Barriers/Safety, *continued*

| Level | Functional Outcome | Treatment Methods | Caregiver Assistance | Precautions |
|-------|-------------------|-------------------|---------------------|-------------|
| | | and applications of positioners. Supervise performance with patient. Adapt home environment to facilitate chair/bed maneuverability. | | |
| | | | | |

Environmental Compensations: Wheelchairs

| LEVEL | FUNCTIONAL OUTCOME | TREATMENT METHODS | CAREGIVER ASSISTANCE | PRECAUTIONS |
|-------|--------------------|--------------------|-----------------------|-------------|
| 6 | Improve mobility through use of wheelchair to reduce locomotor disability. | Selection: Select wheelchair that will best meet patients' needs considering diagnosis, prognosis, age, size, weight, safety factors, method of transfer, and mode of propulsion. Collaborate with patient to consider expense factors, life style, and environment. Introduce optional features. Facilitate active problem solving to consider those features necessary for optimal function. Instruct patient in information regarding repairs and methods to obtain replacement parts. Mobility: Teach patient wheelchair management, facilitating inductive and deductive reasoning to learn to measure space and judge speed and distance with the wheelchair; adapt to viewing the environment form a different eye level. | | |
| 5 | Same as level 6. | Selection: Collaborate with patient and caregiver to consider expense factors, life style, and environment. Introduce and demonstrate optional features. Demonstrate wheelchair maintenance and point out common problems. Mobility: Demonstrate wheelchair | Standby: To check maintenance; check for failure to anticipate safety hazards; cue to unsafe maneuvers. | Write out individualized plan for maintenance, providing information regarding warranties, repairs, and methods to obtain replacement parts, including telephone numbers and addresses of sources. Identify consequences of impulsive or |

Wheelchairs, *continued*

| Level | Functional Outcome | Treatment Methods | Caregiver Assistance | Precautions |
|---|---|---|---|---|
| | | management techniques and point out all relevant safety factors. Facilitate inductive reasoning by demonstrating basic principles of measuring space and judging speed and distance with the wheelchair. Check for failure to anticipate safety hazards; cue for impulsive actions that are not organized and/or are too fast. Teach caregiver methods to facilitate carry over. | | unsafe maneuvers (e.g. doing "wheelies" across heavy traffic or downstairs). |
| 4 | Same. | Selection: Consider patient's desires and collaborate with caregiver to consider expense factors, life style, and environment. Consider only those features that are necessary for optimal function. Teach caregiver maintenance.<br>Mobility: Train patient in wheelchair management by providing step-by-step demonstration. Initiate situation-specific training in discharge setting to determine measurement of space, speed, and distance patient will have to learn in order to maneuver safely and effectively; provide striking visual cues to guide performance (e.g., marks on floor, furniture landmarks, etc.). Provide assistance in identifying and correcting repeated errors and check for compliance of standard procedures (e.g., | Minimum: To continue training; initiate maintenance; solve new problems; cue to reposition body parts; identify potential unsafe situations and remove hazards; provide assistance to maneuver in unfamiliar areas and resistive terrain; cue for compliance with standard procedures. | Caregiver to prevent medical complications (e.g., cue to reposition body parts; repair unsafe wheelchair parts; identify unsafe situations and remove hazards). |

Wheelchairs, *continued*

| LEVEL | FUNCTIONAL OUTCOME | TREATMENT METHODS | CAREGIVER ASSISTANCE | PRECAUTIONS |
|---|---|---|---|---|
| 3 | Same. | locking and unlocking brakes, etc.); position body parts. Teach caregiver home program and supervise performance with patient. <br><br> Selection: Collaborate with caregiver. Teach caregiver maintenance. <br> Mobility: Initiate drilling to facilitate repetitive actions to propel wheelchair forward or back with directive cues. Position weak body parts, have patient imitate locking and unlocking brakes with directive cues. Complete sequence of standard procedures for safety. Provide an open space for patient to maneuver safely in. Train caregiver in home program and supervise performance with patient. | Moderate: To continue drilling patient; manually assist around architectural barriers; complete sequence of standard procedures. | Caregiver prevent medical complications. Keep verbal directions to patient simple (i.e., noun and verb). Provide environmental supports to ensure patient is safely secured in wheelchair. Provide additional locking systems or posterior mounted brakes if patient will be in potentially hazardous situations where he or she may operate wheelchair in an unsafe manner. Provide assistance to stop perseverative actions or use of the wheelchair in an unsafe manner. |
| 2 | Improve mobility to reduce locomotor disability-related patient care. | Selection: Same as level 3. <br> Mobility: Train caregiver to use environmental supports to position patient in wheelchair and reposition body parts as needed. Teach caregiver wheelchair management considering safety and environmental factors. Supervise performance with patient. | Maximum: To position and propel patient; do wheelchair maintenance. | Caregiver to prevent medical complications. Provide environmental supports to ensure patient is safely secured in wheelchair. |
| 1 | Same as level 2. | Same. | Total: Same. | Same as level 2. |

Environmental Compensations: Upper Extremity Orthotics

| LEVEL | FUNCTIONAL OUTCOME | TREATMENT METHODS | CAREGIVER ASSISTANCE | PRECAUTIONS |
|---|---|---|---|---|
| 6 | Improve/protect hand function and/or range of motion to reduce body disposition and/or dexterity disabilities; prevent medical complications. | Teach patient application and use of static or dynamic splints. Establish wear and care schedule. If splint related to surgical protocol, facilitate understanding of underlying mechanism of injury by using verbal, written, and/or diagrammed information. Facilitate sensitivity to changing medical condition that may cause complications (e.g., ischemic, pressure areas, increased pain, edema) and other conditions that may require immediate follow-up. | | |
| 5 | Same as level 6. | Demonstrate to patient correct and incorrect application of static or dynamic splints. Point out potential pressure areas, symptoms of improper fit, systemic changes. Demonstrate underlying mechanism of injury by using three-dimensional models or making concrete comparisons of diagrams to patient's body part. Demonstrate activities patient can do while wearing splint. Initiate craft activity in clinic incorporating desired actions/resistance and cue to correct errors. Point out with what activities patient may need physical assistance. Teach caregiver methods to facilitate carry over. | Standby: To check for treatment compliance. | Provide concrete examples of consequences of treatment noncompliance. Write out individualized wear and care schedule for patient. Avoid abstract medical explanations of underlying mechanisms. Consider conservative approach, opting for slower, safer gains versus relying on patient's judgment to "wear to tolerance," since he or she may be impulsively anxious to achieve gains faster than advised. |

Upper Extremity Orthotics, *continued*

| LEVEL | FUNCTIONAL OUTCOME | TREATMENT METHODS | CAREGIVER ASSISTANCE | PRECAUTIONS |
|---|---|---|---|---|
| 4 | Same. | Train patient in application of splints, one step and body part at a time. If essential to use dynamic splinting, train caregiver in application to ensure proper fit and alignment. Demonstrate familiar activities and/or task-analyzed crafts patient can do using bilateral upper extremities with the splint on. Train caregiver in methods, including activities patient will need assistance with; supervise performance with patient. Provide caregiver with splint wear schedule. | Minimum: To continue training; follow splint wear and care schedule; readjust splint as needed; check for systemic changes; assist with activities patient should not or cannot do. | Caregiver to prevent medical complications. Avoid dynamic splinting to prevent medical complications that may result from improper fit. Avoid splinting if patient demonstrates functional neglect because the splint may reinforce the patient's impression that the part is "sick" and dependent. Patient will need long-term repetitive training to learn neuromuscular adjustments to operate functional dynamic splints (e.g., ratchet splints). |
| 3 | Same. | Train caregiver in application, precautions, and care of static splints. Provide simple adaptive equipment that can be attached to splint to encourage functional use of the affected upper extremity. Initiate familiar activities with repetitive actions using bilateral upper extremities. Supervise caregiver performance with patient. | Moderate: To apply splint; follow schedule for wear and care; make adjustments; check for systemic changes. | Caregiver to prevent medical complications. Avoid use of dynamic splints that would require constant monitoring or new neuromuscular adjustments. Avoid use of splints if patient exhibits tendency to use material objects in an idiosyncratic or dangerous fashion. Apply secure straps with D-rings or buckles to prevent premature removal by patient secondary to non-goal-directed actions. |

Upper Extremity Orthotics, *continued*

| Level | Functional Outcome | Treatment Methods | Caregiver Assistance | Precautions |
|---|---|---|---|---|
| 2 | Prevent deformities and/or protect weak joints to reduce body disposition disabilities associated with patient care; prevent complications associated with joint deformities. | Train caregiver in application and maintenance of splints; prevent medical complications. Provide schedule for wear and care. Facilitate monitoring patient's responses for pain that may be caused by splinting. Supervise caregiver performance with patient. | Same. | Caregiver to prevent medical complications. |
| 1 | Same as level 2. | Same as level 2. | Same as level 2. | Same as level 2. |

Environmental Compensations: Upper Extremity Prosthetics

| LEVEL | FUNCTIONAL OUTCOME | TREATMENT METHODS | CAREGIVER ASSISTANCE | PRECAUTIONS |
|-------|-------------------|-------------------|---------------------|-------------|
| 6 | Compensate for upper extremity amputation through use of prosthetics to reduce body disposition and dexterity disabilities. | Review stump hygiene/care with patient. Identify nomenclature of parts of prosthesis; review or teach maintenance. Teach operation of prosthesis using demonstrated, verbal, written, and/or diagrammed instruction. Teach indicators for improper fit and rely on patient's judgment to notify prosthetist for adjustments. Discuss need for psychological evaluation and vocational rehabilitation. | | |
| 5 | Same as level 6. | Identify nomenclature of parts on patient's prosthesis. Demonstrate maintenance. Evaluate fit and construction, and notify prosthetist regarding inconsistencies. Demonstrate operation of prosthesis. Provide opportunities for practicing new neuromuscular adjustments in activities that patient can generalize from. Provide functional activities, like crafts, in the clinic where standby assistance can be given to correct undesired motions and point out potentially hazardous or ineffective consequences of actions. Teach caregiver methods. Discuss | Standby: To check for treatment compliance. | Provide individualized schedule for stump and prosthesis maintenance. Provide concrete examples of treatment noncompliance. Schedule appointment with prosthetist for readjustments as applicable. Consult with other services regarding mild cognitive disability if applicable. |

Upper Extremity Prosthetics, *continued*

| Level | Functional Outcome | Treatment Methods | Caregiver Assistance | Precautions |
|-------|--------------------|-------------------|----------------------|-------------|
| 4 | Same. | psychological adjustments to a new disability. Assess need for psychological follow-up and vocational rehabilitation.<br><br>Review and demonstrate stump care to patient and caregiver. Identify nomenclature of patient's prosthesis, one part at a time. Notify the prosthetist regarding ill fit. Demonstrate donning and doffing device one step at a time. Train patient in use of device on action at a time in situation-specific tasks. Provide verbal and visual cuing to correct leverage and ineffective or unsafe actions. Train caregiver in home program. | Minimum: To initiate stump care and prosthesis maintenance; continue training; assist with potentially unsafe activities. | Caregiver to prevent medical complications.<br><br>Complicated dynamic terminal devices may not be an effective choice due to the higher demand for making new neuromuscular adjustments. Consult with prosthetist to consider simpler alternatives (e.g., working parts clearly visible, least complicated leverage, etc.).<br><br>*Note: If more complicated device is desired, consult with caregiver and insurance company to start intensive program for at least one month to assess carry over of learning and functional effectiveness.<br><br>Avoid written, diagrammed instructions, use of model or analogies with patient. Training must remain concrete and tangible in task-specific situation with little expectation for generalization of techniques.<br><br>Patient will require long-term repetitive training to learn new neuromuscular adjustments for effective results. |

Upper Extremity Prosthetics, *continued*

| LEVEL | FUNCTIONAL OUTCOME | TREATMENT METHODS | CAREGIVER ASSISTANCE | PRECAUTIONS |
|---|---|---|---|---|
| 3 | Same. | Train caregiver to perform stump care and do prosthetic maintenance. Demonstrate donning and doffing of prosthesis to caregiver. Initiate drilling patient in repetitive activities emphasizing use of affected extremity as a gross assist. Train caregiver in medical precautions and treatment methods and supervise performance with patient. | Moderate: To do stump and prosthetic maintenance; assist with donning and doffing; continue drilling; assist with bilateral fine-motor and potentially unsafe activities. | Caregiver to prevent medical complications. Avoid dynamic terminal devices that require goal-directed actions to learn a series of new steps and new neuromuscular adjustments. Consult with prosthetist for simpler alternatives. Avoid terminal devices that would present a potential safety hazard if used improperly or in a non-goal-directed manner (e.g., hooks). |
| 2 | Prevent medical complications associated with upper-extremity amputation; compensate for loss of function to reduce personal care, locomotor, body disposition, and dexterity disabilities associated with patient care. | Review stump care with caregiver. Demonstrate hygiene and bandage wrapping to caregiver, noting medical precautions. Initiate assisting patient with bilateral postural actions for the purposes of feeding and positioning. Supervise caregiver performing methods with patient. Teach caregiver to observe for improved cognitive ability, and to notify therapists for reevaluation if applicable. | Maximum: To perform stump care; assist with activities that require bilateral postural actions. | Caregiver to prevent medical complications. Patient is not a candidate for terminal devices. Assist initially for potential impaired balance during locomotor activities. |
| 1 | Same as level 2. | Demonstrate stump care to caregiver. Supervise performance with patient. Teach caregiver to observe for improved cognitive ability and to notify therapist for reevaluation if applicable. | Total: To perform stump care; compensate for lost movements. | Same as level 2. |

## Training Procedures

Learning training procedures with new physical disabilities places instructional and biomechanical demands on the patient's information processing system.

The predominant instructional demands are inherent in the person and require that the person:

• recognize the need to learn how to accomplish activities in a new way;

• be capable of learning and retaining a sequence of new actions or making alterations to a familiar sequence of actions;

• be capable of making alterations in normal movement patterns (new neuromuscular adjustments);

• be capable of solving problems for surface and spatial properties that would improve the effects of actions;

• be capable of considering potential secondary effects of actions (e.g., locking wheelchair before transferring; observing total hip or cardiac precautions while doing activities).

Biomechanical demands that increase physical disability and place additional demands on cognitive capacity include:

• impaired sensation

• impaired range of motion

• impaired strength

• impaired coordination

• impaired balance

• pain with movement

• edema

• impaired endurance

Increased physical disability requires increased cognitive ability to effectively compensate for personal care, locomotor, body disposition, and dexterity disabilities in a safe and efficient manner. At level 6, this is no problem. At level 4, training will be long and tedious with the therapist breaking down new learning procedures step-by-step in situation-specific settings and monitoring safety. At level 4.6, the patient can make brief neuromuscular adjustments and be trained to follow a few new steps. Training will require more repetition at level 4.6

than at level 4.8. At level 4.8, the patient can be trained to make several neuromuscular adjustments when the activity is broken down into segments for one new adjustment at a time. Training procedures will require very little repetition at level 5.0. A series of new steps and neuromuscular adjustments are learned, but a caregiver needs to stand by to cue for safety and solve new problems for surface and spatial properties.

Selected ADL training procedures commonly used by occupational therapists will be analyzed by the minimum mode of performance required to learn them effectively. The greater specificity of the decimal system, described in Chapter 5, will be used to further clarify the cognitive complexity of training procedures. Application of the decimal system can be found in Chapter 7. An additional category will be added if caregiver assistance will be needed to provide cuing, observe for safety precautions, and solve new problems.

Sometimes if a patient is very motivated and diligent and has a supportive caregiver who will agree to continue training, provide cuing, and solve new problems, successful results can be achieved with a cognitive capacity below the level of instructional demand. The minimal mode of performance should be regarded as a suggestion that can be overruled by professional judgment.

We have selected common training procedures used with CNS injuries since these are most likely to involve diminished cognitive ability and complicating biomechanical factors.

Instructional techniques, like joint protection and energy conservation techniques, designed for self-administration, will also be analyzed by the minimal mode of performance required to learn and generalize information for everyday use. Caregiver assistance will be included for confirmation of new methods and pointing out potential secondary effects of actions in new situations not originally targeted in rehabilitation.

These categories are not inclusive of the infinite variety of training techniques available to therapists and their patients. It is hoped that therapists will be able to generalize from these examples to analyze training procedures of their choosing based on professional judgment.

| LEVEL | TRAINING PROCEDURE | DEMANDS | CAREGIVER ASSISTANCE |
|---|---|---|---|
| 4.8 | Dressing for the hemiplegic patient:<br><br>Upper Extremity<br>• Position body for stability.<br>• Position garment correctly (inside of shirt up, collar closest to patient, etc.).<br>• Put garment on affected arm first.<br>• Work sleeve on completely.<br>• Pull garment around shoulder with or without adaptive aid.<br>• Attach fasteners.<br>• Reverse sequence to doff. | Capability to memorize a sequence of new actions by rote; imitate new neuromuscular adjustments, one adjustment at a time; note primary effects of actions, correcting any errors without assistance; rotate clothing and correct spatial location difficulties without assistance; respond to cuing to adjust for secondary effects (adjusting tail and collar after donning, slipping finger into belt loop to prevent trousers from falling down while standing up). | To solve problems for surface and spatial properties for different types of clothing and/or environments, giving extra time to memorize new sequences.<br>To assist with small or hard-to-reach fasteners.<br>To cue for secondary effects. |
| Same. | Lower Extremity (sitting position)<br>• Position body for stability.<br>• Cross hemiplegic leg over unaffected leg.<br>• Slip trouser over hemiplegic leg.<br>• Uncross leg.<br>• Slip on opposite trouser leg.<br>• Work trousers up to hips.<br>• Wiggle side to side, pulling pants over hips.<br>• Reverse sequence to doff. | Same. | Same. |
| 4.8 | Transfers for the hemiplegic patient:<br><br>Stand pivot transfers from a wheelchair<br>• Position wheelchair with stronger side at parallel angle with furniture.<br>• Lock both wheelchair brakes.<br>• Position feet evenly beneath body.<br>• Push up from wheelchair arm with stronger side.<br>• Establish balance while standing briefly.<br>• Turn body toward stronger side while flexing knees to sit, stabilizing body on furniture with stronger arm.<br>• Reverse sequence to transfer back to wheelchair. | Capability to memorize a new sequence of actions by rote; imitate neuromuscular adjustments, one adjustment at a time; correct spatial location of wheelchair; learn importance of consistently locking wheelchair brakes before attempting transfer to prevent safety hazards. | To remove safety hazards in the environment.<br>To check for compliance with standard procedures for safety.<br>To retrain in unfamiliar settings, allowing extra time to memorize new solutions. |

| Level | Training Procedure | Demands | Caregiver Assistance |
|-------|--------------------|---------|----------------------|
| 5.4 | Sliding Board Transfers<br>• Position wheelchair with stronger side at parallel angle with furniture.<br>• Lock wheelchair brakes.<br>• Remove wheelchair arm and put in accessible place.<br>• Place transfer board for stability underneath hip and overlapping furniture.<br>• Use stronger side to pull body over, scooting over transfer board and onto furniture.<br>• Remove transfer board and put in accessible place.<br>• Push wheelchair slight distance away.<br>• Hook unaffected leg under hemiplegic leg to pull onto furniture if going into supine position.<br>• Reverse sequence to transfer back to wheelchair. | Capability to consider space between wheelchair and furniture; consider overlap of transfer board in relation to distance between wheelchair and furniture; make fine-motor adjustments to remove wheelchair arm; make postural adjustments for differing transfer heights; heed verbal explanations regarding safety precautions. | To check safety. |
| 5.6. | Joint Protection Principles for the Arthritic Patient:<br>• Target known activities that would cause excessive strain on joints.<br>• Avoid positions that cause deformity.<br>• Learn alterations in familiar deforming causing positions.<br>• Avoid sustained positions; change positions or activities frequently.<br>• Use adaptive equipment as needed.<br>• Get assistance when needed.<br>• Plan actions to use the strongest joint for heavy work.<br>• Apply leverage principles to use joints to greatest mechanical advantage.<br>• Respect pain.<br>• Prioritize needs.<br>• Plan activities to maximize function, range of motion, and prevent deformities. | Capability to compare methods to vary and improve performance; change the pace of actions on request. | To remind patient to change position or activities as needed.<br>To remind patient to respect pain and rest as needed.<br>To identify need to get assistance considering others' schedules.<br>To assist with prioritizing needs, planning actions, and using leverage principles.<br>To point out potential secondary effects to avoid new or unexpected situations. |

| LEVEL | TRAINING PROCEDURE | DEMANDS | CAREGIVER ASSISTANCE |
|---|---|---|---|
| 5.6 | Energy Saving Techniques<br>• Target known activities that would consume unnecessary energy or put patient at risk.<br>• Combine tasks to conserve energy.<br>• Prioritize needs.<br>• Plan actions including use of adaptive equipment, making environmental modifications, and getting assistance.<br>• Monitor medical condition (blood pressure, pulse) as needed. | Capability to compare methods to vary and improve performance; change the pace of actions on request; see relations between parts and whole in three-dimensional space. | To assist with prioritizing needs and planning activities.<br>To remind patient of time constraints.<br>To identify the need to get assistance, considering others' schedules.<br>To assist with planning for long-term needs.<br>To remind patient to monitor medical condition as needed.<br>To point out potential secondary effects to avoid in new or unexpected situations. |
| Same. | Work Simplification:<br>• Target known activities that could be simplified for more efficient performance.<br>• Use both hands to work in opposite and symmetrical motions for gross motor activities (dusting, window cleaning, etc.).<br>• Slide objects to avoid lifting and carrying.<br>• Select equipment that may be used for more than one job; eliminate unnecessary motions.<br>• Avoid holding or unnecessary resistive actions; use adaptive equipment to simplify work.<br>• Use gravity to assist motions.<br>• Organize work areas.<br>• Sit to work whenever possible.<br>• Make environmental alterations for best access to work (adjusting table heights, etc.).<br>• Get help when needed.<br>• Monitor medical conditions as needed. | Same. | Same. |

Six cognitive levels can be used as a general framework for setting treatment goals. Professional judgment is required to sequence treatment goals, identify methods, and estimate the length of time needed to achieve goals. The caregiver is considered as an integral part of the treatment process considering the level of assistance the patient will need after hospitalization. This chapter presents guidelines for what can be achieved given the patient's current cognitive level.

## Acknowledgments

I gratefully acknowledge the occupational therapy department of Glendale Adventist Medical Center, Glendale, California, for allowing me to have their patients perform the ACL task evaluations during my work there. The clinical observations I have made there over the past four years have been contributory and invaluable in the confirmation of this model for patients with physical and cognitive disabilities in a rehabilitation setting.

## References

Allen, C.K. (1985). *Occupational therapy for psychiatric diseases: Measurement and management of cognitive disabilities.* Boston: Little, Brown.

Allen, C.K. (1989). Treatment plans in cognitive rehabilitation. *Occupational Therapy Practice, 1,* 1-8.

Allen, C.K., Foto, M., Sperling, T.M., & Wilson, D. (1989). Outpatient occupational therapy Medicare part B guidelines (DHHS Transmittal No. 565). In *Health insurance manual.* Baltimore, MD: Health Care Financing Administration.

Finger, S. (1988). *Brain injury and recovery: Theoretical and controversial issues.* New York Plenum Press.

Kaplan, P.E., & Smith, H.D. (1986). *Stroke rehabilitation.* Boston: Butterworth.

## Suggested Readings

Abreau, B.C., & Toglia, J.P. (1987). Cognitive rehabilitation: A model for occupational therapy. *American Journal of Occupational Therapy, 41,* 439-448.

Bailey, D.M., & DeFelice, T. (1991). Evaluating movement for switch use in adults with severe physical and cognitive impairments (case report). *American Journal of Occupational Therapy, 45,* 76-79.

Bonita, R., & Beaglehole, R. (1988). Recovery of motor function after stroke. *Stroke, 19,* 1497-1500.

Brandstate, M.E., & Basmajian, J.V. (Eds.). (1987). *Stroke rehabilitation.* Baltimore, MD: Williams & Wilkins.

Duncan, P.W., & Badke, M.B. (Eds.). (1987). *Rehabilitation: The recovery of motor control.* Chicago: Year Book Medical Publishers.

Earhart, C.A., & Allen, C.K. (1988). *Cognitive disabilities: Expanded activity analysis.* Colchester, CT: S & S Worldwide.

Hasselkus, B.R. (1991). Ethical dilemmas in family caregiving for the elderly: Implications for occupational therapy. *American Journal of Occupational Therapy, 45,* 206-212.

Hopkins, H.L., & Smith, H.D. (Eds.). (1988). *Willard and Spackman's occupational therapy* (7th ed.). Philadelphia: Lippincott.

Lee, W.A. (1989). A control systems framework for understanding normal and abnormal posture. *American Journal of Occupational Therapy, 43,* 291-301.

O'Sullivan, S.B., & Schmitz, T.J. (Eds.). (1988). *Physical rehabilitation: Assessment and treatment* (2nd ed.). Philadelphia: F.A. Davis.

Pedretti, L.W., Zoltan, B. (Eds.). (1990). *Occupational therapy: Practice skills for physical disabilities* (3rd ed.). St. Louis: Mosby.

Sabari, J.S. (1991). Motor learning concepts applied to activity-based intervention with adults with hemiplegia. *American Journal of Occupational Therapy, 45,* 523-530.

Silliman, R.A., Wagner, E.H., & Fletcher, R.H. (1987). The social and functional consequences of stroke for elderly patients. *Stroke, 18,* 200-203.

Toglia, J.P. (1991). Generalization of treatment: A multicontext approach to cognitive perceptual impairment in adults with brain injury. *American Journal of Occupational Therapy, 45,* 505.

World Health Organization. (1980). *International classification of impairments, disabilities, and handicaps.* Geneva: Author.

# Chapter 9

# Learning to Use Adaptive Equipment

## Tina Blue, OTR

**A**daptive equipment is the use of material objects to *compensate* for weak or abnormal movement patterns. Most of the pieces of equipment are commercially available and are used to do self-care and situational activities.

Adaptive equipment is used to make alterations in the environment. Alterations are made to:

- Increase accessibility (e.g., widened doorways, elevated toilet seats, portable mirrors);
- Provide stability (e.g., grab bars, tub seats, body positioners, bath mats);
- Ensure safety (e.g., safety straps, posterior-mounted wheelchair brakes, security bars to doors);
- Simplify patient care (e.g., shampoo basins, garments for incontinency, adaptive clothing, hospital beds);
- Prevent further medical problems (e.g., antipressure cushions, medical alert tags, positional splints);
- Conserve energy (e.g., velcro shoe fasteners, extended dispenser handles, reachers); and
- Accomplish tasks in a new way (e.g., button aids, rocker knives, toilet tissue aids, suction hand brushes).

This chapter recognizes the purposes stated above as being of primary importance in doing activities. In this chapter, the modes of performance required to learn how to use the pieces of equipment effectively are analyzed. Assumptions are made that the patient or caregiver wants to fulfill one of the goals stated above and that commercially available equipment will be used whenever possible. Once the assumptions can be reasonably made, the next question is can the equipment be used effectively and safely? Cognitive guidelines for answering that question are suggested.

The uniformity of these pieces of equipment makes it possible to do a detailed analysis of the mechanical and instructional demands placed on the person's information-processing system. The decimal system described in chapter 5 is used to suggest the lowest mode of performance that a person needs to learn to use the equipment.

A general framework for the activity analysis contains the cognitive level, type of compensation that can be achieved, and type of response demanded by the environmental stimuli. An overview of these criteria is provided in Table 9.1.

Pieces of equipment that can be used successfully with severe cognitive disabilities (levels 1 and 2) provide a *passive compensation* for normal movements. Patients do not have to think to be able to use a passive compensation effectively; the compensation is made by external force. Passive compensations do not require a change in normal actions or the formation of new sensorimotor models because the force is external. There is no cognitive demand on the patient. Examples of passive compensations are positioners, safety straps, and antipressure cushions. Pieces of equipment that can be used at levels 3 and 4 require *active compensation*. Patients move these material objects, but they do not have to learn how to change their normal movement patterns. *Dynamic compensations* are learned comfortably at levels 5 and 6. Dynamic compensations place more complex demands on the information-processing system. The differentiation between active and dynamic compensation is based on the cognitive complexity of the information that must be processed to use the equipment effectively.

The information provided by adaptive equipment is divided into three categories: biomechanical, mechanical, and instructional (see Table 9.2). Biomechanical information comes from the musculoskeletal system. At level 1, adaptations are from a totally external force and do not require processing from either a biomechanical or cognitive level. At level 2, biomechanical information can be processed to overcome the effects of gravity and to indicate comfort or pain. Mechanical information comes from material objects and is processed according to usual body movements. Mechanical demands can be processed at levels 3 and 4. Instructional information comes from material objects and is processed comfortably at levels 5 and 6 to change usual body movement patterns to learn a new way of doing things. By processing the information, the individual meets a cognitive demand required to successfully use a piece of adaptive equipment.

## Decimal System

Further breakdown of the cognitive complexity can be achieved with the decimal system described in

Table 9.1 Cognitive activity analysis of adaptive equipment

| Cognitive level | Compensation | Demand |
| --- | --- | --- |
| 1 | Passive | None |
| 2 | Passive | Biomechanical |
| 3 | Active | Mechanical |
| 4 | Active | Mechanical |
| 5 | Dynamic | Instructional |
| 6 | Dynamic | Instructional |

Table 9.2 Information provided by adaptive equipment

### Biomechanical demands (level 2)

(Inherent in the person)

- Sensation
- Range of motion
- Strength
- Coordination
- Balance
- Pain with movement
- Edema
- Endurance

### Mechanical demands (levels 3 and 4)

(Inherent in the device)

- Object has unfamiliar appearance (new sensory cues)
- Object requires use of normal movement patterns in a characteristic manner (includes pushing, pulling, grasping, pinching, turning, lifting, placing)
- Object supplies leverage to simplify actions and overcome resistance
- Object requires set-up (can be done by caregiver)

### Predominant instructional demands (levels 5 and 6)

(Inherent in person)

- Willingness to use equipment versus having caregiver assist with activity
- Capability to learn and retain a sequence of new actions
- Capability to solve problems for surface and spatial properties that would improve effects of device use

chapter 5. Active and dynamic compensations required to operate the equipment are used to orient the reader to the move detailed analysis.

*Active compensations* may require identification of new sensory cues combined with normal action. Normal actions include pushing, grasping, pinching, turning, lifting, and placing. There may be a change in appearance that is normally associated with the material object. Some devices have adaptations built in, as with built-up or weighted utensils, and require normal manipulative actions to operate them, achievable at levels 3.2 to 3.4. Other examples would be use of utensil cuffs (donned with the assistance of a caregiver), enlarged cup handles, and spouted cups. Drilling patients to match a linear cue to attach velcro buttons or modify actions to use a scoop dish may be effective at level 3.6. Active processing may be successful in the 4.0 to 4.4 range if simple mechanical leverage is supplied without requiring a change in normal actions or alteration of a sequence of familiar actions. Examples of these types of equipment would be extended dispenser handles, tab-grabbers, and looped scissors.

*Dynamic compensations* require changing normal actions or learning a sequence of new actions, achievable at level 4.6 and up. Spontaneous neuromuscular adjustments of short duration may or may not be successful at level 4.6. At level 4.8, the patient may be able to memorize a longer sequence of steps (usually more than four) and imitate a series of new neuromuscular adjustments, one new adjustment at a time. However, training results may be inflexible, frustrating, and abandoned at level 4.8 without the benefit of prolonged, situation-specific training and the availability of a caregiver to solve new problems that require continuous neuromuscular adjustments or response to tangible properties in new situations (using a dressing stick to put on different types of clothing). The capability to learn several new steps at one time while making continuous neuromuscular adjustments is learned more comfortably at level 5.0. When a device requires making continuous neuromuscular adjustments in response to surface and spatial properties, the demand for effective learning increases to level 5.4 (e.g., using a button aid). Equipment requiring adjusting to all tangible properties and following a tedious sequence independently, like routinely inspecting potential skin breakdown areas with an adjustable, extended mirror, may be successfully taught at a higher mode of performance of level 5.6.

In the next section, selected equipment representing passive, active, and dynamic compensations will be analyzed by the recommended minimal mode of performance required for use. The minimum level of physical disability inherent in the need for the piece of equipment will be considered. Increased physical disability requires increased cognitive ability to be able to learn how to use the equipment effectively and safely. For example, a patient with shoulder range of motion limitations may only need a cognitive level of 4.6 to be able to learn to use a long scrub sponge to bathe, versus a patient with postural instability who will need to be at 5.4 in order to make the spontaneous postural adjustments necessary to prevent falling while washing hard-to-reach areas.

An additional category will be added if caregiver assistance will be needed to observe safety precautions, do set-up, perform maintenance, provide cuing, or solve new problems. Equipment will be categorized according to the World Health Organization's (1980) two-digit categories for disability.

Some equipment has not been included because it can be used in many different ways and situations. For example, a mouthstick can be used to point to a communication board at level 4.2. Using a mouthstick to operate an environmental control unit demands the cognitive capacity to learn a sequence of new steps by rote at level 4.8. A transfer board can be used successfully by a caregiver to transfer a level 2 patient; however, transferring independently and safely with a transfer board requires a minimum cognitive level of 5. The need to remember vital information, like total hip replacement precautions, also places more complex demands on the information-processing system. Therefore, adaptive equipment needs to be analyzed in the context of an activity because the cognitive ability is dictated by the activity as well as the piece of equipment.

Sometimes if a patient is very motivated and diligent and has a supportive caregiver who will agree to continue training, successful results can be achieved with a cognitive capacity below the level of instructional demand. The minimum mode of performance should be regarded as a suggestion that can be overruled by professional judgment.

## 1. Behavior Disabilities—Learning Acquisition Disabilities (10–13)

| Equipment/Goal | Demand | Compensation* | Cognitive level | With caregiver |
|---|---|---|---|---|
| Security door bars, locks, gates: May be used to ensure safety, prevent wandering of confused, ambulatory patients. | None. | P | N/A | To set up. |
| Soft safety straps, posey jackets: To ensure safety, prevent medical complications of confused, impulsive patients who are weak and unaware of need for assistance with transfers and walking. | None. | P | N/A | To set up. |
| Home intercom system: May be used by caregiver to monitor patient's behavior and/or medical condition from another room. | None. | P | N/A | |

## 2. Communication Disabilities—Listening Disabilities (23–24)

| Equipment/Goal | Demand | Compensation* | Cognitive level | With caregiver |
|---|---|---|---|---|
| Telephone amplifier: Can be attached to telephone receiver when there is a reduction in the ability to receive audible messages. | None. | P | N/A | |
| Flashing telephone light: Can be used when there is a mild/moderate restriction in the ability to hear the telephone bell. (Can be used in conjunction with amplifier.) | Training to scan visible environment for flashing light cue. Can use usual movement patterns to operate telephone. | A | 4.6 | To remind patient to scan visible environment for |

## Seeing Disabilities (25–27)

| Equipment/Goal | Demand | Compensation* | Cognitive level | With caregiver |
|---|---|---|---|---|
| Magnifiers: Used when there is a restriction of the ability to execute tasks requiring adequate visual acuity, such as reading, writing, and visual manipulation. | Training to match perimeter of magnifier with copy, move device over copy in | A | 4.0 | To monitor safety with potentially breakable object; prevent loss by laying down and forgetting placement. Remind |

* P = passive; A = active; D = dynamic.

## Seeing Disabilities (25–27), continued

| EQUIPMENT/GOAL | DEMAND | COMPENSATION* | COGNITIVE LEVEL | WITH CAREGIVER |
|---|---|---|---|---|
| | sequential manner, one segment at a time. Don/doff free-handed version as needed. | | | patient to doff free-handed version before ambulating. |
| Prism glasses: Used when condition prevents neck or postural movement to read, watch television, or execute tasks requiring visual manipulation like sewing or playing board games. | Images are projected parallel with the body and can be disorienting. Capability to have flexibility in estimating spatial relationships, volumes of objects in relationship to space while concurrently manipulating material objects. | D | 5.6* | |

### Other Communication Disabilities (Writing) (28–29)

| | | | | |
|---|---|---|---|---|
| Built-up, weighted writing utensils: Used when there is a reduction of ability to make marks, secondary to weak grasp or unsteady hand. | Capability to accept adaptations that allow dominant hand to be used in a normal manner. | A | 3.4 | To monitor safety with sharp object. |

* P = passive; A = active; D = dynamic.

* Lower-level capability (4.0) required to don for watching television, with caregiver to retrieve and store after each use.

## Other Communication Disabilities (Writing) (28–29), continued

| Equipment/Goal | Demand | Compensation* | Cognitive level | With caregiver |
|---|---|---|---|---|
| Adapted writing utensils (Writing Bird®, Writing Frame®): Used when there is an inability to grasp writing utensils to make marks. | Capability to imitate a modification of a normal action to match device shape to configuration of hand. Normal arm movement patterns required to write. | A | 3.6 | To set up. |
| Writing splints: Used when there is a loss or reduction of ability to execute written messages or to make marks secondary to weak prehension patterns and/or wrist instability. | Capability to match one visible feature at a time to match anatomical shapes and attach preadjusted velcro straps. Normal arm movements required to write. | A | 4.2 | To maintain, replace straps, readjust straps when there is edema. |

## 3. Personal Care Disabilities—Excretion Disabilities (30–32)

| Equipment/Goal | Demand | Compensation* | Cognitive level | With caregiver |
|---|---|---|---|---|
| Raised toilet seats: May be used when standard-height toilet is too low to accommodate stooping and rising disabilities secondary to weakness and/or pain with movement. | None. Device provides external environmental compensation to accommodate normal movement patterns. | P | N/A | To perform hygienic maintenance, set-up. |

* P = passive; A = active; D = dynamic.

**Excretion Disabilities (30–32),** *continued*

| EQUIPMENT/GOAL | DEMAND | COMPENSATION* | COGNITIVE LEVEL | WITH CAREGIVER |
|---|---|---|---|---|
| Toilet support: Used to provide stability and ensure safety when there is a deficiency in balance while sitting on the toilet. | None. | P | N/A | To monitor safety. |
| Chair/bed urinals: (Male) can be used when there is difficulty in transferring to and from lavatory. | Capability to recognize physical disability is restricting access to regular bathroom and accept adaptive equipment that uses familiar action sequence to relieve self. | D | 4.0 | To perform hygienic maintenance. Place device within arm's length. Check for spillage. |
| Bed/chair urinals: (Female) can be used when there is difficulty in transferring to and from lavatory. | Capability to make one spontaneous adjustment in position to place device under body, and follow suggestions to make spatial changes that would improve results and prevent spillage. | D | 4.6 | To perform hygienic maintenance. Check for spillage. |
| Toilet tissue aids: Used for postexcretion hygiene when there is a deficiency in balance and/or upper-extremity ROM/strength. | Capability to recognize loss of ability to clean self | D | 4.8 | To check for hygienic maintenance. |

* P = passive; A = active; D = dynamic.

## Excretion Disabilities (30–32), continued

| Equipment/Goal | Demand | Compensation* | Cognitive Level | With Caregiver |
|---|---|---|---|---|
| | in typical manner. Capability to learn a new series of actions by rote to attach needed amount of toilet paper to device end, perform wiping, evaluate effectiveness by checking striking results, release used tissue in bowl with lever mechanism, and repeat process as needed. After cleaning self, capability needed to detect secondary effects of wiping to clean device after each use. | | | |

### Personal Hygiene Disabilities (33–34)

| Equipment/Goal | Demand | Compensation* | Cognitive Level | With Caregiver |
|---|---|---|---|---|
| Slip-proof bath/shower mats/treads: Used to provide stability, ensure safely during bathing and transfers in the bathroom. | None. | P | N/A | To maintain. |
| Wash mitts: May be used when there is difficulty in bathing self secondary to minimal hand function. | Capability to accept adaptations that allow dominant extremity to be used in a normal manner. | A | 3.4 | To set up; sequence through activity; complete bathing of parts not noticed, like lower extremities and parts of back. |

* P = passive; A = active; D = dynamic.

**Personal Hygiene Disabilities (33–34), continued**

| EQUIPMENT/GOAL | DEMAND | COMPENSATION* | COGNITIVE LEVEL | WITH CAREGIVER |
|---|---|---|---|---|
| Long scrub sponges/brushes: Used when there is difficulty in reaching parts of the body to bathe secondary to limitations in ROM, strength, and/or endurance. | Capability to make brief spontaneous adjustments in position, strength, and duration of movement to use an extended aid in a familiar sequence of actions. Capability to imitate demonstrations of spatial changes that would increase efficiency or effectiveness of washing. | D | 4.6 | |
| Suction hand brush: May be used when there is a difficulty in washing a hand secondary to hemiparesis or amputation. | Capability to follow shape of hand to guide washing actions. Ability to modify actions (e.g., duration, scrubbing fingernails, turning hand over). | A | 3.6 | To set up, sequence through activity (e.g., using soap, rinsing, drying). |
| Suction denture brush: Used when there is inability to wash dentures secondary to loss of bilateral movements. | Capability to imitate demonstrations of spatial changes and rotate dentures for better access to cleaning at an | D | 4.6 | |

* P = passive; A = active; D = dynamic.

## Personal Hygiene Disabilities (33–34), continued

| Equipment/Goal | Demand | Compensation* | Cognitive Level | With Caregiver |
|---|---|---|---|---|
| | unfamiliar angle. Capability to make brief neuromuscular variations to adjust for depth to clean inside cavity of dentures. Normal sequence of actions required to rinse, store, or place in mouth. | | | |
| Shaving cream dispenser handle: May be used when limitations in pinch or hand strength prevent use of dispenser to groom | Simple leverage to overcome resistance. Normal action of pushing required to operate with an ability to grossly approximate amount of foam needed. | A | 4.2 | To set up; monitor liquid amounts. |
| Adjustable angle rotating razor (turns 360° in two different planes to adjust): May be used to shave body parts when there are limitations in grip strength or ROM. | Capability to memorize a sequence of new actions by rote to adjust razor head to positions predetermined by therapist (based on sequence of normal shaving routine, joints, | D | 4.8 | To monitor safety; solve new problems for spatial properties. |

\* P = passive; A = active; D = dynamic.

**Personal Hygiene Disabilities (33–34), continued**

| Equipment/Goal | Demand | Compensation* | Cognitive Level | With Caregiver |
|---|---|---|---|---|
| | angles, and arcs of patient's body). Capability to check razor position by close examination and correct all striking features in an invariant manner. | | | |
| Dressing sticks: Multiple uses to don/doff clothes (upper and lower extremity) with large hook at one end; small hook used for zipping, unzipping large-ringed zipper pulls, untying shoelaces when there are limitations in contralateral strength, and/or limitations in trunk mobility. | Capability to memorize a new sequence of actions by rote for situation-specific activities including: positioning garments, going through new dressing procedures, using appropriate end of device to move clothing, noting primary effects of actions and correcting spatial location difficulties, adjusting for secondary effects (e.g., adjusting tail and collar after donning). | D | 4.8 | Cue for secondary effects of actions and solve new problems for spatial or surface properties of different types of clothing. |

* P = passive; A = active; D = dynamic.

**Personal Hygiene Disabilities (33–34), continued**

| EQUIPMENT/GOAL | DEMAND | COMPENSATION* | COGNITIVE LEVEL | WITH CAREGIVER |
|---|---|---|---|---|
| Button aids: May be used to attach button fastenings when there is contralateral weakness and/or painful and/or weak prehension. | Capability to continuously vary strength, range of motion, make fine-motor adjustments in tight spaces, adjust for surface and spatial properties of buttons and clothes. | D | 5.4 | |
| Sock/stocking aids: May be used to don socks or stockings with either one- or two-handed use. | Capability to learn a short sequence of new actions to put sock/stocking on device, imitate placing device at foot, placing foot into device, and pulling sock/stocking up leg with normal two-handed use. (May require 5.0 capability to make continuous neuromuscular adjustments if using one hand.) | D | 4.6 | Monitor for potential secondary effects of too tight or wrinkled hosiery. |

\* P = passive; A = active; D = dynamic.

| EQUIPMENT/GOAL | DEMAND | COMPENSATION* | COGNITIVE LEVEL | WITH CAREGIVER |
|---|---|---|---|---|
| **Feeding and Other Personal Care Disabilities (37–39)** | | | | |
| Rocker knives: Used to cut food when there is contralateral weakness preventing stabilization of food. | Requires a variation of normal motor actions to cut food ("rocking" versus slicing), which may be effective with cuing to increase downward pressure when cutting more resistive food. | D | 4.6 | To help with cutting resistive food (e.g., tough meat). |
| Extension utensils: Used to convey food to mouth when there are limitations in proximal upper-extremity ROM. | Capability to adjust and correct amount of food in utensil bowl, and correct spatial location difficulties to convey food to mouth from an unaccustomed distance. | D | 4.8 | |
| Swivel utensils: May be used to convey food to mouth with built-in swivel mechanism that keeps food level when wrist or finger motion is absent. | Capability to recognize loss of range of motion and ability to use utensils in typical manner. Learn adjustments by | D | 4.8 | |

P = passive; A = active; D = dynamic.

**Feeding and Other Personal Care Disabilities (37–39),** *continued*

| Equipment/Goal | Demand | Compensation* | Cognitive level | With caregiver |
|---|---|---|---|---|
|  | rate to maintain arm position while allowing swivel mechanism to bring food level with mouth versus making unnecessary and tiring postural adjustments. Capability to correct liquid measures to prevent spillage. |  |  |  |
| Electric self-feeder: May be used to convey food to mouth, select food for next spoonful without the use of arms. | Multimechanical device requiring slight head movement on chin switch to activate motorized pusher that fills spoon and conveys food to mouth. Select food by pressing pedal to rotate plate. Capability to memorize a sequence of new actions, one step at a time, and correct for spatial location (of plate) without assistance. | D | 4.8 | To set up and maintain. |

* P = passive; A = active; D = dynamic.

## 4. Locomotor Disabilities—Ambulation Disabilities (40–47)

| EQUIPMENT/GOAL | DEMAND | COMPENSATION* | COGNITIVE LEVEL | WITH CAREGIVER |
|---|---|---|---|---|
| Offset door hinge: Used to increase accessibility by adding 2 inches to door width for extra wheelchair clearance. | None. | P | N/A | |
| Furniture leg extenders: May be used when standard-height furniture is too low to accommodate stooping and rising disabilities. | None. | P | N/A | |
| **Other Locomotor Disabilities (48–49)** | | | | |
| Walker/baskets/trays: May be used when there is difficulty with carrying objects while operating walker for ambulatory assistance. | Capability to adjust for all tangible properties; considering extra length of protruding aid to walker when negotiating architectural barriers; adjusting pace and making neuromuscular adjustments for transporting heavier objects or a full tray; requiring flexibility with instruction to recognize when additional assistance may be needed to avoid potential hazards (e.g., asking someone else to transport heavy or excess objects). | D | 5.6 | To assist with consideration of weight, size of objects to transport for safety. |

* P = passive; A = active; D = dynamic.

**5. Body Disposition Disabilities—Domestic Disabilities (50–51)**

| EQUIPMENT/GOAL | DEMAND | COMPENSATION* | COGNITIVE LEVEL | WITH CAREGIVER |
|---|---|---|---|---|
| Free-standing, one-handed can opener: Designed for one-handed use to open cans independently. | Capability to alter device to accommodate different sizes of cans before use: Solve problems for spatial properties to set up and stabilize can in relation to device before proceeding to operate with one hand. | D | 5.4 | |
| One-handed cordless can opener: Used to open cans with one-handed use. Recommend placing Dycem beneath can to stabilize before use. | Capability to learn several steps at one time and make continuous neuromuscular adjustments to align cutting mechanism with rims of different sizes of cans, apply and hold effective amount of downward pressure to stabilize can while squeezing lever to allow cutting action. | D | 5.0 | |

* P = passive; A = active; D = dynamic.

**Domestic Disabilities (50–51),** *continued*

| Equipment/Goal | Demand | Compensation* | Cognitive level | With caregiver |
|---|---|---|---|---|
| Zim® jar lid opener: Used for removal of lids on jars and bottles with strong one-handed use or weak two-handed use. | Capability to align jar/bottle lids with device, correct spatial location difficulties, make continuous neuromuscular adjustments to push forward and turn, and repeat procedure until effective results are achieved. | D | 5.0 | |
| Capscrew jar opener: Bell-shaped opening accommodates miniature bottles to jam jars. May be used with strong one-handed or weak two-handed use. | Capability to make brief, spontaneous adjustments in strength. May not be successful if adjustments need to be sustained, as with tightly fitting lids (accomplished at 5.0). | D | 4.6 | |
| Gordon® peeler: Peeling device is stabilized to edge of table for one-handed use to prepare food. | Capability to alter normal movement patterns to peel food with one hand. Capability to | D | 4.6 | |

\* P = passive; A = active; D = dynamic.

**Domestic Disabilities (50–51),** *continued*

| Equipment/Goal | Demand | Compensation* | Cognitive Level | With Caregiver |
|---|---|---|---|---|
| | correct spatial location difficulties with assistance, rotate food to check primary... effects of actions and correct errors. | | | |
| Long-reach sponge mop: May be used with household disability to do manual cleaning when there is limited reach and ROM. | For cursory housekeeping involving a well-learned sequence, capability to effectively vary range of motion and strength while mopping with extended aid to produce better results on striking effects. | D | *5.0 \*If thorough cleaning results are desired, cognitive capacity of 5.4 is required for capability to make spontaneous neuromuscular adjustments in response to all tangible properties (consideration of corners, angles, arches of architecture); make postural adjustments to improve effects of work; adjust actions for surface properties seen at unaccustomed distance | |

\* P = passive; A = active; D = dynamic.

**Domestic Disabilities (50–51)**, *continued*

| EQUIPMENT/GOAL | DEMAND | COMPENSATION* | | COGNITIVE LEVEL | | WITH CAREGIVER |
|---|---|---|---|---|---|---|
| | | | | (dirt), barring impaired vision. | | |

**Body Movement Disabilities (52–57)**

| EQUIPMENT/GOAL | DEMAND | COMPENSATION* | | COGNITIVE LEVEL | | WITH CAREGIVER |
|---|---|---|---|---|---|---|
| Reachers: May be used with retrieval and reaching disabilities secondary to ROM, strength, and/or endurance. | Capability to make continuous neuromuscular adjustments and solve problems for spatial properties of objects with a flexibility in estimating volumes of objects in relationship to space. Requires flexibility with instruction to recognize when additional assistance may be needed to avoid | D | | 5.6 | | To assist with consideration of weight, size of objects to retrieve and move for safety. |

* P = passive; A = active; D = dynamic.

## Body Movement Disabilities (52–57), continued

| Equipment/Goal | Demand | Compensation* | Cognitive Level | With Caregiver |
|---|---|---|---|---|
| | potential hazards (i.e., asking someone else to retrieve or move objects too heavy or cumbersome.) | | | |
| Wheelchair brake lock extension: Extension device fits over standard lock to provide greater leverage to those with pushing/pulling disabilities related to upper-extremity weakness and/or ROM limitations. | Capability to use familiar motor actions (pushing and pulling) to operate. Capability to judge effects of actions when following demonstrations of use, remembering one linear direction at a time associated with movement. | A | 4.2 | To cue when brakes need to be locked for safety and unlocked for mobility. |

## Other Body Disposition Disabilities (58–59)

| Equipment/Goal | Demand | Compensation* | Cognitive Level | With Caregiver |
|---|---|---|---|---|
| CVA arm slings: Used to maintain appropriate relations among different parts of the body by donning preadjusted positioning device. | Training to memorize a new sequence of steps by adding one step at a time. Capability to correct spatial location difficulties without assistance, | D | *4.8<br><br>(*Requires no demand if donned by caregiver—i.e., becoming a passive compensation.) | To check position, readjust for safety, cue for secondary effects. |

---

* P = passive; A = active; D = dynamic.

## Other Body Disposition Disabilities (58–59), *continued*

| EQUIPMENT/GOAL | DEMAND | COMPENSATION* | COGNITIVE LEVEL | WITH CAREGIVER |
|---|---|---|---|---|
| | understand secondary effects of donning before orienting self to parts of sling and/or proceeding unsequentially, resulting in tangled and confusing straps, awkward and ineffective positioning. | | | |

## 6. Dexterity Disabilities—Daily Activity Disabilities (60–61)

| EQUIPMENT/GOAL | DEMAND | COMPENSATION* | COGNITIVE LEVEL | WITH CAREGIVER |
|---|---|---|---|---|
| Car door opener: May be used to open car doors when there is hand weakness or malformation secondary to arthritis, trauma, or deformity. (*Two styles available for either pull-up or push-button handles.) | Capability to align device with door opener latch and follow suggested spatial adjustments to increase effectiveness. (Capability to make one spontaneous adjustment in strength or position to open door. | D | 4.6 | |

\* P = passive; A = active; D = dynamic.

**Daily Activity Disabilities (60–61)**, *continued*

| Equipment/Goal | Demand | Compensation* | Cognitive level | With caregiver |
|---|---|---|---|---|
| Adapted key holders/turners: Used to use keys when there are limitations in hand mobility and/or strength. | Capability to make one spontaneous adjustment in position or strength for better effect when using rigid devices. | D | *4.6<br><br>(*For flexible devices or hard-to-turn keys, may need 5.0 capability to make continuous neuromuscular adjustments to sustain position and pressure while achieving best leverage effect to turn key.) | To cue for change in hand position, if needed. |
| Door knob extensions: May be used to operate door knobs when there are limitations in grasping and turning. | One new sensory cue to act on. Drilling to imitate placement effect of hand on extended handle, and modify normal action of turning to pushing/pulling sideways. | A | 3.6 | |

* P = passive; A = active; D = dynamic.

## Manual Activity Disabilities (62–66)

| EQUIPMENT/GOAL | DEMAND | COMPENSATION* | COGNITIVE LEVEL | WITH CAREGIVER |
|---|---|---|---|---|
| Universal holders: May be donned to hold objects when there is a holding disability secondary to hand weakness, malformation, or amputation. | Capability to match one feature at a time in a short series of steps to slip cuff over hand, attach preadjusted strap, and attach utensil into cuff. Normal movement patterns proximal to hand required to use utensil (e.g., feeding, combing hair, etc.). | A | *4.2 <br><br> (*Lower minimal mode of performance required [3.4] if applied and set up by caregiver.) | To readjust straps, position of utensils, as needed. |

## 7. Situational Disabilities—Dependence and Endurance Disabilities (70–71)

| EQUIPMENT/GOAL | DEMAND | COMPENSATION* | COGNITIVE LEVEL | WITH CAREGIVER |
|---|---|---|---|---|
| Walker seat: May be used when intermittent resting is necessary secondary to disability. | Instruction to demonstrate several steps at one time to stabilize self on walker while clipping seat at four interior corners to use, then reverse | D | 5.0 | To check safety. |

* P = passive; A = active; D = dynamic.

**Dependence and Endurance Disabilities (70–71), continued**

| Equipment/Goal | Demand | Compensation* | Cognitive Level | With Caregiver |
|---|---|---|---|---|
| | sequence, fold seat forward when not in use. | | | |
| **Environmental Disabilities (72–77)** | | | | |
| Lamb's wool padding: May be used for bedding when there is a disability relating to temperature and/or humidity tolerance. | None. | P | N/A | To set up. |
| Clamp-on umbrella: May be used when there is an intolerance to sunlight. | None. | P | N/A | To set up. |
| Antipressure cushions: Used to prevent further medical problems related to intolerance to pressure, especially over sustained periods of time. | None. | P | N/A | To set up. |

* P = passive; A = active; D = dynamic.

## Ethical and Legal Implications

Safety risks associated with operating adaptive equipment should be evaluated to determine if a slight degree of care, ordinary care, or a high degree of care is required for use. Since many of the cognitively disabled can only exercise a slight degree of care, potential ethical problems exist with legal implications. Therapists are legally responsible to accurately determine that a patient's ability to exercise care is commensurate with safety risks when using adaptive equipment. An example would be if a patient with a moderate cognitive impairment (level 4) is issued a reacher and does not have caregiver supervision to monitor safety at home. Theoretically, without the ability to consider leverage principles or generalize situation-specific training in the clinic to different situations in the home, the patient would unsafely attempt to retrieve heavy packages from a cupboard and lose his or her balance, resulting in a fall and the breaking of his or her hip.

To protect the patient from further injury, do not issue equipment that makes cognitive demands above the patient's current level. If future improvements in the cognitive level are expected, the best protection may be offered by asking the patient to come back for more equipment when the cognitive improvement is expected.

## Acknowledgment

I thank Mary Lou Herndon, OTR, and her occupational therapy staff at LAC-USC Medical Center, Los Angeles, California, for their support and for allowing me to access their adaptive equipment.

## Reference

World Health Organization. (1980). *International classification of impairments, disabilities, and handicaps.* Geneva: Author.

## Suggested Readings

Allen, C.K. (1989). Treatment plans in cognitive rehabilitation. *Occupational Therapy Practice, 1,* 1–8.

Allen, C.K., Foto, M., Sperling, T.M., & Wilson, E. (1989). Outpatient occupational therapy Medicare Part B guidelines (DHHS Transmittal No. 565). *Health Insurance Manual.* Baltimore: Health Care Financing Administration.

Allen, C.K. (1985). *Occupational therapy for psychiatric diseases: Measurement and management of cognitive disabilities.* Boston: Little, Brown.

Earhart, C.A., & Allen, C.K. (1988). *Cognitive disabilities: Expanded activity analysis.* Colchester, CT: S & S Worldwide.

Hasselkus, B.R. (1991). Ethical dilemmas in family caregiving for the elderly: Implications for occupational therapy. *American Journal of Occupational Therapy, 45,* 206–212.

Hopkins, H.L., & Smith, H.D. (Eds.). (1988). *Willard and Spackman's occupational therapy, 7th edition.* Philadelphia: Lippincott.

Mann, W.C., & Lane, J.P. (1991). *Assistive technology for persons with disabilities: The role of occupational therapy.* Rockville, MD: American Occupational Therapy Association, Inc.

O'Sullivan, S.B., & Schmitz, T.J. (Eds.). (1988). *Physical rehabilitation: Assessment and treatment, 2nd edition.* Philadelphia: F.A. Davis.

Pedretti, L.W., & Zoltan, B. (Eds.). (1990). *Occupational therapy: Practice skills for physical disabilities, 3rd edition.* St. Louis: Mosby.

## Catalogs

Ableware. (1990). *Aids for daily living, home healthcare, rehabilitation.* Pequannock, NJ: Maddak Inc.

AdaptAbility. (1991). *Designs for independent living.* Colchester, CT: S & S Worldwide.

Enrichments. (1990). Grand Rapids, MI: Bissell Healthcare Corporation.

Rolyan. (1991). *Splinting and rehabilitation products for occupational therapists and physical therapists.* Menomonee Falls, WI: Smith & Nephew Rolyan Inc.

Sammons Catalog. (1991). *Your complete source for rehabilitation and ADL products.* Brookfield, IL: Fred Sammons, Inc., Bissell Healthcare Corporation.

# Chapter 10

# Case Studies

## Introduction

Ten case studies are presented as examples of different ways that cognitive disability theory can be applied. All of the authors are working in post-acute-care settings. One of the cases illustrates a referral to a rehabilitation setting and another assists a parent with planning for long-term care. Seven of the cases are from psychiatric settings but that is not the reason for their selection. The psychiatric cases were selected to illustrate different responsibilities that the therapists assumed. Three physical disability cases are presented to show how these same responsibilities can be fulfilled in a rehabilitation setting. An opportunity to contrast and compare different types of postacute care is provided Two geriatrics cases are located in chapter 4.

The names of all of the patients are fictitious, of course, to protect their confidentiality.

## Collaboration with Physicians

*Catherine Earhart, OTR*

The following case describes how occupational therapy treatment assisted in the clinical management of a patient receiving a course of electroconvulsive therapy (ECT) for intractable depression.

Cindy is a 54-year-old, divorced, Caucasian woman who was transferred to an acute care psychiatric hospital from a state hospital where she had lived for 5 years for a trial of ECT. The patient had not responded to various medication regimens and indeed had worsened to the point where she no longer could feed, dress, bathe, or groom herself, and would lie in bed all day, mute or screaming. Differential diagnosis was major depression with mood-congruent psychotic

features, R/O schizoaffective disorder, R/O schizophrenic disorder, chronic paranoid type.

## Patient History

Cindy grew up in a close, Italian family. Her father abused alcohol and likely had bipolar disorder. She was a well-adjusted and popular child who excelled in music and dance. After graduating from high school, she earned a BA in English and Dramatic Arts at a New York university. She worked briefly as a dance and music therapist for developmentally disabled children before her marriage at age 19, and later after her first hospitalization. During most of her marriage, she did not work, instead raising three sons. Both she and her husband abused alcohol according to the mother. Cindy's psychiatric problems began around age 28, after an affair and abortion. She began to feel guilty and depressed. She required a brief hospitalization at age 30 and again 2 years later. During the next 5 years she worked as a dance therapist, then was hospitalized again, this time for 1 year. Her husband left her at this time. At discharge, Cindy went to live with her mother. Though not able to work, Cindy was able to care for her own needs, and saw an outpatient psychiatrist for the next 8 years. At age 49, symptoms of psychosis and depression worsened, resulting in hospitalization for the next 5 years. Cindy's mother visited her in the state hospital on weekends during this time. Cindy had not responded to many different trials of neuroleptic and antidepressant medications; one effective medication caused a dangerous reduction in white blood cell (WBC) levels and had to be discontinued.

## Course of Treatment

ECT was given three times a week (Monday, Wednesday, Friday) in the morning. Initial estimate was for

8 to 12 treatments, with others to be scheduled if the patient demonstrated improvement. At the start of treatments, Cindy lay in bed all day, either nonresponsive or screaming for hours at a time. She was cooperative with being fed and taken to the bathroom by staff and swallowed medications given to her (Thiothixine, 10 BID.) Verbalizations suggested presence of nihilistic delusions ("I am dead," "I have no face"). Cognitive disability was estimated by the occupational therapist to be at level 1.8.

Over the next 2 weeks (seven treatments) screaming lessened and finally stopped. Cindy walked to the bathroom on her own and to the day room to feed herself when she was told. She did not dress, bathe, or groom herself. She was socially withdrawn. Cognitive level was estimated by occupational therapist to be at 3.0 and an occupational therapy evaluation was requested by the physician.

## Occupational Therapy Initial Evaluation

The occupational therapy initial evaluation consisted of an interview and administration of the Allen Cognitive Level (ACL) test. Cindy could answer specific questions about her past history but was unable to state that she had a mental illness or to judge the severity of her disability. She had no future goals or any opinion about what she would prefer to do in the present. Delusions about having no face, hands, and feet were expressed. Cindy's mood was depressed and psychomotor retardation was severe. The patient worked slowly and with great effort to produce a score of level 3.8 on the ACL.

## Occupational Therapy Treatment Plan

Short-term treatment goals were as follows:

1. Monitor changes in disability associated with ECT treatments by daily assessment of cognitive level in clinic groups.

2. Monitor for changes in acute symptoms, specifically delusions, psychomotor retardation, affect, subjective mood.

3. Monitor for side effects of treatment, specifically confusion and memory loss.

Long-term treatment goals were as follows:

1. Identify level of assistance needed when treatments are completed based on residual disability to assist with discharge planning.

## Occupational Therapy Treatment Methods

Since Cindy did not state preferences for her treat-ment groups but did state a willingness to comply with whatever the therapist suggested, she was scheduled into two groups: Grooming group (morning on off-treatment days) to observe performance of self-care tasks and Basic Crafts (daily in the afternoons) to observe performance in standardized tasks with high accuracy in detecting small cognitive changes. Both groups lasted 1 hour. Changes were made in this schedule as needed. Progress was noted in daily rounds with the physician and other staff and documented weekly in the chart. Symptoms and side effects were rated as follows: (+++) = very severe; (++) = marked; (+) = present; (0) = absent.

### Weeks 1 and 2 (Treatments 8–12)

• Cognitive level: Varies from 3.6 to 3.8 in Crafts group (Cindy picks up tools spontaneously but needs to be sequenced through the actions to complete the tasks.) Cindy seemed to do less well in grooming (needing prompts to pick up comb or brush and to continue actions, refusing to look in a mirror) and delusions about her missing face, etc., were suspected to be interfering with her using her capacity. This group was discontinued and the work group substituted.

• Symptoms:
  - Delusions (+++)
  - Psychomotor retardation (+++)
  - Sad affect (+++)
  - Subjective mood ("miserable")

• Side effects: None observed

• Ward behavior: Feeds self, remains in bed throughout day, no spontaneous bathing, grooming, dressing.

The physician decided to extend the number of treatments to a possible 16 based on positive response in behavior and symptoms.

### Week 3 (Treatments 13–15)

• Cognitive level: Increase to 4.0 observed in both Crafts and Work groups. Cindy now collates a series of three forms without prompting, and goes on to the next step in crafts. Indicates she realizes she is making an object like the sample in crafts but can't see matching errors.

• Symptoms:
  - Delusions (O) None verbalized
  - Psychomotor retardation (++) works slightly faster

- Sad affect (++) less grim
- Subjective mood ("constant turmoil")
- Side effects: None observed
- Ward behavior: Gets out of bed spontaneously during day, dresses self 1 day during the week, no grooming, bathing.

### Week 4 (Treatment 16)

- Cognitive level: By end of week, increase to 4.2 and occasional 4.4 is seen in Work and Crafts groups. Cindy is aware of matching errors and asks for assistance in work tasks and attends to two cues in crafts at times. She is more aware of her deficits, especially how slow she is compared to others. Agreed to begin a third group where she decides what to do (Sewing).
- Symptoms:
  - Delusions (0)
  - Psychomotor retardation: (+)
  - Sad affect (+) Less sad
  - Subjective mood: ("Not good") (but less bad)
- Side effects: None observed
- Ward behavior: Dresses every other day, better grooming noted by staff.

The physician decided to continue treatments and to space them out based on continued improvements in cognitive level and symptoms.

### Week 5 (Treatments 17–18)

- Cognitive level: Dips at beginning of week to 4.0, when patient has flu symptoms, then returns to 4.2; by end of week back to 4.4 with some spontaneous variations in actions observed (4.6) when Cindy shifts papers to produce more efficient outcome in work.
- Symptoms:
  - Delusions: (0)
  - Psychomotor retardation: (+)
  - Sad affect: (+) Brief spontaneous smiling
  - Subjective mood: ("Still not good")
- Side effects: None observed
- Ward behavior: Dresses daily and grooms self (combs hair, no make-up), bathes when encouraged.

### Week 6 (Treatment 19)

- Cognitive level: maintains at 4.4 to 4.6 in Work,

Crafts, Sewing groups (Cindy checks for errors against a sample and makes an adjustment such as recutting a length of ribbon without prompting, or removing and redoing a sewing stitch.) Works without stopping for 30 minutes before fatiguing. Still very indecisive and prefers others to make decisions for her about what tasks to do.

- Symptoms:
  - Delusions: (0)
  - Psychomotor retardation: (+)
  - Sad affect: (O) Now blunted but smiles when greeted and taking leave and at jokes.
  - Subjective mood: "Fair;" remarks to RT that "What I make in OT makes me feel good."
- Side effects: (+) memory loss for recent events noted on treatment days only.
- Ward behavior: Continues to dress and groom self. Nurses note spontaneous short conversations with others. Bathes with encouragement.

### Week 7 (Treatments 20–21)

- Cognitive level: Drops to 4.4 only, and 4.0 on treatment days. Patient seems mildly confused on treatment days in the afternoon and begins to show spatial disorientation (cannot find the occupational therapy bathroom down the hall) even on nontreatment days.
- Symptoms:
  - Delusions (+) patient says the ECT is "changing the shape of her ears" and the ears of another patient.
  - Psychomotor retardation: (+)
  - Sad affect: (O) Continues to be blunt
  - Subjective mood: "Fair"
- Side effects: (++) memory loss for recent events, spatial disorientation, mild confusion on all days.
- Ward behavior: Unchanged except for confusion.

The physician decided maximum benefit of ECT was reached based on the adverse effects of side effects and the drop in cognitive level and, as a result, discontinued treatment.

### Week 8 (No Treatments; Patient Receiving Same Medications)

- Cognitive level: maintained at 4.4 with some evidence of 4.6. Still works more slowly than normal, makes decisions reluctantly and tenta-

Figure 10.1 Functional changes during Cindy's ECT

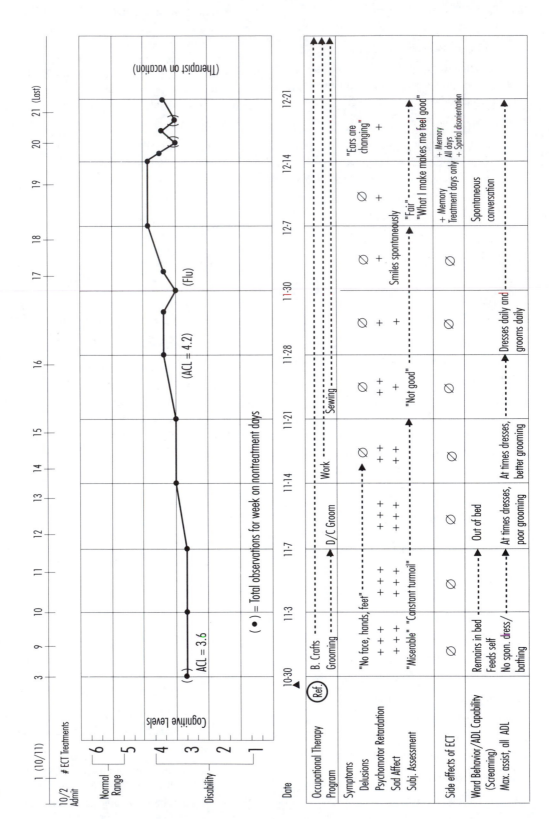

tively, but says she likes to come to groups. Has few preferences about activities and cannot state any future plans except to state that maybe she would like to return to live with her mother.

- Symptoms:
  - Delusions (+) but doubted by patient. Psychomotor retardation (+)
  - Sad affect (O)
  - Subjective mood: "Fair;" "Ready to leave"
- Side effects: memory loss diminished, spatial disorientation resolved.
- Ward behavior: Unchanged

Cindy's cognitive disability was judged to have stabilized at 4.4, a marked improvement from her initial status yet far from her highest level of function of more than 15 years prior. With this degree of impairment, it was expected that she could perform routine daily self-care (dressing, bathing, grooming, eating) without prompting when needed objects were in usual, visible locations. New or potentially hazardous activities such as traveling in the community, shopping, preparing food, managing money, and taking medications would need to be supervised by others. Cindy was made anxious by having to make decisions about the use of her time, and was eager to accept assistance in this area. Cindy's compliance with assistance suggested that she could be cared for at a lower level of care than that of a state hospital, such as a home environment with caregiver supervision, or an unlocked board and care home.

These recommendations were communicated to Cindy's mother in family meetings with the social worker. Cindy's mother expressed willingness to provide the needed level of supervision for Cindy and was judged by the staff to be capable of doing this. The patient was transferred back to the state hospital, which discharged her to her mother's home. Follow-up was arranged with a private psychiatrist. Both Cindy and her mother were pleased with these arrangements.

## Sensitivity to "Blind" Medication Changes

*Nancy G. Adams, OTR*

Dimitri (not his real name) signed himself in as a research volunteer in the Neuropsychiatric Research Hospital (NRH). It seemed like the best thing for

him to do. After all, he could not continue working. He was too busy "listening" to concentrate. A problem with his concentration could result in an accident, and he didn't want to be responsible for anyone being injured. So, he signed in and agreed to testing, various research protocols, and participation in the NRH program.

The NRH is part of the Intramural Research Program of the National Institute of Mental Health (NIMH). Because the NRH is supported by the federal government, participation involves minimal cost to the family or patient. Currently, the research at NRH focuses on four patient populations: those with chronic schizophrenia, persistent tardive dyskinesia, schizoaffective disorder, and dementia occurring in early adulthood. Dimitri was accepted to participate in the studies about schizophrenia.

Dimitri is a single, African-American male in his early 30s. He was born and raised in the middle Atlantic states. He is from a middle class background. He has strong religious beliefs. His family lived close enough to NRH for him to make occasional visits without incurring excessive time or expense.

In program planning for occupational therapy, the model of cognitive disability was selected for this facility for two reasons. First, the Allen Cognitive Level (ACL) test provides a quantitative measure that can be used to identify changes, including those that may accompany participation in the research. Second, the model is compatible with the philosophy of the Hospital.

> Definition: A cognitive disability is a restriction in voluntary motor action originating in the physical or chemical structures of the brain and producing observable limitations in routine task behavior. (Allen, 1985)

The NRH is the inpatient part of the NIMH Neurosciences Center. Various research methods are employed at the Center in order to gain information about the brain and its functions. Kirch used the words "Research Windows on Schizophrenia" as a way of conceptualizing how each of these methods contributes to the study of the brain and schizophrenia (Darrell Kirch, MD, NIMH, oral presentation and personal communication, July 3, 1991). The "windows" are: phenomenology; biochemistry; immunology; radiology; electrophysiology; neuropathology; epidemiology; pharmacology; genetics; and neuropsychology. Although

Dimitri's illness was severe, these windows did not reveal striking abnormalities.

When Dimitri was admitted to the NRH, his positive symptoms were: paranoid delusions, auditory hallucinations, thought insertion, and thought control. His negative symptoms were: affective flattening, mild blocking, increased latency of response, mild anhedonia, and social isolation.

In the categories of biochemistry and immunology, he had a lumbar puncture, and his cerebral spinal fluid studies were all normal.

In the category of radiology, his computed tomography (CT) and magnetic resonance imaging (MRI) scans were both read as normal. The MRI scan showed that his ventricles were normal in size, even in terms of the schizophrenia research literature. He also participated in the regional cerebral blood flow study while both on and off medication. During the procedure, he was asked to perform a task known to place a demand on the dorsolateral prefrontal cortex, namely, the Wisconsin Card Sort. This study showed that, as a group, the individuals with a diagnosis of schizophrenia had a decrease in the blood supply to that area when more circulatory activity was needed, whereas the control group had an increase there.

Dimitri's electroencephalograms (EEGs), done while he was drowsy, asleep, and awake, were all normal. He participated in research involving evoked potentials and Brain Electrical Activity Mapping (BEAM).

Psychopharmacology was accompanied by hourly ratings of activity involvement and twice-daily ratings on the Psychiatric Symptom Assessment Scale (PSAS) (Bigelow & Berthot, 1989). The latter evolved from additions and other modifications to the Brief Psychiatric Rating Scale (BPRS) of Overall and Gorham (1962). The PSAS assesses patient statements and behaviors. These ratings showed that Dimitri had higher (worse) scores during drug-free periods and thus that neuroleptics did benefit him.

He showed a genetic vulnerability for schizophrenia with one first-degree relative with the illness.

The initial neuropsychological testing resulted in a full-scale IQ of 90 with a verbal IQ of 93, and a performance IQ of 88. He scored a high 12 on the block design, a measure that has been found to correlate with the ACL test. On the Halstead-Reitan,

he had an average impairment rating of 1.42, which is suggestive of mild neuropsychological impairment. Retesting on an extensive battery did not support a possible learning disability, showed no evidence for focal neuropsychological deficit, and showed the same or slightly better cognitive functioning than on admission.

His predischarge neuropsychological summary was that he "continues to demonstrate impressive cognitive abilities in light of his chronic illness." The testing showed the following: He performed within normal limits on the Hooper Visual Organization Test and the Boston Aphasias subtest involving comprehension of complex oral language, and recall and recognition memory were adequate on the California Verbal Learning Test. During the same predischarge period, his score on the ACL was 5.6.

The initial occupational therapy evaluation consisted of a semistructured interview, a questionnaire, and two tests of performance. Dimitri had not had any previous experience in occupational therapy. He described tactile as well as auditory hallucinations. In terms of occupational performance, he received assistance in budgeting. He had difficulty reading some words. Because of "bad thoughts," he had difficulty carrying out one of his home maintenance responsibilities, washing the dishes. He hoped to work in the future. He had few leisure interests and they were all solitary. In terms of the performance component of sensorimotor functioning, he reported poor balance and posture. The problems in cognitive functioning that he identified were concentration and memory. He did not consider his symptoms to be a mental illness. He felt isolated from others. He was unable to name any of his strengths but did identify his positive symptoms as problems. Given a list, he was able to select goals toward which he wanted to work in occupational therapy.

Dimitri's initial score on the ACL was 4.5. Note: The 1986 scoring revision is used for continuity in data collection for research. Also note: Occupational therapy is now being included in many of the research protocols. During the "testing windows," the ACL is readministered, and the patient is rated on the Comprehensive Occupational Therapy Evaluation Scale (Brayman & Kirby, 1976).

The initial occupational therapy plan was: Problem—social and occupational impairment. Initial occupational therapy objectives were: He will contribute spontaneously to group discussion; he will participate in activities that require intellectual skills; and he will name one or more assets in the area of task performance, indicating a reduction in his negative attitude about himself. Dimitri was rated on each objective after each session. In addition to the monthly progress notes, a group of ratings was studied by the physician to further assess the effectiveness of one of the medication studies. The occupational therapist was "blind" during all of the double-blind studies. That is, the therapist did not know whether the patient was on active medication or a placebo at any given time in order to avoid bias in the ratings. Fluctuations in cognitive level may or may not occur as the medications are changed.

Dimitri primarily participated in the Occupational Therapy Task Skills Group and the Social Skills Group. The former focuses on cognitive functioning as shown in task performance, such as ability to follow instructions. It has a parallel group format, partly because that is the most effective for observing subtle changes in cognitive level. The Social Skills Group focuses on clarity and self-confidence while communicating a sense of group membership. This Group has an egocentric cooperative group format (Mosey, 1970).

He also participated in several time-limited occupational therapy groups: money management, Work Process Skills, Safety, Social Judgment, and Sensory Integration. Posttesting for the Sensory Integration Group showed some improvement on a few items, but these could not be attributed to the Group rather than other activities. The greatest change was in Standing Balance: Eyes Open.

In applying the model of cognitive disabilities in this setting, each patient is allowed the maximum independence to function within his or her cognitive level with standby supervision to anticipate difficulties that may arise, for example, by attempts to do part of a process that may be above the individual's cognitive level or by fluctuations in cognitive level occurring due to the illness or changes in medication.

In occupational therapy, the location of supplies, activity selection, and modification follow the cognitive levels. Given the evidence of inadequate circulatory, electrical, and chemical input to the areas of the brain involved in problem solving, etc., the patients with a diagnosis of schizophrenia are supported in taking "breaks" of no more than 5 minutes each. An attempt is made to treat these patients more like those with other types of insults to the brain, for example, by avoiding stress and fatigue.

Dimitri was encouraged to make decisions and to select an activity from suggestions or a list corresponding to his then-tested level of cognitive disability. He was encouraged to subjectively report day-to-day changes, such as an increase in what he "heard" or "ideas coming into [his] head" that interfered with his concentration. Easier activities were suggested as required, and he was encouraged to participate to the extent of his ability. In keeping with the treatment team's plan to improve the appropriateness of his remarks in specific situations, he was not supposed to write or talk about his delusional system during occupational therapy.

Dimitri was rated on the Comprehensive Occupational Therapy Evaluation Scale several times. The items that were more sensitive to changes in functioning due to changes in status were Nonproductive Behavior and Punctuality. At times he was nonproductive for up to one quarter of the session. Some days his symptoms were so severe that he could not get out of bed in order to arrive on time, if at all. Usually, he remembered and was punctual for those appointments for which he was highly motivated. When his symptoms were worse, he was able to concentrate on the task for only one half of the session. He was rated as having moderate problems on the item relating to Attention to Detail: "He may be so precise that the project will take twice as long as expected." In addition to being overly precise and working very slowly, he became so absorbed in what he was doing that he did not stop and allow time for cleaning up before the end of the session. This problem with time is described in the section on sanding and level 5.0. His appearance usually reflected level 4. His shirt was often tucked in in front but not in back. The back of his hair was not recombed after he had been lying down.

In addition to occupational therapy, he participated in recreational therapy, Re-entry Group, group psychotherapy on the unit, individual psychotherapy with a member of the nursing staff and his ward physician, shared responsibilities on the unit, and participated in unit and buildingwide activities. He participated in Industrial Therapy until his delusions and auditory hallucinations worsened.

During one session he made repetitive movements characteristic of level 3, rather than working in a goal-directed manner. For months, he functioned at level 4. During 1 month he was unable to resume spontaneously after stopping work on a task due to his preoccupation with psychotic thinking. At this time he was making a pair of leather moccasins, following oral instruction plus demonstration. His performance was more characteristic of level 4.8 than a decline in cognitive functioning to level 4.0. Later, a test score of level 5.0 led to hope that he would return to that level. By beginning to make a few variations and exploring new ways of organizing a process, the beginning of the transition to level 5 was signalled. The frequency of variations increased. Dimitri experimented with different media over and over again. For example, he made several pairs of ceramic earrings by hand, each with a different crystal glaze with different placement of the crystals to create a pattern. He did similar experimentation with mixing and using leather dyes on an embossed belt. In a facility that used another frame of reference, such long-term experimentation might not have been tolerated.

His score on the ACL was 5.0 on the day that he was given the Scoreable Self-Care Evaluation (Clark & Peters, 1984). His slowness affected his evaluation. Each of the four subscores was below the norm for males. His total score was even lower. (Patients who score at levels 4.9 and below are given the Kohlman Evaluation of Living Skills [McGourty, 1979].)

Dimitri was well-liked by other patients throughout the Hospital. Although he was tall and heavy, he was soft spoken and had a gentle manner. He valued being able to help others.

The following was the occupational therapy plan and status at the time of discharge:

Problem: psychotic symptoms

• Occupational therapy objective 1: He will concentrate well enough to participate in an activity without causing undue delays.

  Patient's response: He did so during 9 out of 10 applicable sessions (90%). Status: not achieved. During one session he expressed psychotic and paranoid ideation that he had not previously expressed.

Problem: social isolation.

• Occupational therapy objective 2: He will arrive within 5 minutes of the starting time.

  Patient's response: He did so 4 out of 10 applicable times. Status: not achieved.

• Occupational therapy objective 3: He will speak to a peer once each session.

  Patient's response: He did so during 8 out of 11 sessions (73%). Status: not achieved.

  He responded to peers with less prompting than previously. Assessment: His social functioning had improved.

**Cognitive functioning:** While mending his clothes he showed more exploratory behavior and overt trial-and-error problem solving. Assessment: This behavior suggests improving cognitive functioning. Once he was able to solve a mechanical problem for occupational therapy. As described in chapter 3 for level 5.6, he used both overt and covert trial-and-error problem solving to solve a new problem that combined neuromuscular effects with the surface, interior, and exterior properties of two objects. He did feel "good" about his accomplishment and contribution. Assessment: Dimitri's negative symptoms were less, and he was less delusional. In the past he denied making any worthwhile contributions.

Successful methods:

1. He was advised to assess his performance based on observable behavior, regardless of the cause, after he expressed psychotic and delusional material.

2. Rating a few specific behaviors each day was eventually successful. After several months, he tried hard to improve his ratings.

  His scores on the ACL test were sensitive to changes in medication status (see chart on page 312).

*Note:* A higher number on the ACL test indicates a higher level of one type of cognitive functioning. A higher number on the Psychiatric Symptom Assessment Scale indicates more severe signs and symptoms. A correlation would be negative. The last PSAS mean listed may have partly reflected anxiety about discharge. He was stabilized on the Decanoate injection form of his medication prior to discharge because of his ambivalence about taking medication.

The ACL test score of level 5.6 contributed to his community placement plans, and he was discharged to a supervised apartment program in the community. He continues to do well and participates in a day treatment program.

His discharge diagnosis was schizophrenia, paranoid, chronic. There were no other diagnoses. Axis V, Global Assessment of Functioning was 40+, major impairment in several areas, such as work, judgment, and thinking.

Dimitri's medication status

| ACL test scores | Dates | Open trials and research medications | PSAS mean |
|---|---|---|---|
| 4.5 | 1/11/89 | Prolixin and Cogentin | 1.232 |
| 5.0 | 10/18/89 | Haldol* and Cogentin* | 0.791 |
| 4.8 | 3/14/90 | Moban liquid and Cogentin | 2.045 |
| 4.8 | 5/16/90 | Moban*, Cogentin*, and Sinemet** | 2.200 |
| 5.6 | 9/19/90 | Haldol | 1.755 |

\* Coded during research protocol: active.

\*\* Coded during research protocol: placebo.

In summary, the model of cognitive disability served as a framework for interpreting changes in behavior and for promoting improvement in cognitive functioning. The ACL test gave useful information to the treatment team and researchers. Combined with the Routine Task Inventory (RTI), it provided a basis for realistic expectations for the staff, patient, and family.

## Acknowledgments

I thank present and previous staff of the NIMH Neuropsychiatric Research Hospital and the NIMH Neurosciences Center at St. Elizabeth's for their contributions to this case study.

## References

Allen, C.K. (1985). *Occupational therapy for psychiatric diseases.* Boston: Little, Brown.

Bigelow, L.B., & Berthot, B.D. (1989). The Psychiatric Symptom Assessment Scale (PSAS). *Psychopharmacology Bulletin, 25*(2), 168–179.

Brayman, S.J., & Kirby, T.F. (1976). Comprehensive Occupational Therapy Evaluation Scale. *American Journal of Occupational Therapy, 30*(2), 94–100.

McGourty, L.K. (1979). *Kohlman Evaluation of Living Skills.* Seattle, WA: KELS Research.

Mosey, A.C. (1970). *Three frames of reference for mental health.* Thorofare, NJ: Slack.

Overall, J.E., & Graham, D.R. (1962). The brief psychiatric rating scale. *Psychological Reports, 10,* 799–812.

Wyatt, R.J., Alexander, R.C., Egan, M.F., & Kirch, D.G. (1988). Schizophrenia, just the facts— What do we know, how well do we know it? *Schizophrenia Research, 1,* 3–18.

## Postacute Patient without Social Support

*Nancy Gierut-Wicker, MA, OTR*

Harvey was admitted to the adult acute inpatient psychiatric unit after an exacerbation of his chronic paranoid schizophrenia. The psychiatric unit has a 17 bed inpatient service in a community hospital. The average length of stay is 6.5 days, and the service goals are primarily evaluation, crisis stabilization, and referral to community resources.

This 33-year-old divorced white man was admitted involuntarily as gravely disabled from a residential treatment center where he had been living for the past year. His current stressor was impending dental surgery that involved extraction of most of his teeth resulting from poor dental hygiene.

He began to feel threatened when surgery was planned and developed the delusion that people were plotting to maim and kill him. He became fearful of another resident whom he accused of throwing objects and destroying property. Staff denied any such incidents, but Harvey was afraid to attend the program and was planning to escape to a city 60 miles away where his parents lived. His parents were unable to care for him, and he was admitted for treatment. Harvey had been diagnosed with schizophrenia at age 21 and had one previous hospitalization when he needed dental care. He was currently being treated with Halperidol and Cogentin.

The day after admission, Harvey was screened for cognitive functioning with the Allen Cognitive Level Task Evaluation, revised.. He was able to imitate the sewing stitch but was unable to imitate the whip stitch. He refused to attempt the whip stitch after a second demonstration and stated "I can't do that." The cognitive level score was 3.2, which indicated a severe cognitive impairment requiring a moderate level of cognitive assistance, to safely accomplish routine tasks of living. However, clinical observations did not support the ACL-90 score.

While Harvey had refused to attend the occupational therapy group, observations of behavior on the unit suggested cognitive level 4 functioning as described in the revised Routine Task Inventory (RTI 2). He was able to initiate self care independently, but was unkempt, appearing with hair combed only partially, and shaving just the clearly visible parts of his face. His clothing was rumpled, slightly soiled, and ill fitting. He was goal directed in seeking out cigarettes and food. He denied the need for medical intervention and resisted taking medications. When interacting with others, he was interruptive and unaware of his impact on them, (Earhart & Allen, 1988). He repetitiously told the story of his dental problems during the community meeting. At this point, the occupational therapy treatment goal was to involve Harvey in a basic craft group to clarify cognitive functioning and develop more specific treatment goals.

Performance in the first craft group Harvey attended confirmed suspicions of level 4 functioning. While doing a copper tooling project he requested an exact match of the sample. He was unable to vary the amount of pressure he used on the tool, resulting in a poorly detailed product. He bent the copper while removing the tape from the mold, and removed the clay from the copper impression before affixing the project to a plaque, (Earhart & Allen, 1988). He was attentive to objects adjacent to his immediate environment suggesting level 4.2 functioning.. With this additional information, further treatment goals were developed and communicated to the multidisciplinary team via chart documentation and verbally in team meetings.

A checklist format was used for the written documentation. The format included, but was not limited to, information about ACL performance, observations in basic craft groups, an assessment section, and a checklist of potential social consequences for the patient based upon his cognitive level 4 functioning (Allen & Allen, 1987). This checklist of potential social consequences for each cognitive level was developed to expedite documentation and provide clear, practical information for the team (see Figure 10.2).

The assessment section included information about expected difficulties with abstract thinking, inability to generalize information, and difficulties initiating new learning and with problem solving.

Recommendations were made for nursing staff to monitor follow through with activities of daily living (ADLs), to provide simple visual cues with any new information, to anticipate potential safety hazards, and to include the patient in concrete task groups rather than verbal process groups.

Since the patient was expected to return to the residential treatment center, longer-term recommendations were made about follow-up treatment approaches. It was suggested that any new activity be taught one step at a time with visual demonstrations and an expected training period of 3 months.

Treatment goals were stated as follows:

1. Patient will attend occupational therapy once a day, 6 days a week, to verify and monitor cognitive level.

2. Patient will participate in familiar activities safely and successfully with staff supervision to identify safety hazards and provide set-up for activity and step-by-step visual demonstrations for instructions.

3. Patient will be discharged to residential treatment center where staff provide supervision for recognition of potential safety hazards, assistance with money/medication management, and ongoing training in routine tasks of living.

During the course of his hospitalization, Harvey attended the basic craft group once more. At that time he again demonstrated goal-directed behavior and unsuccessfully attempted to initiate a diagonal tile pattern. He recognized spacing errors but could not solve the problem and requested help from the therapist. His awareness of the environment expanded as he left his chair to search for supplies. Based on this behavior he was recognized as improving from level 4.2 to 4.6 (Allen, 1991).

While Harvey did show improvement in functioning over the brief course of his hospitalization, the initial occupational therapy recommendations were applicable at discharge. Copies of the occupational therapy documentation and the level 4 portion of Allen's "Profiles of the Cognitive Levels" (Allen, 1988) were included in the discharge packet for the residential treatment center. The treatment center staff had been educated regarding use of the cognitive disability theory and were familiar with its application in community living.

Figure 10.2  Checklist of potential social consequences for each cognitive level

ADDITIONAL INFORMATION: _____

_____

_____

_____

_____

COGNITIVE LEVEL:_____

_____

_____

_____

ASSESSMENT: _____

_____

_____

_____

_____

_____

_____

**COGNITIVE LEVEL FOUR**
Potential Social Consequences (Checked areas pertain to patient)

_____ Peculiar use of make-up;

_____ Miss spots shaving;

_____ Neglect back of head/body, uncombed hair, unrinsed shampoo, unwashed back of body, holes/dirt in clothes;

_____ Color/pattern of clothes mismatched, wrong size;

_____ Money management: lose, gets stolen, need to limit daily allowance;

_____ Heat, chemical reactions, electrical hazards not recognized;

_____ Neglect safe storage of possessions, need for trash removal not recognized;

_____ Need visual, not verbal directions if lost;

_____ Eat whatever's seen, cannot follow restricted diet;

_____ Problems driving: parking tickets, violations, accidents, get lost on new routes;

_____ Don't recognize disability - refuse support;

_____ Refuse medications - don't understand why prescribed;

_____ Cannot sustain work beyond one to two months;

_____ Requires live-in or frequent check-in support.

PLAN: _____

_____

_____

_____

_____

This case was selected to illustrate the point that the cognitive disability model must be used as an integrated system using the ACL task evaluation, the RTI–2, and craft group observations concurrently. In this case, reliance on the ACL score alone would have provided an inaccurate picture of the patient's abilities and needs. By observing behavior on the unit and performance in basic crafts, the therapist was able to note progress and to develop a plan that allowed the patient to function safely at his capacity. By educating the residential treatment staff and sending occupational therapy documentation, important information about follow-up care was provided for ongoing treatment.

## References

Allen, C.K. (1991). *Change within the Allen cognitive levels 3, 4 and 5.* Paper presented at the annual conference of the American Occupational Therapy Association.

Allen, C.K. (1990). *Allen cognitive level 9ACL) test manual.* Colchester, CT: S & S Worldwide.

Allen, C.K. (1988). Cognitive disabilities. In S. Robinson (Ed.), Focus. Rockville, MD: American Occupational Therapy Association.

Allen, C.K. (1985). *Occupational therapy for psychiatric diseases: Measurement and management of cognitive disabilities.* Boston: Little, Brown.

Allen, C.K., & Allen, R.E. (1987). Cognitive disabilities: Measuring the social consequences of mental disorders. Journal of Clinical Psychiatry, 48, *185–191.*

Earhart, C.A., & Allen, C.K. (1988). *Cognitive disabilities: Expanded activity analysis.* Colchester, CT: S & S Worldwide.

## Postacute Rehabilitation Patient with Social Support

*Mark S. Austin, MS, OTR*

### Admission and Other Relevant History

Matt was a 22-year-old white male admitted to the hospital secondary to his parents' complaints of "patient talking to himself; bizarre behavior" and general concern that the patient was "doing nothing" except isolating in his room all day. Attempts by the parents to involve the patient were met with aggressive and verbally abusive behavior from the patient, which ultimately led to the patient's hospitalization. The parents reported that Matt had stopped taking his medications (Halperidol) about 3 weeks prior to hospitalization. This was Matt's fourth psychiatric admission in the past 3 years. The patient's diagnosis (Axis I) was chronic paranoid schizophrenia (Axis II— 6; Axis III— 0; Axis IV— psychosocial stressors included interpersonal/family conflict and unemployment; Axis V— current = 30, past year = 50).

Matt had completed high school with a 3. 5 grade point average. Soon after graduation, he left home to attend a community college. It was during Matt's first semester of college that he experienced his first psychotic episode and subsequent hospitalization. Following this hospitalization, Matt left school and returned to his parents' home to live. He continued outpatient therapy (medication management) through the public mental health system and was maintained "reasonably well" on psychotropic medications until age 20 when severe symptoms presented requiring a second hospitalization. Subsequent hospitalizations, including the most recent, typically were associated with Matt's periodic discontinuation of his medication (not medically supported) and an associated increase in difficulties within the family, at work, etc.

Matt had acquired several jobs after his withdrawal from college, all as a beginning worker in fast-food outlets. The maximum length of service within the same competitive employment environment was 4 weeks. Matt was reportedly "slow" at learning routines and unable to shift from one work responsibility to another as expected in fast-food service jobs. When approached by supervisors regarding these difficulties, Matt would typically claim that he was being "picked on" and would subsequently quit or be fired from the position. Matt emphasized that he wanted to work and identified a desire for assistance with finding and maintaining employment. Matt reported no income except a small weekly allowance from his parents.

As reported by his parents and ward nursing staff, Matt was able to independently accomplish personal self-care, though he frequently presented as dishevelled. According to his parents, Matt "should" have been able to independently address community living needs as well; however, they reported that Matt did not typically "choose" to do these tasks. For example, mother identified that although Matt knew how to do his laundry, he did not independently wash his clothes unless someone told him that his clothes were dirty or smelly . Because of her son's "unwillingness" to independently take responsibility for life skills, mother identified that it "was just easier to do things for him."

Matt reported that he did not want to live with his parents anymore due to continuous conflict and feeling like he was "treated like a baby." His parents also reported high levels of stress and frustration associated with Matt living at home.

## Hospital Plan

Based on Matt's presentation, history, and identified needs, the following areas were identified for intervention: .

1. Stabilize his medical condition through reintroduction of psychotropic medication (Halperidol).

2. Provide supportive and structured programming to facilitate optimal patient functioning while stabilizing his medical condition and assessing patient response to medical interventions.

3. Initiate disposition planning to address: (a) Parent education; (b) patient living situation after discharge (with parents versus alternative); (c) medication monitoring; (d) patient's financial resources; (e) daily structure in postdischarge environment (work versus other).

## Occupational Therapy Interventions

Initial cognitive level assessment—The initial cognitive level screening, using the Allen Cognitive Level test (ACL) was administered on the 2nd day of hospitalization. Initial screening yielded a cognitive level score of 4.2. Occupational therapy records from a prior hospitalization at Colorado Psychiatric Hospital indicated that the patient had achieved a cognitive score of 4.6 at the time of discharge.

Occupational therapy treatment plan—The following problems and goals were established based on the general treatment plan for hospitalization, specific occupational therapy assessment, and the patient's current and anticipated cognitive levels:

1. *Problem:* Acute exacerbation of psychiatric illness/symptoms with an associated cognitive decompensation.

*Patient goal:* Patient will complete at least one concrete task (craft project) during cognitive-task groups in occupational therapy, 4X/week until discharged, and will acknowledge relationship between medication and cognitive level improvement as a result of occupational therapy.

*Outcome:* As anticipated, with the reintroduction of psychotropic medication, Matt's cognitive level improved to 4.8 by the 9th day of hospitalization. During discussions with the occupational therapist, the patient acknowledged a "possible" positive contribution of medication to his improved level of functioning.

2. *Problem:* Parent education needs and patient living situation.

*Goal:* The occupational therapist, patient, and Matt's parents will meet for 1 to 2 1-hour sessions in order to review assessed patient strengths and limitations and to determine/formulate realistic expectations for the patient within his parents' home. Based on these sessions, Matt and his parents will make a decision regarding his return home (with parents) versus an alternative living situation prior to discharge (program social worker also involved in meetings).

*Outcome:* Matt and his parents expressed relief following discussion of Matt's abilities and establishment of expectations based on those abilities. Agreement was reached for Matt to return home to live with parents. At the same time, Matt agreed to attend a life-skills training program offered through the public mental health system and to initiate involvement in a state-sponsored work program.

3. *Problem:* Need for structure in postdischarge environment.

*Goal:* Patient will agree to involvement in public mental health "Life Skill Training Program," Monday through Friday, for at least 3 months following discharge from the hospital.

*Goal:* In occupational therapy, prior to discharge, patient will contact State Vocational Rehabilitation Services and establish an appointment for intake to this service.

*Outcomes:* As patient involvement in the "Life Skills" program had been presented as a potential way to improve skills required for independence, Matt agreed to become involved in the program for 2 to 3 months. Matt was very enthusiastic about vocational rehabilitation involvement and continued to express a high level of motivation for work. Based on Matt's cognitive level at discharge and with Matt's approval, the occupational therapist recommended a supportive work environment and job coach to the vocational counselor completing Matt's intake.

(Medication management and financial resources for Matt were addressed by other disciplines during Matt's hospitalization.)

## General Discussion

This case involved interventions during both the acute and postacute phases of illness and involved planning for the rehabilitation phase. Initial occupational therapy interventions were directed toward assessment in order to determine the level of cognitive ability and disability associated with the acute phase of illness. In addition to providing data to guide initial interventions, the initial cognitive level score was used for comparison to subsequent clinical cognitive level assessments for the purpose of monitoring and measuring changes (cognitive) associated with primary medical treatment (medication).

As Matt entered the postacute phase of his illness, emphasis shifted to interventions and recommendations consistent with his need for environmental (external) adjustments/ modifications in order to function optimally within the community. Family education regarding patient strengths, limitations, and realistic performance expectations addressed this need and led to increased confidence related to Matt's return home. Referral to the independent life skills training program, emphasizing repetitive experience with tasks associated with self-care, community living, and communication was accomplished as part of Matt's postacute and rehabilitation program and addressed World Health Organization ICIDH Code 2, "Physical Independence Handicap," and Code 5, "Social Integration Handicap." Matt's parents agreed to work closely with the independent living program in order to reinforce rote learning and provide structured practice at home. The patient's involvement in this program would be primary, at least until vocational rehabilitation eligibility was determined (typically 2 to 6 months).

The vocational rehabilitation referral, with a recommendation for supportive employment and a job coach, is consistent with abilities at cognitive level 4.8 and was directed toward the rehabilitation phase of Matt's illness. This referral addressed Matt's "Occupational Handicap" (ICIDH Code 4) as de-

fined by the World Health Organization and, indirectly, Matt's "Economic Self-Sufficiency Handicap" (ICIDH Code 6). The patient's mental health center therapist, working with the patient and vocational counselor, agreed to track the progress of the patient with regard to work and Matt's potential for successful competitive employment.

All postacute interventions and postacute and rehabilitation-phase recommendations were based on the theoretical proposition that patients who achieve or stabilize at cognitive level 4.8 may be successful with new learning *if* new behaviors are concrete and are repeated numerous times with clear support from the environment (amenable to rote learning).

## Consulting for Long-Term Care

*Sarah P. Skinner, MEd, OTR/L*

Paul was admitted to the psychiatric unit following recent recurrent episodes of pulling a butcher knife on his mother in their family home. The patient was 33 and had been hospitalized three times due to exacerbations of psychotic behavior. His diagnosis was schizophrenia.

Paul was seen by an occupational therapist and assessed with an interview and the Allen Cognitive Level (ACL) test. His ACL score was 4. The patient was assigned to the structured track of group treatment sessions with goals of further assessing cognitive level in daily life activities and in task completion. He performed consistently at a level 4 in these groups, which his mother stated was consistent with performance at home.

During a family conference, it was decided to administer the Routine Task Inventory (RTI) to gather specific information related to the issue of referral postdischarge as the patient's mother was no longer willing to have him live in the family home full time.

Paul's mother was a professor in a nearby university. She had been able to meet most of her son's needs for structure in recent years by assigning him tasks each day, which she felt confident he could do. On further discussion with the mother, it became clear that the key was *familiar* tasks. Tasks Paul has previous expertise doing and locations he had been to many times and was comfortable navigating to provided him with a variety of meaningful tasks he could do for the family. When he was having a bad day, his mother simply defined tasks within the home. Sometimes he remained in bed all day; however, until recently, Paul had not acted out in a violet manner. This recent behavior had frightened his mother and made her feel unable to handle her son at home, although the family would remain involved with Paul.

The idea of placement was highly conflictual for the mother. She saw this as her failure to care for her son. The family conference began with ample time for her to discuss her guilt and concerns. Among questions asked by other professionals, the occupational therapist gathered RTI information from the mother as she had first-hand knowledge of her son's functioning in the home. Following are the results.

## Physical Scale

- **Grooming: 4**—Paul was able to initiate most grooming tasks as part of his daily routine; however, he occasionally neglected combing the back of his hair and shaving was incomplete.

- **Dressing: 4**—Paul was independent in dressing; however colors were not attended to, resulting in poorly matched dress. He did not seem to attend to wrinkles or missing buttons when not clearly visible when he checked himself in the mirror.

- **Bathing: 4–5**—Paul generally was independent in bathing. On those bad days, however, he tended to avoid showering. He used deodorant but often used excessive cologne.

- **Walking: 4**—Paul was able to navigate in familiar surroundings. If given written or verbal instructions to a new location, he consistently got lost.

- **Feeding: 3**—Paul's table manners were not socially acceptable; the family had stopped eating in restaurants due to this.

- **Toileting: 4**—Paul was independent using familiar toilets but needed assistance locating bathrooms in new locations.

## Instrumental Scale

- **Housekeeping: 4**—Paul, under instruction from his mother, was able to dust, put dishes away, vacuum, and make his own bed. Frequently his mother noted he did miss cleaning areas not clearly visible and never noticed silverware that had fallen through to the bottom of the dishwasher. At one point several years ago, the mother had moved the glasses to a different cabinet in the kitchen and Paul was unable to locate them. She then returned them to their original location to avoid frustrating him.

- **Preparing food: 4**—Paul was able to make sandwiches if his mother had placed everything he would need on a tray in the front of the refrigerator. He also scrambled eggs and could heat up canned or frozen food but often neglected to turn off burners on the stove. He left the oven on more often and burning food was a problem.

- **Spending money: 4**—Paul was given money each day and was able to handle simple transactions at the grocery and drug stores near his home. The neighborhood business people had come to know Paul and assisted him.

- **Taking medications: 3–4**—Mother had taken responsibility for administering Paul's medications as he was unable to follow the regime independently. His mother would set Paul's medications out each morning for the time she would be gone and administer afternoon and evening medicines when she got home. An aunt who lived two doors down would take over for mother when needed.

- **Doing laundry: 3**—Paul had never learned to do his laundry as a child. His mother had tried to teach this skill after his psychotic break at age 18, thinking this would be a fairly safe homebound activity he could do. She had written instructions, drawn pictures, and attempted in a step-by-step manner, with poor results. Therefore, she did his and the family's laundry.

- **Traveling: 4**—Paul is able to navigate via public transportation to familiar places. He has not driven since age 24, when his parents decided this was too high a level of responsibility. Paul routinely ran out of gas, would get out of the car, and be found wandering the streets. He had several minor traffic violations.

- **Shopping: 4**—Paul shops for several familiar items at familiar locations. If the store is out of the brand usually purchased, he becomes confused.

- **Telephoning: 4**—Paul successfully calls familiar numbers. He routinely uses 411 with mixed results as he also tends to transpose numbers when writing down the number from directory assistance. He no longer attempts to look numbers up in the telephone book as "it was too frustrating."

While gathering information from Paul's mother during the family conference, she made several "ah haaa" exclamations. She was being educated about the levels and what limitations an individual at a level 4 would be expected to experience. She also heard that this most likely would be a lifelong situation and was able to come to terms with placement for her son. She now saw placement as a positive situation for her 33-year-old son who needed to live out of the house for self-esteem reasons as well as the obvious safety reasons facilitated by the butcher knife episodes. In a professionally structured living environment, the patient might with repetition learn some new independent living tasks. He would still be an integral part of the family, visiting on weekends and holidays and maintaining telephone contact. The family could be relieved of their constant caretaking role and not feel guilty that they had not done enough.

This is an unusual case, but important in several ways. It illustrates the accuracy of the ACL as a screening tool and gives specific information on daily life tasks that can substantiate the need for supervised living situations for the chronically mentally ill. An extra benefit in this case is illustrated when family members gain better understanding of the disease and subsequent limitations.

## Functional Consequences of Cognitive Disability

*Greta Traugott Binkley, OTR*

### Admission Circumstances and History

Lisa is a 43-year-old black female whose family dropped her off at the psychiatric emergency department without staying to give further information. She was disorganized, disheveled, and malodorous. She mumbled nonsensically to herself and was unable to communicate with others due to selective mutism and hostility. Her primary diagnosis was Axis I: schizophrenia, chronic undifferentiated type. Although Lisa was an unreliable historian and the family was unavailable at first, much information and background was already known about her due to her long history of multiple psychiatric hospitalizations—most at this facility.

Lisa was born and raised in another state until her late 20s. She completed the 9th grade and had no further training or education. Her work history consisted of sporadic unskilled jobs in early adulthood, lasting up to 3 months at a time. She was supported by Social Security Insurance (SSI).

Lisa had three sons, ages 25, 22, and 21, who were raised predominantly by relatives and lived independently at this point. Her oldest son had tried to function as caregiver to Lisa in recent years, but was sporadic and unreliable due to his own problems and responsibilities. Lisa's mother and sister were supportive but not supervisory and not able to care for Lisa full time.

Lisa's history of mental illness onset began at age 18. She was hospitalized for psychotic behavior reportedly following unintentional ingestion of LSD. It was clear that this began a course of repeated psychiatric hospitalizations but the frequency and durations were not known until her late 20s when she moved to this area. From age 28 to 43, Lisa had over 20 known admissions to this hospital plus an unknown number of stays at other facilities including other acute hospitals, long-term (state) hospitals, and special treatment programs.

Following the natural course of her mental illness, Lisa had exhibited more frequent and severe decompensations and less cognitive recovery post-acute as years went on. Occupational therapy records and observations indicated that Lisa's behavior dropped to Allen's cognitive level 2 or even 1 when acutely ill. At times she would not respond to stimuli in her environment at all; at other times, momentary automatic purposeful actions such as a few strokes with a hairbrush could be guided. Familiarity and documentation also indicated that Lisa historically responded well to psychotropic medications in that symptoms would decrease and functional/cognitive capability would increase with treatment. When Lisa first became known at this hospital, she would reconstitute to level 5 capability by the time of discharge (prior to 1983). In the last 6 to 7 years, however, assessments were within the level 4 range (recently 4.4).

Two of Lisa's premorbid strengths and interests were socializing/interacting (i.e., church activities) and her personal appearance. Because of these interests and rote familiarity with the skills of these activities, Lisa could—once symptomatically stable—give a superficial impression of higher capability than she could exhibit in actual task behavior. Unfortunately, this resulted in family, caregivers, and legal professionals forming unrealistic expectations and situations for Lisa after her last several discharges. Several years prior, Lisa had secured a rare and valuable commodity—subsidized housing. Lisa and her caregivers shared a reluctance to relinquish it. This also contributed to the "give her another chance (to live independently)" strategy of prior discharge planning. During this hospitalization, occupational therapy cognitive level assessments were used by the treatment team to supplement her history of repeated and increasingly frequent admissions as evidence to prove grave disability, and to pursue conservatorship and long-term placement for Lisa. Eventual family contact further supported this plan since her son, sister, and mother had acknowledged that Lisa could not manage her mental illness outside of a structured facility, and they could not provide her with adequate supervision.

## Treatment Team Agenda

1. Stabilize acute schizophrenia by resuming and titrating psychotropic medications (Prolixin, Cogentin, Tegretol).

2. Observe, assess, and monitor status before and throughout titration process to justify initiation and continuation of treatment.

3. Gather and document all pertinent information for proper care and legal concerns.

4. Provide safe and structured environment to compensate for Lisa's disability and protect her from unintentional self-harm.

5. Initiate disposition planning.

6. Provide family services.

## Occupational Therapy Agenda

• **Phase I:** Severely symptomatic status

  - Observe and assess Lisa on the ward.

  - Provide information regarding current observations and previous history to treatment team.

  - Begin to explain to team members (resident physician, psychiatric social worker) consequences of level 4 disability as evident in Lisa's function prior to admission.

• **Phase II:** Beginning symptom control

  - Administer Allen Cognitive Level (ACL) standardized task evaluation.

  - Assess and evaluate Lisa's ability to perform various tasks in occupational therapy groups.

  - Share initial evaluation with treatment team.

• **Phase III:** Symptom stabilizing

  - Continue observation and assessment of Lisa's

symptoms, possible medication side effects, and cognitive level on the ward and in occupational therapy groups.

  - Provide frequent verbal and weekly written reports of current assessments and implications for medication titration, behavior management, and beginning disposition plans.

• **Phase IV:** Subacute symptoms diminished

  - Continue observation and assessment on ward and in occupational therapy groups.

  - Continue verbal and written reporting of assessments and implications.

  - Confer with psychiatric social worker regarding pertinent cognitive level information for family.

  - Confer with medical case worker regarding pertinent cognitive level information for placement.

## Course of Treatment

### Phase I

During the first phase of Lisa's hospitalization, she was severely withdrawn, paranoid, agitated, responding to auditory and possibly visual hallucinations, and was unable to participate in any meaningful activity, even basic self-care. She was incontinent and refused most food and water. Her spontaneous behavior was bizarre and unpredictable, such as hiding under her bed, in her closet, or wrapping herself up in sheets, talking to or destroying other patients' belongings, disrobing in the hallways and common rooms, masturbating, and smearing feces and urine around when incontinent. Lisa needed primarily nursing and medical care at this phase. She was inappropriate for occupational therapy participation.

The treatment team's focus at this time was to manage Lisa's behavior and care, provide medication when emergently justified (she refused to consent), pursue legal authority to treat without consent (Reese hearing), and gather further information to aid in planning Lisa's treatment and disposition.

The occupational therapy focus, though not directly involved at this time, was to provide historical information from previous admissions and explain the significance of Lisa's cognitive level to her dysfunction outside of the hospital. Lisa had a history of having decompensated to ACL 3.2 or even 1 on admission. Recent recoveries, as mentioned, had not reached capability 4.4, but Lisa could present a misleading superficial impression. At cognitive level 4.4, she should not have been expected to manage independent living. She was not capable of maintaining medication or follow-up treatment compliance, managing her financial affairs, or problem solving through any sudden or emergent change that would arise during the course of daily routines. Although family members were involved with Lisa, their visits were too infrequent and social (i.e., shopping, visiting) to provide adequate supervision for Lisa. Her son's previous intention to live with and care for Lisa did not work out.

## Phase II

Lisa had rebuffed all early attempts at interaction by the occupational therapist. As her symptoms began to decrease, Lisa had begun acknowledging previous acquaintances and responding briefly but more appropriately. She could not tolerate sufficient interaction for an interview, refused to perform the ACL screening evaluation, but did agree to go to the grooming group.

Once there, Lisa continued to be intermittently distracted by symptoms and had to be prompted to interact with objects in the environment. She used only supplies given to or placed immediately in front of her. She became more interested in the effect she could create than any reasonable or social standard. She applied cosmetics without concern for their purpose and followed the perimeters of shapes and contours of her face. The result was white racoonlike circles around her eyes and a "T" of pink lipstick across her forehead and down her nose. Once prompted, Lisa wiped or blended the pink with a tissue, and followed a demonstration to put lipstick on her lips. Moments later, however, she reapplied the "T."

Lisa was assessed at level 3.6 at her best. Similar performance in two more grooming groups confirmed this. Lisa refused other activities. Assessments were shared with the team and documented in the chart (i.e., initial evaluation write-up).

## Phase III

By this time, Lisa was taking routine medications without incident or refusal. Her symptoms were diminishing and cognitive level improving. Lisa began to participate in Basic Crafts and occasionally the Sewing Group, as well as Grooming. Assessments improved incrementally over several weeks:

3.6, 3.8/4.0, 4.2, as she became more organized and aware of her environment. On the ward, she had increasingly become more appropriate and interactive, following ward routines and socializing with staff and peers.

As Lisa improved, updated assessments were shared with the treatment team with particular emphasis on her disability and its implications. Though seemingly negative in focus, it was important not to let improvement overshadow the reality of her functional limitations.

Further information was provided by the family and landlord via the psychiatric social worker during this time as well. It was through family meetings and therapy that her family finally acknowledged the extent of Lisa's disability and their inability to provide adequate supervision. Additionally, Lisa's landlord evicted her because of the increasingly frequent and severe nature of her exacerbations and numerous complaints from neighbors.

## Phase IV

During the last week or two of hospitalization, Lisa continued to participate in groups and interact appropriately on the ward, with the exception of her psychiatrist whom she blamed for losing her apartment. Her symptoms were diminished, and her cognitive level plateaued as she stabilized. Legal procedures had been completed, and conservatorship was granted with a public guardian for Lisa.

Assessments in occupational therapy were predominantly 4.4, occasionally 4.2 in various task groups. Lisa would work diligently to replicate a sample or conform to a given standard. She would try to determine her course of action by comparing her supplies or project to the sample and would often ask for confirmation such as "is this right?" Lisa could usually consider two to three striking visual cues such as shape, color, and size but occasionally would need to look at just one feature at a time, particularly when trying or being prompted to recognize or resolve an error.

Occupational therapy's documentation and verbal reports continued. It was explained that although persons functioning at Lisa's level can typically do well in an open, supervised environment, recommendations for Lisa would be for continued locked and structured placement, given her history of repeated treatment noncompliance and resultant decompensations. Special effort was made to communicate specifically with the psychiatric social worker and medical case worker. The social worker was provided a description of typical functional consequences to aid the family in understanding and providing future compensations for Lisa's cognitive level. Placement alternatives and their inherent expectations in comparison with Lisa's cognitive capability were discussed with the medical case worker. As it turned out, an opening at a locked long-term-care facility (state hospital) occurred before other placement could be achieved, and she was transferred there.

The point in this case study is the importance of considering a patient's cognitive capability in treatment and disposition planning, as well as to describe a history of the natural course of a mental illness.

## Sensory Integration and Cognitive Disability

*Sandra K. David, OTR, MHE*

Two case studies are presented that reflect the grading of the clinical experience to the cognitive level of the patient. These particular cases were selected because they involved successful treatment of dissimilar patients. The two patients whose treatments are described were of different ages; one was medicated and one was not; and only one had prior experience with occupational therapy. In order to provide a proper perspective on the case studies, we start with a detailed portrayal of the psychiatric occupational therapy clinic where the case study patients were treated.

Cabinets in the occupational therapy clinic are organized according to the cognitive levels. Three cabinets are opened during treatment sessions, one containing patients' projects in progress, another dedicated to ceramics samples, and the last displaying nonceramic samples and supplies for projects. The nonceramics cabinet is centrally located. Displayed at eye level are sample items with sharp contrasts in color and shape. The other shelves in this cabinet contain ready-to-use supplies divided into sections for leather, tile, wood, copper, beads, stenciling, and handwork. Bins in each section are organized by the standard task sequence. Both the shelves and bins are identified with large, brightly colored labels with large black lettering. General supplies, including stain brushes, stains, and tools, are kept in labeled low-walled bins located on a shelf directly below the samples.

The ceramic samples cabinet contains projects appropriate for a patient functioning as low as cognitive level 4.0. The samples serve as a standard of performance. The patient is first given a sequence of directions with the therapist providing guidance as difficulties arise. The choice of ceramic projects is based on usefulness and the simplicity and visibility of the joint seams. The ceramic molds are of objects that are functional or a part of everyday life. An example project is the shell salad bowl. It is 10 inches across and has only one joint seam. This seam runs along the edge of the shell and across the back. Ridges on the back of the shell run perpendicular to the joint seam, creating a sharp contrast. This area requires some guidance by the therapist for an accurate execution of cleaning. Often the shell is placed on a cleaning stand to improve visibility of the seams. This is an example of matching the task requirements to the patients' cognitive abilities to provide the successful task execution needed to build self-competence. After cleaning, the ceramic project is fired and the patient selects the glaze from colors applied to the exterior of a canister, which is labeled on the bottom.

The ceramics room is therapist-guided with the exception of the counter. Patients work cooperatively with the therapist to bind and pour the ceramic molds. The counter section is set up for level 4 with an opened small ceramics brush case and a large and a small basket. The large basket contains glazes that are labeled on the lids. The small basket contains dividers with cleaning tools and sponges, as well as an underglaze section with a small tile underglaze color sampler. A drawer below the counter contains a ceramics brush bin with adjacent water cups for easy visibility and access.

Items pertinent to daily living motivate adults for engagement in gross motor and larger movements. Activities promoting sensory integration are selected using criteria that include deep proprioceptive input, repetition, tactile variety, fine- and gross-motor coordination, and linear vestibular acceleration. Woodworking kits must have at least one piece of wood that is a minimum of 14 inches in length. The mixed porcelain tile is brought out in a bucket 8 inches in height and 9 inches in diameter. The average size of the ceramic pieces is 10 inches in at least one dimension. Copper tooling and copper punch items are tacked to the usable wood projects.

## Case 1

Janice was a 28-year-old female admitted by her family for evaluation. Her family reported significant social stressors including 2 years of physical and sexual abuse by her boyfriend and strained relationships with her family of origin. Her diagnosis was major depression. She reported headaches and insisted that she did not feel depressed or have reason to be depressed. In her interactions with others she was very defensive, guarded in conversations, often emphasizing that she was not under any stress. However, she displayed psychomotor retardation, sad affect, and sloppy grooming and dressing. She wore no make-up and appeared to give no attention to her hair either by washing or brushing.

Janice's Allen Cognitive Level (ACL) was 4.5, she was right-hand dominant, and avoided crossing midline during tasks where it was necessary. She was not on any psychotropic medications at the time of admission and was not started on any during her 14-day hospital stay. She was seen in the occupational therapy clinic for 14 sessions of 1 hour each over her admission period of 10 working days.

During her treatment, she chose woodworking and ceramics projects, which she worked on alternately during her admission. She focused on the task for 4- to 5-minute periods during the first session. During the first few sessions she had difficulty attending to task and making decisions without encouragement. She was given demonstrated instruction on solving task problems when asked. By the third session her attention span had increased to 25 minutes. The patient was encouraged to produce 1/4 cup of sawdust before staining or painting. Her questions about the tasks focused on the physical aspects and techniques required to execute the project and clean up. Janice produced approximately 1 cup of sawdust per wood project without redirection.

During her admission she completed a total of three woodworking projects. All of these were stained with the same color stain. She chose not to put decorations on the wood projects (e.g., copper tooling) and was not interested in making the wood projects look different from each other although the projects had varying uses. She only interacted with others when not engaged in the task execution.

Janice began working on her ceramic greenware project during the fourth session. She received one demonstration of the procedure to clean ceramic joint seams. She attended to the seams of the visible areas only but required only one instruction to turn the project to inspect for further areas to be cleaned. Only after initial orientation to the ceramics room, did she locate project materials. Ceramics glazes are selected because their raw color contrasts sharply with the bisqueware. It was significant that she needed reminders to turn the ceramic project to apply the three coats of glaze without leaving areas uncovered. She needed reminders to completely clean up her area. Often her ceramics brushes were only rinsed, with raw glaze still visible within the core of the brush (level 4.6). Her cognitive level did not change during hospitalization.

Janice appeared visibly improved 2 days prior to discharge. Her appearance and grooming were neat, her hair clean and styled, and she had applied make-up. At discharge, her attention span had increased to 45 minutes, she displayed a bright affect, and her motor speed was within normal limits. She had been headache-free for 3 days. She frequently crossed midline during engagement in activities.

Also at the time of discharge, Janice engaged other patients and family members in conversation without defensiveness. When asked by her therapist if she was feeling better, she replied that she had felt fine all along. Her occupational therapist also asked her if she felt that any of the activities were stress reducing for her. She responded that she wasn't under any stress. This inability for self-observation is typical of a patient at level 4.

## Case 2

Emma was a 60-year-old woman with a history of psychiatric admissions to private hospitals. Her diagnosis was major depression and general anxiety disorder. Her most recent hospitalization had been 3 months previous. Emma had a delusion that she was unable to and did not care for herself unless a family member was around. Her anxiety revolved around the fear of her husband having an accident. The physicians were readjusting her medications to decrease her anxiety and improve her depression.

Emma was dressed neatly but casually in blouse and pants with her hair clean and brushed; no make-up was applied. She had mild arthritis, and endured moderate levels of activity for 5 to 7 minutes before complaining of fatigue. Emma was right-hand dominant, avoided crossing midline, and tended to move slowly through space. She was goal directed, her ACL was 4.8, and her initial attention span was 2 to 3 minutes. She had decreased self-esteem and was highly anxious and distractible. When Emma entered the clinic, she remarked that she had been in occupational therapy many times and could not do "creative artsy things." The crafts she chose to execute during her 16-day stay were copper tooling, woodworking, and ceramics. Copper tooling was her first project. She used a detailed sample in front of her to effect an exact match without redirection by the therapist. She was directed to reduce the size of the stick as soon as she was not getting detail to show, which she did. The samples are sharply contrasting and display a great deal of detail. During the antiquing process she remarked about the effect the liver of sulfur had on the copper. She was careful to examine the copper and commented that she was unable to get the corners to blend exactly. The therapist told her that these areas could be removed if needed. During the third session, Emma had chosen a wooden peg rack on which to tack her copper project. Sanding blocks were used to assist in promoting joint protection and to allow the patient to engage in a repetitive deep proprioceptive activity. She produced 1/2 cup of sawdust in preparing the wood for the staining process when only 1/4 cup is encouraged. Emma had the therapist cut the copper to fit onto the wood project. She had no difficulty centering the copper on the wood or tacking it exactly the way the instructions were given.

Ceramic cats held a special appeal for Emma as cats were an important part of her life at home. In cleaning the ceramic project, she needed prompting once to check the seams and put her initials on the bottom. But even with visual and verbal cuing, she missed the rough areas on the bottom of the project. She asked the therapist to execute the underglazed details of the cat. Instead of the therapist doing her details for her, part of the preparation of the patient for guidance in a new technique is the gathering of supplies needed from different locations in the clinic. This usually consists of three short trips between the ceramic room counter and the work table to gather the needed supplies (linear acceleration) and strategic unfolding of the paper towels to prepare the area (spatial orientation). Emma was very successful in following the instructions precisely on areas that were visible. She was directed to

turn the object over and inscribe her initials. Orienting the cat in this way visually exposed the seam and a roughened hole. The therapist asked her if she saw any seams or rough places that needed cleaning. She indicated that she did not and put her initials on the cat. Emma did not recognize the surface properties of the base of the project (the seams and rough areas). She attended to the visible details of her cat, including filling in the cat eyes and making the pupils. She completely filled the iris area without either being short of or extending beyond the eye line; the pupil was appropriately located. Emma used different-sized brushes for these details with only verification of her execution. She received consensual support from the other patients regarding the execution of her completed project. However, when the first cat was complete, Emma continued to try to convince the therapist she had not executed the eyes of the cat.

The next cat met with similar success, as she exactly followed the procedures she had done before. She checked with the therapist to see that she had indeed followed the correct procedures (firing ceramic prior to glazing, technique on completing the eyes). But this time she seemed to quietly accept her task execution. Emma took a greater risk on the last cat by attempting a replica of one at home. She brought in photographs and talked about this cat, sharing during treatment sessions some of the history of this animal. Emma did an excellent job of attending to the sharp visible details during the cleaning process. She also noticed and corrected mistakes made in visible areas of her ceramic projects. However, she still did not attend to the seams or rough places concealed on the base of the project. Her cognitive level had improved to 5.0.

At discharge, her attention span was 45 minutes. She would spontaneously cross the midline during task execution as necessary. Emma tolerated 40 minutes of moderate activity without complaint. Her motor movement was within normal rate. She appeared neatly groomed and dressed, with her hair styled. Emma displayed pride in her work. The most remarkable event of her admission occurred during her last session. She reported that she never before believed that she could do such fine work. She felt that she actually could be independent and had intentionally spent time home and in various other locations alone for several hours at a time. Emma reported that this was due to her treatment sessions in the occupational therapy clinic. She maintained that she "didn't know what it was but that what we did was very different from all the other occupational therapy clinics" she had been in before. She reported feeling like a competent person because of the success in completing the tasks to her standards, which she could never do before.

The following commentary speculates about why both of these patients improved, in order to encourage others to study possible explanations for the behavior. Is this natural healing? Does engagement in any type of activity have healing properties? Do we as therapists facilitate natural healing through the application of activity analysis? Is there additional benefit to be gained by combining the cognitive modes of performance with sensory integration?

Several processes are taking place during the engagement in an activity. The primitive sensory systems of movement, touch, and pressure organize the brain for function as part of the body's survival mechanisms. This organization may be promoted by providing opportunities during activities for deep pressure, tactile variety, linear movement in space, and the range of motion used to complete the steps in the task. The key to providing an increase in the efficiency of brain functioning lies in the amount of input into the nervous system. Small, refined movements contribute too little information to the nervous system and hence tend not to optimize the integrative effect of multisensory systems. In contrast, larger and gross-motor movements supply substantial amounts of consistent information that increase the efficiency of brain functioning. An adaptive response reflects the accuracy of the individual's spatial orientation and multisensory integration during a perceptual motor task.

The patient's engagement in craft activities allows an adaptive response to be observed in an environment in which the functional capacities of the patient are optimized by the grading of the steps to match the capacity of the person. Janice's activity choices may reflect Ayres's statement that "a human being is designed to enjoy things that promote the development of his brain and therefore we naturally seek sensations that help organize our brain" (1979, p. 7). Perhaps Janice's choices of woodworking and ceramics activities reflected self-organizing behavior. Improved organization may have increased her access to already existing functional capacities or it may have reduced frustration in attempting to function above her capacity.

The second case is harder to interpret because of medication effects. Emma may demonstrate that relevant activities that promote efficiency of sensory processing may result in improved use of already existing capacities. Her feelings of self-competence may reflect the additional energy available to recognize successful performance. That she associated her improvement with these particular activities merits further investigation.

### Reference

Ayres, A.J. (1979). *Sensory integration and the child.* Los Angeles, CA: Western Psychological Services.

## Craniotomy—Postacute

*Tina Blue, OTR*

The following is an example of how the Allen Cognitive Levels (ACL) were used to monitor a patient in the postacute phase of healing after a craniotomy secondary to a nonmalignant brain tumor. Confirmations of the ACL task evaluation done at 2 1/2 and 3 1/2 weeks status postsurgery were done through observations of task performance in grooming and clinic activities.

### Brief History

Jill is a 43-year-old married woman with no previous medical history. She lives with her husband and two young children, ages 3 and 5, in a two-story townhouse. She was working as a secretary before her surgery. Avocational interests included reading and cooking. She plans to return home after discharge from rehabilitation.

### Presenting Condition at 2 1/2 Weeks Status Postsurgery

Jill had functional range of motion and mildly impaired strength and coordination of her left upper extremity with selective movement, mild hyperflexia with resistive maneuvers, and impaired reflexes. Left grip strength was 30 pounds. Her right dominant upper extremity was functional with good strength, selective movement, and normal tone and reflexes. Her affect was blunted with restricted range. She was distractible and could not remember what therapy she was in or what she had done in therapy on the previous day. She appeared to be apathetic regarding her disability and answered open-ended questions with short phrases or one-word answers.

When asked what she would like to work on first, she blandly answered, "Whatever you want." Her treatment plan in occupational therapy included grooming, left upper-extremity strengthening and coordination activities, and cognitive/perceptual tasks. Her ACL score was 3.3.

After being given a demonstration of the running stitch, she impulsively began making random stitches, going in and out, skipping holes and modifying actions without checking her effects. When errors were pointed out, she became frustrated and abandoned the task by saying, "I don't want to do this anymore."

### Observation of Task Performance

*Grooming:* Jill was able to apply make-up (eyebrow pencil, mascara, lipstick) in a habitual manner, with set-up. She followed the general outline of her eyebrows with a line above the brow in an uneven arch; mascara was splotchy and uneven; lipstick was uneven where she had attempted to follow the shape of her lips (over and under the lip line in areas). *Bilateral sander with weight:* Jill kept wanting to take the cylindrically shaped weight out of the sander to "roll" it back and forth with both hands instead of holding onto the handles to push and pull the sander in a repetitive linear direction, despite several demonstrations. *Minnesota Rate of Manipulation Test (MRMT):* She was instructed to perform maneuvers with her left upper extremity to turn the discs over to reveal a differently colored side and then place them in a forward slot. She spontaneously began using both hands to turn or place the discs in a random fashion despite repeated verbal cues and redemonstrations to the contrary. She could use one hand for brief periods of time and would either forget to turn the disc over or place it in a forward slot without judging her effects to recognize the errors. *Form board with 12 shapes:* Jill was able to successfully pick up and match the larger-sized square, circle, and triangular shapes, but had difficulty with matching variations of sizes and more complicated shapes like octagons and pentagons. With probing, she was able to modify her actions to turn pieces around to match the form board perimeters after initially trying to repeatedly force shapes into random slots. (Note: This might look like a focal-perceptual deficit.)

### Analysis of Task Performance

Performance in a familiar grooming activity was consistent with cognitive level 3.6, which was higher than the ACL score of 3.3. Task performance with the bilateral sander was consistent with criteria for 3.2 (e.g., spontaneous initiating back and forth movement with the weight, which she may have associated with a familiar object like dough or a rolling pin). She was unable to retain a demonstration or guide her actions by looking at the object while performing the MRMT exercise, which is also consistent with 3.2. She was, however, able to follow shapes to guide placement of simple recognizable shapes with cuing, which is consistent with 3.6. Overall assessment for the session was that she could function at 3.5 (high 3) in familiar activities (grooming, matching familiar shapes) and 3.2 (low 3) with unfamiliar, or new-learning activities (sander, MRMT).

## Presenting Condition at 3 1/2 Weeks Status Postsurgery

Overall strength and coordination were improved in Jill's left upper extremity, with more normalized tone and an increase to 36 pounds of grip strength. Her affect was still essentially blunted, but brighter with improved range. She was noticeably more verbal and asking goal-directed questions like: "What do you want me to do?" She was less distractible, but still had difficulty remembering what therapy she was in. She did not remember this therapist from working with her a week prior.

Jill's ACL score was now 4.2. She was able to complete three whip stitches with one demonstration, but was unable to correct twists in the lacing. She refused to attempt the single cordovan.

### Observation of Task Performance

Jill was able to set up her own familiar grooming supplies, and application effects were noticeably improved. She was able to perform the bilateral sanding and MRMT exercises without demonstration, and could match the 12 shapes without assistance or cuing within a near-normal pace.

### Analysis of Task Performance

Jill's performance was consistent with the ACL score of 4.2. She was spontaneously goal directed and was able to judge the effects of her actions by matching features for shape, color, and linear direction, as well as being able to independently keep up with a prescribed count of actions to perform exercise sets with the bilateral sander.

The improvement in Jill's cognitive/perceptual tasks paralleled the improvement in her mode of performance. The advantage of the measurement of the mode is the association with Jill's intended activities after discharge. At level 4.2, the therapist would not recommend independent care of her children or returning to her job as a secretary.

## Stroke: Comparison of Impairment- versus Disability-Driven Models for Treatment

*Tina Blue, OTR*

A single case is used here to present two different approaches to rehabilitation. The impairment-driven model is commonly used in current practice. The disability-driven model is suggested by this text as more meaningful to the patient and the social support system.

### History

John is a 74-year-old retired male with a diagnosis of 11 weeks status post–cerebral vascular accident with right hemiparesis. His medical history includes: diabetes myelitis, hypertension, chronic myelogenous leukemia, past colonectomy for diverticulosis and gastrointestinal bleeding, status post-old-right cerebrovascular accident with mild left residual upper-extremity weakness. He is left-hand dominant, wears bifocals, and has mild bilateral hearing loss. John lives with his wife in a one-story house with two front porch steps. Previous interests included cooking and gardening. John was unable to state his rehabilitation goals, but his wife stated that she would like for him to be able to help with dressing and transferring himself.

### Presenting Condition at 2 Weeks Status Postonset

John's medical condition was stable. His right upper extremity was flaccid with impaired deep tendon reflexes and no reaction to pin prick. His left-dominant upper extremity had functional range of motion and strength with good grasp and pinch to manipulate objects that were placed in his hand. His right lower extremity had increased extensor tone with passive range but no spontaneous movement. Left lower extremity range of motion and strength appeared to be within functional limits with selective motor control, based on observation of spontaneous movements. Sitting and standing balances were poor, and endurance was very poor. There were no problems with chewing or swallowing, and head control was good. He did not feed himself. Sensation or perception could not be adequately assessed due to the severity of John's cognitive and communicative limitations. He did not speak, but grimaced or gestured to indicate needs that were not understood. Handwriting was barely legible and nonsensical. He was, however, able to follow demonstrations of gross up and down movements with his left upper extremity. He was both bladder and bowel incontinent. In occupational therapy, he needed maximum cognitive assistance to initiate movements with his intact extremity for exercise and manipulating material objects. For brief periods of time, he was able to imitate postural movements to bat beach balls and throw bean bags to hit a target. Basic self-care required maximum assistance to elicit attempts to participate. He was able to grasp safety rails with guidance but needed assistance to release them. He was unable to perform the Allen Cognitive Level (ACL) test, but task performance was consistent with criteria for *cognitive level 2.8.*

### Impairment-Driven Rehabilitation Course

John underwent rehabilitation for 9 weeks with occupational, physical, and speech therapies. *Occupational therapy goals* focused on: increasing activities of daily living (ADL) skills (i.e., independent dressing, standby assistance bathing, independent grooming, independent transfers, and supervised functional mobility); improving self-feeding; facilitating normal postural reactions and normal muscle tone; preventing deformity; increasing endurance and sitting–standing tolerance; improving perceptual/cognitive skills; improving awareness of and/or compensation for sensory deficit; increasing patient/family education about rehabilitation program.

*Treatment methods* included: self-care activities (including learning one-sided dressing, using adaptive equipment as applicable); transfer training (including to and from bed, toilet, shower bench, mat, and other furniture from wheelchair in a safe manner); community reorientation (including field trip to hospital cafeteria, restaurant, if possible, and home visit); feeding activities (including use of adaptive equipment as applicable); functional activities in clinic to reinforce objectives (e.g., crafts, kitchen activities, bean-bag throw, beach ball toss, etc.); therapeutic exercises (including passive, active, and active-assistive range of motion, teaching self-range of motion, Swedish sling); progressive sitting and standing activities (e.g., hydraulic table, standing box while doing functional activities, etc.); neurodevelopmental and facilitation techniques; splinting and positioning; perceptual/cognitive activities (including sequencing tasks, design blocks, puzzles, pegs, cognitive worksheets, and compensating for residual deficits); sensory stimulation; adaptive equipment (including use of wheelchair, safety rails, transfer board, shower bench, dycem, dressing stick, button aid, etc.); patient/family teaching (regarding home program, use of adaptive equipment, environmental alterations, community reorientation, assistance needed, and safety).

*Discharge planning:* John's wife wanted to care for him at home with the assistance of a private nurse's aide and a supportive family who agreed to visit frequently and help with his care. A home visit with John and his wife was done a week before discharge to assess his needs. Equipment was issued and in place when John arrived home, including a standard hospital bed. Adaptive equipment included: standard wheelchair with removable arms and leg rests; wheelchair arm tray, transfer board, bedside commode, urinal, shower bench, safety rails, shower hose, spasticity hand split, and sling. A wheelchair ramp to the front porch was built by the family. Follow-up treatment included home health nursing, and occupational, physical, and speech therapies two to three times a week to continue working on rehabilitation goals.

## Disability-Driven Rehabilitation Model

*Short-term goal:* Verify cognitive level 2.8 with activities the patient can do (e.g., placing comb, toothbrush, wash mitt in hand and guiding movements; see if patient will move intact extremities to cooperate with positioning, bathing, dressing, transferring with tactile cues; imitate postural movements for exercising, batting beach ball, throw bean bags to hit a target, etc.).

*Educate caregiver:* Explain the physical and cognitive assistance currently needed and predict the amount of assistance the patient will need in approximately 2 months, based on knowledge of the natural course of healing (Bonita & Beaglehole, 1988; Dombovy, et al., 1987; Reding & Potes, 1988). (That is to say, the most obvious improvements with stroke patients occur within the first 6 weeks status postonset if there are no complications. John is already 2 weeks status postonset with severe cogni-

tive and physical impairments. Realistic expectations predict that he will probably improve cognitively into the level 3 and possibly the level 4 range of ability with at least moderate residual physical limitations. There are, of course, exceptions.)

*Assess caregiver's willingness to assume long-term-care responsibilities:* John's wife and family want to care for him at home and assume the responsibility of carrying over treatment methods and preventing medical complications when professional therapy has been discontinued.

*Negotiate activities that the caregiver would like the patient to do:* John's wife would like him to be able to help with dressing and transfers.

*Set up training procedures that improve physical impairments, prevent medical complications, and improve personal care locomotor and body disposition disabilities:*

- Sensory stimulation techniques to right upper extremity.

- Passive and active-assistance range of motion exercises to right upper extremity; educate caregiver in methods that prevent medical complications, including protecting flaccid shoulder.

- Apply sensorimotor/neurodevelopmental techniques to normalize tone and facilitate postural actions (e.g., Rood techniques; mat/bed activities with Bobath or Brunnstrom methods); train caregiver in methods for purposes of positioning/patient care, including use of positioners.

- Compensate for impaired sitting and standing balance to prevent safety hazards; teach caregiver compensations.

- Facilitate functional use of intact extremity for self-feeding, transfers using adaptive equipment, and to cooperate with dressing and bathing (e.g., facilitating postural actions).

- Collaborate with nursing to train caregiver regarding patient's basic self-care (e.g., effective positioning, eliciting attempts to cooperate, facilitating postural actions, monitoring and dealing with patient's incontinence).

- Train caregiver in safe transfer techniques with adaptive and safety equipment (e.g., operation of wheelchair, transfer board, use of safety belt, safety rails).

- Train caregiver in use of adaptive equipment that increases patient's comfort, prevents medical complications, and expedites patient care (e.g., splints, positioners, sling, shower hose, etc.).

- Monitor for change in cognitive level; probe for next even number (i.e., 3.0 and up as applicable) and adjust training procedures as improvement occurs.

- Teach caregiver adjustments in level of assistance as improvement occurs.

- Assess sensation and perception as able.

- Collaborate with nursing, physical, and speech therapies to integrate methods.

- Collaborate with social worker regarding patient/family's psychosocial adjustment to potential residual physical and cognitive disabilities.

- Collaborate with caregiver to begin thinking about potential home modifications, community resources.

Disability-driven treatment involves getting the caregivers involved earlier than is typical with impairment-driven methods. This in no way is meant to discourage hopes for the patient's improvement, but begins to set up realistic expectations for the level of assistance that the patient may need after discharge. By being involved early in the treatment process, they are learning how to give effective assistance in order to maximize capabilities, prevent medical complications, and ensure the safety of the care receiver (Evans, et al., 1988).

## Condition at Discharge

John's condition at discharge would probably be the same with the impairment- and disability-driven models. The difference is in the preparation for his discharge and the prevention of injuries to him and his caregivers.

John's right upper extremity is nonfunctional, with pain and spasticity throughout passive range of motion. He cannot bear weight into his right upper extremity and has a potential to sublux his shoulder. He can bear weight into his right lower extremity but actively moves it in a strong extensor pattern. Right upper- and lower-extremity cutaneous and kinesthetic sensations are impaired. Left upper- and lower-extremity sensations appear to be intact. There is moderate pitting edema in his right hand. Sitting balance is fair and standing balance is poor. Overall endurance is fair. He has decreased spontaneous attention to his right side and does not scan the environment. He is confused, easily distracted, and impulsive. He is expressively aphasic and may be receptively aphasic as well. His written communicative skills remain poor. He has difficulty following demonstrated and verbal directions consistently.

There is possible motor apraxia present, and probable visuospatial problems. *Activities of daily living:* John requires moderate cognitive and physical assistance from his caregiver for toileting, transfers, hygiene, dressing, and grooming. He is able to feed himself with set-up and precut food, and is most successful with feeding himself finger food. His caregiver needs to sequence him through his self-care routine and compensate for his physical disability. He frequently resists exercise and positioning attempts with his painful right upper extremity, and does not like to wear his sling. He cannot follow a self-range-of-motion sequence when attempts are elicited. He uses his left upper extremity spontaneously to grasp and manipulate objects that capture his interest. He is impulsive and unsafe in kitchen activities. He has been unsuccessful in attempts to learn to use adaptive equipment that requires goal direction and neuromuscular adjustments with his intact side (e.g., dressing stick, button aid, shoe horn, rocker knife). He requires constant cuing and physical assistance to accomplish safe transfers with and without a transfer board. He is inconsistent with bowel and bladder functions. He is wheelchair bound with a posey restraint. He attempts to propel himself in the wheelchair but frequently runs into walls and furniture. He has fallen out of bed when not restrained. ACL was performed with a score of 3.2, which is consistent with his task performance.

## Recommended Assistance

John needs 24-hour care to monitor his behavior and remove safety hazards; compensate for residual physical disability; place objects needed for activities of daily living in front of him and complete motions for an acceptable result; and, one-on-one supervision to complete the activity with an acceptable result. The caregiver must provide the physical assistance needed to complete transfers with adaptive equipment in a safe manner. The caregiver must also ensure postural stabilization, prevent medical complications by positioning, adding posterior-mounted brakes to the wheelchair, and restraining John as needed. Medical complications must be prevented and John's comfort with modalities, splints/positioners, gentle range of motion, neurodevelopmental, and edema control techniques increased. John must be monitored for incontinence and probed for cognitive level 3.4 as able. The therapist should be notified of John's improving abilities for reevaluation if applicable.

## References

Bonita, R. & Beaglehole, R. (1988). Recovery of motor function after stroke. *Stroke, 19,* 1497–1500.

Dombovy, M.L., Basford, J.R., et al. (1987). Disability and use of rehabilitation services following stroke in Rochester, Minnesota, 1975–1979. *Stroke, 18,* 830–836.

Evans, R.L., Matlock, A.L., et al. (1988). Family intervention after stroke: Does counseling or education help? *Stroke, 19,* 1243–1249.

Reding, M.J., & Potes, E. (1988). Rehabilitation outcome following initial unilateral hemispheric stroke. *Stroke, 19,* 1354–1358.

## Suggested Readings

Earhart, C.A., & Allen, C.K. (1988). *Cognitive disabilities: Expanded activity analysis.* Colchester, CT: S & S Worldwide.

Hasselkus, B.R. (1991). Ethical dilemmas in family caregiving for the elderly: Implications for occupational therapy. *American Journal of Occupational Therapy, 45,* 206–212.

O'Sullivan, S.B., & Schmitz, T.J. (Eds.). (1988). *Physical rehabilitation: Assessment and treatment, 2nd edition.* Philadelphia: F.A. Davis.

World Health Organization. (1980). *International classification of impairments, disabilities, and handicaps.* Geneva: Author.

## Postacute in a Rehabilitation Facility

*Lori Bridges, OTR*
*Karen Richardson, OTR*

## Introduction

Familiar activity cannot be done in the routine manner given the profound motor and perceptual deficits seen in the patient who has had a cerebrovascular accident (CVA). Even basic self-care requires the learning of new sensorimotor patterns. The learning process is complicated by change due to spontaneous clearing. The occupational therapist considers changing medical, motor, perceptual, cognitive, and volitional factors in the treatment to facilitate learning new ways of doing familiar activities. Cognitive impairment is frequently the limiting factor in the process of new skill acquisition in rehabilitation.

In this case study, a range of cognitive levels is given that corresponds to the performance seen in a given week. Some behaviors fall outside of the range to one extreme or the other due to factors of volition, familiarity, or the particular perceptual and motor challenge of the task. Specific weekly changes in the patient's status can be inferred from the descriptions of performance and intervention.

## Case Background

The patient is a 65-year-old female status post–right CVA with dense left hemiparesis. She has a history of hypertension and cardiac problems. The patient lived with her husband, who has cardiac problems himself. The couple lives in New York and was enjoying Space Mountain with their family when the patient experienced a sudden onset of dizziness and left-sided weakness.

The bedside evaluation revealed an alert but confused female with flaccid left side with poor endurance, and trace/poor sitting balance. Functional tasks revealed perceptual deficits, with severe left inattention and possible homonymous hemianopsia Maximum cognitive and physical assistance were required to perform self care tasks. The Allen Cognitive Level screening test (ACL) was administered with adaptation to compensate for hemiplegia. The ACL score was 3.2, suggesting severe cognitive deficits. The patient's performance of routine tasks such as grooming and dressing corresponded to Allen's Routine Task Inventory (RTI) Level 2. Significant impairment was noted in the ability to spontaneously initiate and sustain repetitive motion, such as hair brushing. The patient was unable to make effective gross neuromuscular adjustments in dressing, such as altering position, so the therapist could put on her shirt. The patient demonstrated no awareness of the results of her actions.

The family, present during the evaluation, demonstrated poor insight regarding the functional implications of the patient's deficits. The children work full time; the grandchildren are attending college out of town. The patient's husband nonchalantly stated "we'll get along fine;" but the daughter noted her father's health problems, and declining participation in activities of interest.

Prior to admission, the patient was independent in all activities, including driving. Heavy housework was done once a month by hired help. The patient and her husband are involved in managing their rental properties and investment portfolio, church activities, and entertaining.

## Discharge Goals

- Discharge to daughter's home with 24-hour assistance from husband and daughter.
- Minimum cognitive/physical assistance for basic self-care.
- Minimum cognitive/physical assistance for functional transfers to toilet, tub bench, bed, chair, and car.
- Family demonstrates ability to provide appropriate assistance and protective environment for patient in home.

## Treatment Plan

- Self-care retraining
- Functional transfer training (toilet, tub bench, bed, chair, and car). Adaptive equipment instruction. Therapeutic functional activity (home tasks, games, crafts)
- Neuromuscular therapy
- Family training
- Functional assessment in home

## First Week

### Introduction

Self-care and functional transfers (to toilet) require maximum physical and cognitive assistance. Assistance (ACL 2.8–3.0) consists of facilitated proprioceptive cues by positioning and controlling the trunk and extremities; tactile cues of guiding, hand over hand; visual cues of placing objects in the hand one at a time; and verbal cues of directing with single words. The environment is made distraction free. The therapist's objectives are to enhance postural control and the ability to focus on the immediate action of the task ( rather than the task step sequence).

The patient is interested in cooperating with the therapist to complete basic self-care such as grooming. She is resistive to redirection needed to get the job done adequately. The patient is unaware of the therapist's positioning of the flaccid extremities for weight bearing and protection.

The only adaptive equipment needed are a lap tray, for positioning the left arm to reduce risk of injury by pinching or dangling due to left neglect, and a commode chair.

The therapist's objectives in family training are

to establish rapport, obtain information about the patient's premorbid life, and to orient the family to the functional implications of CVA and occupational therapy services. The family is given suggestions for adaptive clothing (velcro shoes, large sweat suits).

### Self-Care

## Typical Performance

Patient ignores provided grooming set-up and states "you do it" when presented with hairbrush. Patient strokes right side of hair and face three times with back side of brush. Patient resists physical guiding and verbal cues to continue brushing. Patient waves toothbrush in sink, missing stream of water, then pokes it in her eye. In dressing, patient pushes right hand into neck opening and talks about her daughter, oblivious to therapist's attempts to stop the motion. In the bathroom, patient careens toward the toilet, oblivious to physical guiding and verbal cues given by the therapist. Patient attempts to stand in the normal manner without noticing that her feet are still on leg rests. Patient resists practice of toilet transfers, but will accept assistance if there is an urge to void. If a toilet is seen, patient may request to use it.

### Intervention

- *Room environment:* Close door to reduce distractions.
- *Dressing:* Don pants in bed for safety and ease; don shirt in wheelchair. Position garment next to appropriate body part and guide patient's movement through technique sequence.
- *Grooming:* Place wheelchair in front of sink. Prepare objects and hand to patient (Maximum set-up, e.g., water in cup, toothpaste on brush). Provide hand-over-hand guiding and continuous contact between the patient's arms and surfaces (such as sink edge and trunk) when moving toothbrush into running water and mouth. Limit verbal interaction to brief directives.
- *Toileting:* Protect patient and facilitate normal movement patterns by maximal control. Place and set up wheelchair (brakes, footrests, armrests) and position patient's body for safe transfer. Control patient for safe pacing of transfer and restrain patient from lunging toward toilet target, especially if there is a sense of urgency. Capitalize on patient's urgency to void to derive maximum motor learning from natural cooperation in facilitated normal movement to the toilet.

## Second Week

### Introduction

Moderate physical and cognitive assistance is needed. Cognitive assistance (ACL = 3.0–3.2) continues to emphasize guiding, but demonstration and verbal cues are also used. The occupational therapist's objectives are to ensure safety; promote a sense of competency and independence by facilitating effective interaction with objects; introduce compensatory techniques through repetitive exposure in routine; and facilitate normal postural control.

The patient recognizes gross errors, especially dressing errors that restrict movement, but cues are required to correct them. The patient is aware of the position of the left arm only when the therapist directs attention to it. The patient demonstrates ineffective gross neuromuscular adjustments during transfers in her attempt to compensate for impaired mobility. Safety becomes a greater concern during transfers motivated by a sense of urgency (e.g., to toilet, bed). Due to patient's increased initiation and poor awareness of motor skill limitations, vigilance is essential to quickly control the patient's increased impulsivity.

Adaptive equipment needed at this stage includes the lap tray, an elevated armrest for edema control, and a commode chair.

The family has limited awareness of the potential consequences of cognitive/perceptual deficits. Their current expectations regarding discharge are unrealistic. Their full-time jobs limit availability for family training. Family training consists of observation of treatment, verbal instruction, and minimal practice. Instruction is given in positioning and activity selection to promote normal tone and cognitive/perceptual skills. The therapist introduces the family to functional considerations of having the patient in the home.

### Self-Care

#### Typical Performance

Patient dresses right side and stops, leaving the left breast and back exposed. When cued, and assisted to start sleeve over wrist, patient attempts the technique of pushing the left sleeve onto the arm, but perseverates, pushing the wristband over the shoulder. Patient puts both legs all the way into one pant leg and says "That's not right," then with cue, pulls right leg out and looks at pants with a puzzled expression. The bra, buttons, zippers, socks, shoes,

and ankle-foot orthosis (AFO) are abandoned immediately. At the sink, the patient applies too little toothpaste or misses the brush entirely. Patient is unable to locate items placed on the left side of the sink. In the bathroom, patient attempts transfer with pants lowered. Patient lunges for toilet grab bar or arm rest and pulls or pushes herself off balance, roughly hitting the wall. After toileting, patient pulls up the right side of pants and says, "lets go to therapy." Her left arm falls off the lap tray without the patient recognizing it, and it is pinched between the door jamb and wheelchair as patient exits.

#### Intervention

- *Room environment:* Close door. Limit verbal interaction.
- *Grooming:* Place wheelchair at sink. Place objects within a 2-foot radius of patient. Select objects that are very familiar, used daily, and easy to discern, for placement on the left side to reduce "left neglect." Direct attention to these objects by guiding patient's reach for them as they are needed.
- *Dressing:* Place wheelchair facing clothes that are laid out in the correct orientation on the bed. Guide with less control; increase demonstration and simple verbal cues in repetitive task sequences. Teach techniques that involve obvious cues to guide action: e.g., look for labels, pull up pant leg until you see the foot.
- *Toileting:* Set-up of wheelchair (oriented at correct angle and distance from toilet, footrests aside, brakes locked). Because verbal cues are ineffective to curb impulsivity, guide by strong physical assistance to control unsafe movements that could cause a fall (e.g., lunging and grasping for grab bar). Give basic verbal directives and physical assistance to retrieve left arm and place on lap tray.

### Home Activity: Stirring/Wiping

#### Typical Performance

Patient stirs without noticing obvious unblended parts of mix. When asked what she is making, patient states, "I don't know." Patient stops stirring and chatters about her family. Patient wipes table in a circle, directly in front of her, without noticing obvious dirty spots.

#### Intervention

Busy kitchen clinic. Group task at large table. In distracting environment, reduce task demand to repetitive motion such as stirring, wiping, spreading. Provide total set-up within field of view. Stabilize bowls with Dycem or by holding for patient. Provide maximum guiding to ensure adequate quality, and redirect to sustain participation in busy environment.

## Third Week

### Introduction

Self-care and functional transfers require moderate/minimal physical and cognitive assistance. Cognitive assistance (ACL 3.4–3.6) shifts toward increased demonstration and verbal cues and decreased guiding. Verbal cues are delayed to facilitate basic problem solving in routine tasks. Guiding continues to facilitate perceptual, motor, and cognitive skill integration. Repetitive practice of dressing and transfer sequences continues.

Following a demonstration, the patient can imitate and continue a compensatory technique motion, but needs review in subsequent treatment sessions. The patient uses practiced methods to correct gross errors in dressing. As skills improve, the patient begins to tolerate and master greater task demands in physical scale, object feature complexity, sequence complexity, and perceptual–motor complexity. The patient can resume a step in a familiar sequence after a wheelchair trip to access materials in the same room. Improved neuromuscular adjustment skills support more control in transfers and wheelchair use in functional contexts.

The family demonstrates increased understanding of the functional consequences of current deficits, but insight regarding long-term status and consequences is limited. The family begins to ask pressing questions regarding anticipated functional problems and assistance needs after discharge such as bathroom equipment, time required for assisted routines, and prognosis for resumption of former roles. Family training consists of supervised participation in self-care and functional transfers, identification of environmental hazards and distractions, selection of appropriate home activity, and review of positioning and adaptive equipment. This experience also provides the caregiver with a clearer idea of how much time and assistance are required to achieve satisfactory results. Functional home assessment and instruction emphasize application of guidelines to maximize patient's safety and independence in the discharge environment.

### Self-Care

### Typical Performance

When asked "What do you want to wear?" the patient selects favorite soiled top and pants and argues when asked to change selection. While dressing, the patient finds self with two legs inserted into single pant leg and corrects mistake, as practiced. The left sleeve cuff is pushed unnecessarily far up onto upper arm but this problem is not noticed until after the shirt is pulled over the head. The patient looks at the exposed left forearm and pulls the sleeve over it, as practiced. After breakfast, the patient states, HI want to clean my teeth." With cue to gather supplies, the patient looks for key items at bedside table, and on left and right side of sink. The patient slips the tube of toothpaste into her left hand, tries to apply it to brush for some time, then switches tube to more effective right hand, as practiced daily, but squeezes too much out. In toileting, the patient says, "I'm in a hurry," checks brakes, and waits for additional cues and set-up. After using the toilet, patient wipes but stops before effective results are obtained. Patient does not ask for help to get to sink to wash hands. During a tub bench transfer, the patient suddenly overreaches to the far side of tub and nearly loses balance. The patient slowly maneuvers wheelchair through doorways using only the strong side, and corrects position when left rim hits doorjamb. The patient often cradles the left arm with the right hand on the lap tray, but occasionally, the arm slips off the tray, and dangles to the side. The patient sometimes retrieves it when pain is felt.

### Intervention

- *Room environment:* Decrease structure. Open door. Increase scale to include nightstand, closet, edge of bed. Increased length of time for interruptions of task sequence to access items and for nursing procedures. Self-care performed in wheelchair. Remove armrests that interfere with movement.

- *Dressing:* Cue patient to name needs and provide assistance to access and return to bedside to dress. Provide limited appropriate clothing choices. Put clothes in a pile on bed for patient to sequence and orient as needed. When obvious mistakes occur, allow time for patient to initiate practiced technique to solve problem. Continue daily use of simple verbal cues and demonstration for easier items, but guide patient through fasteners, bra, socks, shoes, and AFO that would otherwise be abandoned. Facilitate balance and guide manipulation of clothing while patient performs difficult "hemi" techniques such as crossing leg to reach foot. Assist with balance to stand and pull up pants.

- *Grooming:* Cue patient to gather needed items and take to sink. Place objects within view to left and right to encourage attention to the left and to visually cue patient to perform grooming steps (cloth, comb, toothbrush, cup). Guide normal movement patterns of the left extremity functioning as an assistive gross grasp in bilateral tasks such as washing dentures and opening containers. Provide tactile and verbal cues to stop when enough toothpaste or lotion has been dispensed, and to change hand position to get missed areas of teeth, face, hair.

- *Toileting:* Check quality of toilet hygiene and cue patient to check results or modify technique. Cue to wash hands. Increase physical and cognitive assistance for unfamiliar transfers to curb impulsivity.

### Home Activity: Microwave Mix

### Typical Performance

Patient looks at box and says, "I can't do this. I don't use this kind." When cued to get hot water for the mix, patient gets water without waiting for it to run until warm from the tap. The patient stops in the middle of task. The patient leaves dry unblended parts, distributes batter unevenly in pan, and leaves globs on pan edge. The patient runs spatula along pan edge to spread chocolate frosting on brownies, but does not notice missed areas. Patient suddenly licks utensil in the middle of task.

### Intervention

Use small-scale mix-in-the-pan mix with striking visual contrast, such as yellow mix with chocolate frosting, to provide color and edge cues for coverage. Assist to wheel to opened cupboards to access supplies. Cue/explain to wait for water to get warm from hot tap. Provide general cues to facilitate sequencing to completion. Guide effective incorporation of left hand.

## Fourth Week

### Introduction

In the final week of rehabilitation the therapist promotes skill refinement with minimal physical and cognitive assistance (ACL 3.8–4.0), and identifies the specifics of caregiver/family assistance. The therapist reduces assistance overall, but minimum assistance, in the form of guiding, is required for bilateral manipulation, functional mobility such as

standing to pull up pants or to transfer, and wheelchair mobility. No physical assistance is needed for balance in mixing activity. The left hand's rudimentary grasp and pinch precludes effective bilateral manipulation of tight lids and small fasteners within a practical time frame. The patient now initiates steps in routines, but makes small errors in step sequence (such as forgetting to rinse toothbrush) as opposed to last week's gross errors (pants before underwear). The patient misses gross details that don't interfere with the goal (e.g., hair and shirt disheveled in back). There is carry over of techniques, but effectiveness of efforts to correct errors falls short of adequate. The patient is assisted in techniques to increase self monitoring of gross details and quality.

Family training is specific and intensive. The family is given a home program that meshes with the family's routine, willingness, and capacity to provide appropriate guidance. The family's ideas for home/community activities are supported with tips to maximize safety and success. Continuous supervision is emphasized for safety to prevent impulsive attempts to transfer or smoke alone.

A bell worn around the patient's neck is recommended as "adaptive equipment" to signal a need for assistance to transfer, but its limitations in ensuring safety are emphasized.

### Self-Care

### Typical Performance

While dressing, the patient finds the left sleeve but does not prepare it adequately before pulling it onto the arm. The left hand becomes stuck, and the patient makes small ineffective pulling motions to correct it. Patient spends 5 minutes on one button. After dressing, patient appears disheveled with collar sticking up, shirt bound up around left shoulder, buttons misaligned, underwear elastic exposed in back, and hair swooped up in back. Patient stands to pull up pants on both sides, and loses balance, and falls into chair. Patient falls to one side while struggling with socks and AFO but keeps at it for 10 minutes. Patient found standing, facing bowl, with legs crossed hanging on to grab bars, and she states, "Can you help me with my pants?".

### Intervention Techniques for the Family

Advise family regarding safety hazards, typical errors, and compensatory strategies to implement in the home.

- *Room environment:* Offer appropriate clothing choices or set out clothes for patient.
- *Dressing:* Use short-sleeve shirts to make dressing easier. Provide guiding assistance for difficult manipulation and set a limited goal, such as one button, before completing step for the patient. Follow a set routine of self-care sequences. Delay telling patient about obvious errors. Provide cue to use mirror to check for less obvious errors of hair/clothing alignment, then demonstrate motion to correct. Assist with dynamic balance when pulling up pants, and donning socks, AFO, shoes.
- *Toileting:* In the home bathroom, supervise positioning set up to ensure safety (brakes, body position) and assist transfers. For home safety, provide 24-hour supervision and check on patient in adjacent room frequently. Drill patient to ask for assistance (neck bell) rather than attempting transfers independently, and provide help cheerfully. Be aware that the prevention of a fall necessitates continuous availability of assistance in response to the bell. Do not expect the patient to make an adequate judgment regarding bell use, since the patient is likely to risk a fall to avoid "bothering" the caregiver, or to refuse to wear it at all.

## Home Activity

### Typical Performance

When getting supplies to make a sandwich, patient wheels to refrigerator, reaches for handle, and opens door into legs. Patient backs up, slamming into table behind her while clearing a path for the refrigerator door. Door swings into cabinet, and salad dressing crashes to floor.

Patient talks generally about familiar business matters and her intention to resume full participation when she gets home.

### Intervention: Techniques for the Family

Provide minimum assistance with functional wheelchair mobility involving opening doors and carrying objects. Set up containers, select safe utensils (no machines, knives). Provide complete set-up or have patient name needed materials and assist to access one at a time. Use adaptive equipment such as a suction cup bread board with sandwich guard rails. Choose high contrast materials, several ingredients, steps, and types of action (spread, layer, alignment, assembly sequence) to challenge patient. Redirect patient not to talk. Encourage family to include patient in simple kitchen tasks such as preparing microwave dishes, cold cereal, and sandwiches. Assist patient in writing down shopping needs as patient recognizes them during routine tasks. Assist patient to perform basic business-type tasks, such as dialing the telephone, sorting mail, signing checks. Include patient in private discussion of business. Encourage socializing and community activity at a basic level (friendly greetings and brief visits, attending church services, dining out) and assess ability to engage in familiar activity, such as cards, before attempting it in social group.

## Afterword

The patient was discharged to her children's home with supervision from her husband. The former patient and her husband returned home to New York after several weeks. Months later, the daughter reported that the former patient had suffered a traumatic brain injury and broken hip in an attempt to use the toilet unassisted.

# Chapter 11

# Rehabilitation and Learning

## Claudia Kay Allen, MA, OTR, FAOTA

he unique knowledge and skill of the therapist is set in a theoretical context. The treatment goals suggested in this text are influenced by our current understanding of how the normal brain functions, how abnormalities occur and can be corrected, and how people can mentally adjust to limited abilities. Universal agreement about how the brain works does not exist as of this writing. Choices are available and decisions must be made. Theoretical positions that guide the format of the book are discussed in this chapter.

Safety in doing ordinary activities is the primary treatment goal. Ordinary activities are based on the uniquely human abilities to walk on two feet in an upright position, speak and use language, and manipulate objects with human hands. To be safe, one must acquire knowledge of the external environment. The conscious mind processes information from the external environment and directs movements within that context. Movements are safe when the relevant sensory information is processed and combined with motor actions. The sensorimotor system is regarded as the primary determinant of safety in doing ordinary activities.

A functional safety scale (the cognitive levels) describes degrees of safety according to the individual's ability to acquire and apply knowledge of the environment. A functional safety scale, then, is largely determined by the sensorimotor models that the person is able to learn and use.

## Learning

Learning is done by *attending* to sensory cues, *forming* sensory associations that give meaning to external substances, *recalling* sensorimotor models that

provide a purpose for acting, discovering and storing sensorimotor models, and *inventing* speculative sensorimotor models. Attention is drawn to sensory cues that introduce novelty. The sensory cue adds a little bit of information to the information currently being processed. If too much information is present, it may be ignored so that even though the information is present, it is not processed. Not attending to available sensory cues is the primary problem of the cognitively disabled.

Sensory associations bring the cues into focus and establish a context that compares the cues with past experience. Recognition of safety hazards requires the formation of sensory associations. Sensory associations are formed in the cerebral cortex, and therapists cannot be sure that the association has been formed unless the patient acts on the association. Sensorimotor models are patterns of acting on sensory associations. Motor skills are sensorimotor models learned and practiced while doing something. Internal or external feedback may be used to improve performance by refining the sensorimotor model (Miller, 1981). The discovery and refinement of a model is based on an inductive inference, going from a specific to a general pattern (learning by doing, or by trial and error).

Speculative sensorimotor models are invented to improve premeditated performance. Speculative models are based on deductive inferences, using general sensorimotor models to project specific effects (Miller, 1981). Speculative sensorimotor models are imagined courses of action that might be applied to material objects. The imagined actions may be represented by images, words, or diagrams. The speculation is done in reference to perceivable

Figure 11.1  Cognitive ability and disability

| Input | Throughput | Output |
|---|---|---|
| **Conditions of uncertainty** | **Learning** | **Ordinary activities** |
| Out of the ordinary | Ability | Safe |
| Hazards | Fluctuation | Competent |
| Emergencies | Motivation | Independent |
| | Disability | Unsafe |
| | | Incapacitated |
| | | Assistance needed |

problems presented by material objects; the supposition is concrete rather than abstract. The material object need not be present, but it is referenced with a tangible, imagined change in the object. The deductive inference is built on the memory of inductive inferences that are stored sensorimotor models (Miller). Speculative models also incorporate reference to social standards of performance. Speculative models exclude imperceptible problems and intangible properties of objects.

When the individual is able to process all forms of sensorimotor information, the capacity to learn to do activities safely is present. It is assumed that deductive reasoning, using language and symbols to reach a conclusion, is built on an ability to form deductive inferences. The literature of psychology and philosophy is rich with discussions of reasoning, and further study is not attempted here. The descriptions of the sensorimotor system conclude with the formation of deductive inferences as a prerequisite to deductive reasoning.

There is a close relationship between consciousness and learning that is affected by biological abnormalities. The experience of consciousness involves an inner subjective awareness as well as the formation of memories. The subjective sense of self as an integrated whole person is a conscious experience, and one learns from conscious experiences. Just as medical problems can affect consciousness, they can also affect learning. The degree of disability is measured by drawing an inference about the kind of information that can and cannot be processed.

An ordinal scale of 6 cognitive levels is used to classify the complexity of the information pro-

cessed while manipulating material objects. Level 1 begins with an elementary sensation, a noxious stimuli that has meaning, as inferred by a withdrawal from the noxious stimuli. Information processed at level 2 is thought to be a sensorimotor response to gravity (sitting up) and architectural barriers (climbing stairs), including stored models for gross motor movements. Level 3 information includes associations with objects that can be manipulated with the hands and stored models for doing so (a toothbrush). Out-of-the-ordinary situations, hazards, and most emergencies are not recognized at levels 1–3. Out of the ordinary is recognized at level 4 when presented by striking sensory cues, usually visual. Stored models are used to solve noted problems, and new models are imitated. New models for new motor skills are formed at level 5. Stored, new, and speculative models are judged according to an anticipated outcome at level 6. The deductive inferences drawn at level 6 are seen as prerequisites for learning through the use of language.

At cognitive levels 1 through 5, humans share sensorimotor processes with animals. Information processed at level 6 involves the ability to plan and judge projected events and may be uniquely human. An assumption that people always engage in uniquely human processes is rejected. Many of the events of ordinary life are done by using mental processes that are shared by other species. An assumption is made that the human brain is conservative, using no more information than necessary to do routine activities. Effective object manipulation can be done at cognitive levels 3 through 5 by ordinary people during a large portion of the day. I suspect that people prefer functioning at these lower levels, and that we are often annoyed by situations that require planning. The important thing is that we can if we must—the uniquely human aspect is that the average person can function at level 6 when the need/desire is present.

Throughout the scale an emphasis is placed on safety—on the associations, models, and judgments needed to reduce danger to self or others. A distinction is made between the storage of learned models and the formation of new models. Safety in unexpected situations often requires the formation of new models. The external environment is in a constant state of flux and one predictor of safety in the community is the ability to form new sensorimotor models. New learning, however, is not at the top of the scale; forming new sensorimotor models occurs at level 5. To prevent accidents a person must be able to speculate that an accident might occur. At level 6 people use judgment to anticipate and avoid problems. Problems can be solved before they occur, and accidents and injuries can be avoided.

The focus on the sensorimotor aspects of thought has been broadened to include associated verbal abilities (Allen, 1985). Speech pathologists have helped describe communication abilities that are consistent with the cognitive levels (C. Hagen, personal communication, 1987). The addition of speaking and communicating meaning makes it easier to describe the occasional dichotomy between verbal and motor abilities. The addition may also make it easier to evaluate the learning abilities of patients who have limited motor abilities, like spinal cord injuries or arthritis.

Timing abilities receive a new emphasis that emerged out of the expansion of the 6 cognitive levels. Orientation to the passage of time, awareness of sequences of actions and activities, and the pacing of one's actions seem to be bound up in a subjective sense of conscious performance. Timing may provide another avenue for evaluating the learning abilities of those with limited motor abilities.

The cognitive requirements for doing ordinary activities continues to direct the focus of study. Ordinary activities require a surprising amount of information processing. Most adults process information with ease and take the capacity to do it for granted. When the capacity is lost, the amazing information-processing capacity of the human brain is apparent.

## Open System

Within an information-processing context, the input is a condition of uncertainty in the external environment; the throughput is learning; and the output is safety in doing ordinary activities. This view of the information processing system represents an effort to put former descriptions into more functional terms (Allen, 1985). Information processing is regarded as the internal command center that directs human behavior. Learning determines the person's safety when conditions of uncertainty occur. An increase in safety in doing more activities is expected with an increase in the cognitive level.

When one is doing one's ordinary activities, sensory associations may be formed but not stored. Laying down your car keys and not being able to find them later is an example. An ability may be present, but it is not always used. Some fluctuation in the degree to which the system is used is regarded as normal. Situations that demand an individual's full capacity to process information are required to evaluate a person's ability. Normal fluctuations tend to use less than full capacity.

The uncommon event that occurs while doing a common activity displays the need to be able to operate at full capacity. The uncommon event presents a novelty, a condition of uncertainty about what to do. The individual must go through the learning process when different things happen during the course of daily activities. The out-of-the-ordinary events are the situations that jeopardize the safety of the cognitively disabled.

To some extent people have a natural instinct to learn and protect their safety as well as the safety of others. Attending to some cues, like food, seems to be instinctive, or hard-wired into the brain. The meaning and purpose of one's safety, however, introduce alternative explanations for information processing. Suicides and homicides do occur. Cognitive levels 4 and 5 are associated with troublesome questions about motivation; the difference between what the person wishes to do and what the person can do is often fuzzy. Methods for eliminating plausible explanations for a choice not to process information are required. The truth is that motivational explanations cannot always be eliminated.

## Maximum Functional Level

Level 6 is regarded as the maximum functional ability required to do ordinary activities safely. There are, of course, higher cognitive abilities required to manipulate objects, like engineering. Those abilities are regarded as beyond the scope of ordinary activities. It is assumed that the average person can function at level 6 when safety is at stake. It is also assumed that the average person experiences temporary inabilities to function at level 6 secondary to illness (fever or headache), fatigue, over- or understimulation, and motivation. Everyone shares the experiences of functioning at levels 1 through 5. The difference is that the cognitively disabled cannot draw on higher level capacities when the need arises. The maximum functional ability is elicited when therapists match the disabled person's highest remaining abilities to the demands of the activity.

A sequence of abilities outlines the behaviors that seem to reflect an increased ability to process information. The original 6 cognitive levels have been maintained, but a decimal system has been added to increase the sensitivity of the scale. The sequence of abilities described is based on experience in teaching adults with mental abnormalities. Some associations with the normal learning of children are expected, but differences are also expected. A learning theory for abnormal adults must consider prior learning and limited learning capacity.

Each decimal point is a mode of performance, which is a pattern of behaving or problem solving. The modes range from 0 to 6.0, providing 52 modes for moving, speaking, and timing during the performance of an activity. Each cognitive level contains 10 modes, from .0 to .9 (level 4.0 to 4.9). Informa-

tion is added according to the numerical sequence, which is an ordinal scale. When information processing is impaired, the highest mode of performance is used to predict what type of cognitive assistance the disabled person is going to need and the information that the person can still process without assistance.

## Value of Rehabilitation Services

The description of the cognitive levels has been fraught with difficulties in explaining change within a paradigm that recognizes residual limitations. Fortunately, I am not alone with this difficulty, and major assistance is provided by the World Health Organization (WHO). WHO offers two typologies (see Figure 1.2) that correspond with my prior attempts to divide health problems into acute and stable conditions (Allen, 1985, 1987). To promote universal understanding of terminology, I will change my language to conform with the WHO classifications, as much as possible. WHO has published two classification systems. The first system is commonly called the medical model and is published in the *International Classification of Diseases* (ICD9), 9th edition (1991). ICD9 enjoys the benefits of decades of thought and is subdivided into three categories: etiology, pathology, and manifestations. The second typology is called the *International Classification of Impairments, Disabilities, and*

Figure 11.2 The value of rehabilitation services

### Components of the medical model

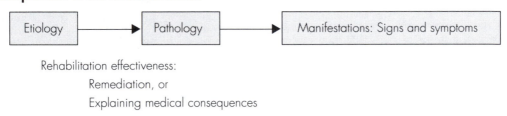

### Components of the consequences model

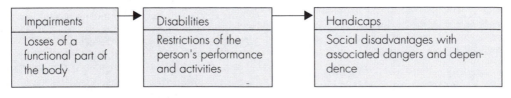

## Table 11.1 Definitions of treatment outcomes

- *The medical model* is driven by the cause of a disease, which is effective with conditions that are self-limiting or amenable to prevention or cure. The patient's thoughts and feelings may have little to no significant effect on treatment outcome. Health care providers have the primary responsibility for selecting treatment methods. Rehabilitation of the cognitively disabled has three major ways of explaining medical changes:

- *Recovery* is a theoretical construct for the complete return to normal. Recovery means that there are no residual manifestations or impairments.

- *Sparing* is a slow process of recovery, with the greatest return to normal occurring within 3 to 6 months, with smaller improvements detectable within the 1st year after onset. Improvements after the 1st year are rarely reported, and the causative factors are unknown. Residual manifestations and impairments are expected.

- *Remediation* switches from normal processes to different internal effectors, receptors, or mental strategies to overcome pathology. The outcome is measured by a reduction in manifestations or impairments, with the assumption that these reductions will also reduce disabilities and handicaps. The assumption is seldom tested and largely unsubstantiated (Finger & Stein, 1982).

- The *consequences model* is driven by losses of function that are a result of a disease process. Consequences are residual limitations that remain after medical treatment and natural healing are complete. The burden of living with consequences is reduced by rehabilitation therapists who maximize the patient's remaining abilities. The feelings and thoughts of the patient and the people in their social support system can have a significant effect on treatment outcome. The treatment methods are a shared responsibility between the health care provider, patient, and long-term caregiver. There are two ways of maximizing remaining abilities:

  - *Environmental compensations* use material objects as substitutes for lost abilities. Adaptive equipment, memory logs, and structured living and working conditions are common examples. Many environmental compensations must be put in place by other people at the beginning of or throughout the process of task performance, but are still less labor intensive than social assistance. When these material objects are in place, the disabled person can overcome limitations and use remaining abilities.

  - *Social assistance* is dependent on the supervision of other people throughout task performance to substitute for lost abilities. Initiation of activities, continuous cuing or verification, removal of hazards, and corrections of errors are common examples. A high potential for injury or other unfavorable effects exists; therapists must warn patients and other caregivers about these possibilities. When the necessary instructions are given and precautions taken, the patient can use his or her remaining abilities to do activities safely.

*Handicaps* (ICIDH) (1980). ICIDH is divided into the three categories contained in the title and is referred to as the consequences model. The consequences model recognizes residual limitations. Some of these limitations require long-term care while others do not. Providing long-term care for those who need it is another measure of the quality of a nation's health care system. These two typologies are designed to fulfill entirely different purposes and have very different expectations for change. Therapists need to understand the pros and cons of both typologies.

## Medical Model

The medical model is driven by the cause of the disease, which is effective with diseases that are self-limiting or amenable to prevention or cure. The medical model aims at explaining the cause of health problems by, for example, identifying brain pathology. The medical model takes an objective view of the patient. As a whole, medical authors do not write about the subjective meanings and purposes people attach to medical procedures. The expected outcome is a return to health by eliminating the etiology, correcting the pathology, or reducing the manifestations. In the early rehabilitation literature, medical views of change were adopted. Indeed, medical views of change were the only accepted values in rehabilitation services for many years, and the influence is still apparent.

Medical information is helpful background information for therapists, providing an understanding of why a disability occurred, how long the disability can be expected to last, and whether the need for assistance can be expected to lessen or not. The location of a brain lesion or the cause of a mental disorder is of primary importance within the medical model but is less important to rehabilitation therapists. Rehabilitation therapists can deliver many effective treatments without any information about the cause or the location of the pathology. This text attempts to be logically consistent with the neuroscience literature. The presence of some sort of brain pathology is assumed.

Signs and symptoms are medical model terms that are associated with a specific cause of a disease. Signs and symptoms are used to guide differential diagnosis and to evaluate the effects of medical interventions. Many of these manifestations are listed as impairments in ICIDH. Impairments and manifestations link the therapist's observations to the concerns of the medical team.

Within the medical model, treatment aims at correcting the biological abnormality: etiology, pathology, signs or symptoms. Recovery, sparing, and remediation are treatment objectives that fit into a medical model view of change and are a part of acute and postacute care in this text. Because these terms are often used with some ambiguity, clarification of precisely what is being avoided is required (Table 1.1).

Recovery is a theoretical construct for the complete return of functions that were lost or impaired. Acute or temporary medical conditions are associated with a complete and identical return of function. Recovery means that there are no residual manifestations or impairments (Finger & Stein, 1982). Recovery is a term that is often misused to describe any improvement, which is especially cruel when used to describe treatment programs to families. A highly selective use of this term is recommended to clarify realistic outcomes of rehabilitation programs for the cognitively disabled. Recovery means that the person regains the cognitive capacity that he or she had before the onset of injury or illness.

Sparing is a slow process of recovery that is associated with the natural healing process of the brain. Manifestations that are present after brain damage are gradually diminished. The greatest improvements are seen 3 to 6 months postinjury, but smaller improvements may continue for several years (Finger & Stein, 1982). The 52 modes of performance presented in chapter 5 may be used to detect the sparing that occurs without rehabilitation services. Descriptive longitudinal studies are badly needed to get a better understanding of the natural healing process.

Recovery and sparing are possible explanations of change in the cognitive level. The position taken here is that rehabilitation services may be associated with the change, but in all probability they are not the sole cause of the change. The possibility that a change in the cognitive level would occur without rehabilitation services is accepted.

Remediation is a switch to different effectors, receptors, or other biological locations that serve as alternative biological mechanisms for the pathology of the brain. Remediation aims at reducing signs and symptoms and assumes that such a reduction will generalize to a reduction in difficulties in doing many or all functional activities. The remedial assumption has seldom, if ever, been tested. Many early rehabilitation conceptual models were framed in this view of change. As people in the neurosciences become more sophisticated about residual impairments and disabilities, there is less adherence to remedial explanations in the rehabilitation literature (Finger & Stein, 1982).

The remedial approaches to treatment such as sensory integration and neurodevelopmental treatment give a causal explanation for change. Within the medical model, treatment must cause the change. There is no evidence to support a medical model view of change, that rehabilitation services cause a change in brain pathology. Random assignment to treatment and control groups would be required to support a causal explanation for change. The control group could receive rehabilitation services by doing activities that match the current maximum ability.

The expanded description of the cognitive levels in chapter 5 may be sensitive enough to detect change that is produced by these remedial approaches. If so, the extent, significance, and conditions required to produce the change need to be identified. If not, alternative explanations for the value of rehabilitation services are required. Even if so, alternative explanations provide a way of comparing treatment outcomes.

Within the medical model, alternatives include

helping to evaluate the effectiveness of medical care, aiding in the determination of when the medical model should be discontinued, and assisting with the adjustments to any consequences of a disease. Within these alternatives, the unique knowledge of the therapist is derived from the therapist's understanding of how losses are apt to affect the individual and his or her social support system.

## Consequences Model

The consequences model is driven by losses of function that are a result of a disease process or injury. Consequences are residual limitations that remain after medical treatment is finished or the natural healing process has stabilized. The treatment goals suggested in this text are designed to match the demands of the activity to the patient's remaining abilities. The burden of living with the consequences is reduced by rehabilitation therapists who maximize the patient's remaining abilities.

It would be interesting to see what differences, if any, can be detected between remediation and consequence approaches. I do not know if remediation works better than matching maximal abilities. I think that these two treatment methods need to be subjected to investigation. The outcome of treatment should be measured in functional terms, which I interpret as the quality of activity performance. I have the greatest confidence in group studies, with control groups, that can be replicated. I have much less confidence in single case studies. The work done in this text, then, aims at getting rehabilitation professionals ready to do group studies with sensitive measures of the quality of activity performance.

The consequences of medical problems are being recognized by many people in the health care delivery system. An international, interdisciplinary effort to cope with the problem was started by the World Health Organization during the 1970s. Overlaps between ICD9 and ICIDH are expected and exist, particularly in the lists of manifestations and impairments. Manifestations are diagnosis specific, and related to the cause of the pathology. Impairments are "concerned with abnormalities of body structure and appearance and with organ or system function, resulting from any cause; in principle, impairments represent disturbances at the level of the organ" (ICIDH, 1980, p. 14). Impairments are experienced by the individual as a loss; the loss may be temporary and of little consequence or long term

and severe. Furthermore, individuals may have a loss, such as a loss of a limb, and not regard themselves as sick or in need of medical attention. Brain impairments include mental retardation, memory, thought processes, thought content, consciousness and wakefulness, perception and attention, emotive and volitional functions, and behavior patterns. Measures of these impairments are found in the psychology literature.

Most of the current cognitive rehabilitation literature is impairment driven. I have not followed that approach for two reasons. Psychologists have already developed many evaluation instruments and treatment methods. More importantly, the relationships between reduced impairments and improved activity performance are assumed, but largely unknown. The result is that the value of cognitive rehabilitation is open to question. Occupational therapy's traditional focus on activities is used to suggest ways of answering these questions.

WHO suggests that disabilities are the primary focus of rehabilitation services, and I agree. Disabilities reflect "the consequences of impairments in terms of functional performance and activity by the individual; disabilities thus represent disturbances at the level of the person" (ICIDH, 1980, p. 14). Impairments divide the individual's losses into pieces that can be measured relatively easily. Disabilities put the impairments and abilities back together during the complex process of doing activities. The meaning of an impairment is easily over- or underestimated, because it is an isolated part of performance. With an inaccurate understanding of the meaning of an impairment, people are unclear about the consequences of health problems.

The sense of self, as an integrated whole person, occurs while a person is doing an activity. Activity provides a context that gives meaning and purpose to one's actions. The subjective impressions formed can compare performance with the process of doing past activities to understand a difference in the quality of performance. Safety hazards take on a real and immediate concern while doing activities that make warnings meaningful. Activities also raise motivational questions. The feelings and thoughts of patients and other people in their social support system can have a significant effect on treatment outcomes. Treatment methods and goals, therefore, must be a shared responsibility among therapists, patients, and long-term caregivers. The cognitively disabled may have an inaccurate understanding of the social meaning of and safety hazards that produced their disability. A closer liaison between therapists and long-term caregivers is suggested when this occurs.

Handicaps are "concerned with the disadvantages experienced by the individual as a result of impairments and disabilities; handicaps thus reflect interaction with and adaptation to the individual surroundings" (ICIDH, 1980). Handicaps place people at a social disadvantage in fulfilling ordinary role expectations. WHO suggests that handicaps are the primary concern of the social welfare system. Therapists can expect to have some involvement with impairments and handicaps; the degree is often determined by their place of employment. Therapists working in hospitals are more involved with impairments, while community-based therapists are more concerned with handicaps.

Environmental compensations and social assistance are the two major ways of maximizing the patient's remaining abilities. Environmental compensations use material objects as substitutes for lost abilities. Adaptive equipment is the most common example; this text offers substitutes for cognitive abilities. The social assistance required by the cognitively disabled includes initiation of activities, continuous cueing or verification, removal of hazards, and correction of mistakes. Therapists help long-term caregivers understand the realistic demands on their time and energy so practical plans can be made for available resources. These resources are directed toward having the patient use his or her remaining abilities as much as possible, within the constraints of his or her long-term-care situation.

Long-term caregivers need to be asked about their priorities in selecting activities that would ease their burden of care. Therapists work with the caregivers to design long-term-care programs that realistically use the caregiver's resources. Caregivers are instructed in how to carry out therapeutic techniques that are effective with the patient, remove hazards, and carry out the necessary drilling of any desired training procedures.

Working with a caregiver who is also adjusting to a new cognitive disability is difficult. The dreaded loss of a part of the patient's personality is objectified during the process of doing ordinary activities. Tears of grief are to be expected. Many people cling to the hope that the condition will improve. These people may choose to think that the adjustment is temporary. As a therapist you may not share that opinion, but you will probably not be able to talk caregivers out of their hopes. Short-term treatment goals are often met by sticking to the present tense and leaving discussions of the future alone.

The difficulty occurs when therapists avoid discussions of the future until the hour before discharge. Clinical experience indicates that patients and families can pay a high price for avoiding the realities of long-term care. The caregivers are not only emotionally unprepared for their new realities, but a lot of costly decisions are made based on unrealistic expectations. Families may agree to take on burdens of care that they cannot sustain or escape. Limited insurance benefits and personal financial resources may be squandered on treatment approaches with poor rehabilitation potential. Therapists have a moral obligation to at least try to provide an objective picture of the functional difficulties that are apt to continue into long-term care. Hopefully, cognitive levels can be developed to improve the therapist's predictive validity in this particularly difficult area of practice. Descriptive research studies that use the cognitive levels to measure the degree and rate of change could be a big help in predicting rehabilitation potential and setting long-term treatment goals.

Therapists should not assume that all caregivers are able to learn at level 6. Instructions may need to be adjusted for those learning at level 5. Caregivers learning at level 4 may need connections with the social welfare system or a family member to protect the patient and the caregiver.

The Institute of Medicine (IOM) (Pope & Tarlov, 1991) has recently published a nomenclature that differs from ICIDH in the way that disability is defined and drops the use of the term handicap. An additional category, functional limitations, has been added. Functional limitations are produced by impairments and restrict performance capacity. The cognitive levels could be regarded as a measure of performance capacity, but the principal focus on limitations is troublesome. To improve performance, the focus must be on the identification of remaining abilities. My major concern is with the deletion of handicap and the claim that disability is a social concept. IOM replaces handicap with quality of life concepts that never have been adequate in defining the burden of care placed on the social support system. Quality of life and the performance of personally valued activities occur at the level of the individual. IOM's goal is to develop a nomenclature that prevents disability, and prevention can be done without considering demands on social support systems (Pope & Tarlov). Rehabilitation's goal is to help people adjust to the presence of a disability. Many people with disabilities are dependent on other people for assistance and on the social welfare system. The evaluation of treatment effectiveness must attend to reductions in the social burdens of care.

## Teaching as a Treatment Method

Rehabilitation therapists vary their teaching techniques in response to the learning abilities of patients and their primary caregivers. The teaching objectives suggested throughout this text use the following definitions of teaching methods. Teaching is a method of imparting knowledge, guidance, or counsel through the use of language. Teaching assumes that learning ability is within the normal range of ability and uses educational materials written and taught by a wide range of health care professionals. As of this writing most third party payers do not reimburse therapists for conducting educational programs because teaching does not require the unique knowledge and skill of the therapist.

Instructing, drilling, and training are the methods used by rehabilitation therapists that do require special knowledge. Instructions provide specific directions about doing an activity with expected generalization. Instructions are given to people learning at levels 5 and 6. Training is situation specific and does not generalize at cognitive level 4. Drilling is the most repetitious and requires constant supervision while the individual practices the new ability at cognitive level 3. Standardized, routine steps are drilled. Learning is not a treatment objective for a person functioning at cognitive levels 1 and 2; at these levels, teach the caregiver.

## Problems in Identifying a Cognitive Disability

Any effort to identify departures from normal must be done with caution. People have a way of using labels in a prejudicial manner that does not tolerate deviance from the normal or ideal. Labels can be used in unreasonable and unfair ways, and safeguards are required to prevent misuse. This section suggests safeguards.

Labels, on the other hand, are required to mobilize social support systems. People require labels to understand when and what kind of assistance is needed. Societies require an explanation of what the social disadvantages are before societies can be held accountable for helping individuals overcome disadvantages.

## Stigma: To Label or Not to Label

Some people will argue that one should not use numbers or anything else to label a disability. I will argue that vague or ambiguous labels perpetuate and even enhance the abuse of cognitively disabled people. My hope is that more responsible health care planning will emerge from the delineation of levels of care required by people with a cognitive disability.

Therapists have an obligation to advocate for the protection and assistance needed by those disabled people who cannot be cured. Because therapists do use labels, they have a corresponding responsibility to carefully explain the meaning of terms and prevent misuse. The safest way to prevent misunderstanding is to use lay language to objectively describe observed behavior, which is done throughout this text as much as possible. An effort to specify behavior, identify warnings, and recommend precautions is present in chapters 3, 5, 6, 7, 8, 9, and 10. The authors offer these specifications with the understanding that these are our best guesses of what might happen. Feedback about errors and omissions is requested. Clinicians should also note this potential for error and use judgment in applying these descriptions.

A discussion of additional factors that can confound the assessment of a disability follows. The objective is to avoid labeling a person as disabled if there is another plausible explanation for poor performance.

## Normal Fluctuation or Disability

A view of normal cognitive ability is required to set a standard for normal performance of ordinary activities. The quality of human function is largely determined by the quality of thought required to do functional activities. The difficulty is that we all know from our experience that we do not operate at full capacity all of the time. The full capacity of the brain is not used all day long, but the full capacity may be needed at any time during the day that the environment changes or becomes hazardous.

Fluctuation in the quality of thought used during the course of a day is regarded as normal. The human brain seems to conserve energy and uses the minimum amount required to do a particular task. If a task can be done on automatic pilot, we usually do it that way. A cognitive disability affects the range of ability available to a person at a specific moment in time. It is assumed that all people experience a temporary cognitive disability, usually in response to fever or fatigue. Most temporary cognitive disabilities are of little personal or social consequence. We adapt by taking an aspirin, going to bed, taking time off from work, and avoiding dangerous situations. Social allowances are made for temporary disabilities. Disabilities that extend beyond the usual social allowances, like 2 weeks of sick time, require more social support.

Frequent denial of the presence of a cognitive disability is confounded by the recognition that there is a normal fluctuation in the amount of thought people use during the course of an average day. A standard for when people are expected to use their full capacity is required to differentiate between a normal fluctuation in thought and a cognitive disability. The source of social agreement that is suggested in this text is a law dictionary, representing socially agreed on expectations placed on the average citizen. When therapists use the law to identify situations that demand level 6 problem solving, they can avoid the difficulties of placing their own value judgments on patients.

The full range of all 6 levels of cognition should be available to normal adolescents and adults; the actual age of normal onset for level 6 is uncertain at the present time. Clinical experience suggest that adolescents can reach level 6, but children are not legally responsible until the age of 18. A study of normal children is in progress that aims at increasing our understanding of the range of application (T. Turgov, personal communication, 1991).

## Disability or Motivation

Cognition is an umbrella term that can be used to signify two alternative explanations for behavior: motivation and ability. The cognitive levels seek to eliminate motivational explanations in order to permit a clearer evaluation of ability. Motivational explanations may be eliminated by having the patient select the activity that he or she would like to do. The patient must agree with the meaning and purpose of the activity. When a therapist imposes an activity selection on to a patient, motivational ex-

planations are valid reasons for poor performance. The evaluation of ability/disability is based on the assumption that the individual's performance is the best of his or her present abilities. That assumption cannot be sustained when the activity lacks meaning and purpose for the individual. Therapists often need to be very resourceful to suggest activities that will elicit the cooperation of cognitively disabled people.

Information processing goes on inside a person's head. An outside observer will always be in the position of drawing an inference about what is going on in the other person's mind. To keep the level of inference as objective as possible, the sensory cues that capture attention and the resulting motor actions are used to describe the levels. Observations of behavior are used to identify the patient's ability to process information. A distinction must be made between *will not* and *cannot*. Difficulties in doing an activity are often explained by not liking the activity. To further confound the matter, people do not like activities that they cannot do. The patient must agree to do the activity; the purpose for doing the activity must be meaningful to the patient. Otherwise motivational questions can obscure the therapist's assessment of the patient's ability to function.

The worst case scenario does happen; the patient refuses to do anything that the therapist suggests. When the patient will not try, one cannot make a distinction between ability and motivation. The cognitive level cannot be evaluated when the patient refuses to try anything. This tendency to refuse stretches a therapist's knowledge of activity analysis. Therapists need to be prepared to analyze any activity that the patient might be willing to try. I have long suspected that frequent refusals were behind occupational therapy's traditional use of crafts. Patients functioning at levels 3 and 4 will often try to do crafts when they refuse to try everything else. Computers may replace crafts as great motivators. One thing is clear—the selection of the activity matters a great deal to the patient, and therapists have to work around what is agreeable to them.

## Selecting Activities

ICIDH provides a comprehensive list of the activities that might be limited by the presence of a physical disability. Chapters 8 and 9 use this list to apply the cognitive levels to the physically disabled. Unfortunately ICIDH has a major flaw. The behavior disabilities that are associated with a cognitive disability are not related to activities. The meaning of the disability is lost without the activities. A typology of activities for the cognitively disabled is required to correct this deficiency.

Many of the activities affected by a cognitive disability are the same as for a physical disability, like dressing and eating. Everyone does these activities. There are, however, vast differences in the difficulties experienced by people who have physical versus cognitive disabilities. One cannot really rate dressing and eating with arthritis and Alzheimer's disease on the same scale with any degree of clinical precision. Separate rating scales and typologies are required. Some overlap in the list of activities is to be expected, because there are basic human activities. Some different difficulties found only with the cognitively or physically disabled are also to be expected.

In ICIDH, the two-digit codes listed under behavior disabilities are intended for the cognitively disabled and need to be changed to include activities. Different headings are suggested to help differentiate between physical and cognitive disabilities, which may be helpful when reporting research data or in documentation. In practice, and in this text the terms may be used interchangeably. The term "behavior disabilities" has been changed to the following headings with a number system that follows the ICIDH pattern:

1.    Behavior disability
10.   Self-awareness disability
11.   Situational awareness disability
12.   Occupational role disability
13.   Social role disability

There are a few activities that almost everybody has to do, and those activities are analyzed and fit into the self-awareness and situational awareness categories. Self-awareness and situational awareness disabilities list 16 activities found on many functional inventories that enjoy general agreement in the rehabilitation literature. The overlap in activities done by the physically and cognitively disabled is intended; the problem is mental. Mental, cognitive, and behavior are used interchangeably.

Self-awareness disability is a mental disturbance in the ability to meet the natural demands of one's body. Self-awareness activities include grooming, dressing, bathing, walking and exercising, feeding, toileting, taking medications, and using adaptive equipment. Self-awareness can be used to differentiate these activities from the self-care activities of a physical disability.

Situational awareness disability is a mental disturbance of the capacity to register and understand relationships between objects and persons within the context of daily living. Activities done within the context of daily life include housekeeping, preparing and obtaining food, spending money, doing laundry, traveling, shopping, telephoning, and adjusting to change. Activities of daily living (ADLs) or instrumental activities of daily living (IADLs) refer to activities restricted by a physical disability.

"Occupational role disability is a mental disturbance of the ability to organize and participate in routine activities connected with the occupation of time, not only confined to the performance of work" (ICIDH, 1980, p. 152). The disturbance may be noticed when one is planning and doing major role activities and spare time activities. The mental processes required to do these activities included timing, exerting effort, judging results, and speaking. These mental processes are used because it is impractical to analyze the enormous list of major role and spare time activities that people do. Occupational role also includes following safety precautions and responding to emergencies.

Social role disability is a mental disturbance in the ability to meet social expectations when interacting with other people. The disturbance is apt to be observed while doing the following activities: communicating meaning, following instructions, contributing to family activities, caring for dependents, cooperating with others, supervising independent people, keeping informed, and engaging in good citizenship.

An effort has been made to develop a comprehensive list of activities that most people do, as a heuristic devise to limit the number of activities that therapists must analyze. There is no intent to define what people ought to do. Such an intent would be contrary to the traditions of rehabilitation that recognize individual differences and personal choice. The activity analysis criteria are provided with the expectation that therapists will analyze unusual activities. While an attempt has been made to make the list of activities as comprehensive and universal as possible, the problems of individual and cultural differences will require professional judgment.

## References

Allen, C.K. *Occupational therapy for psychiatric diseases: Measurement and management of cogni-*

*tive disabilities.* Boston: Little, Brown.

Allen, C.K. (1987). Activity: Occupational therapy's treatment method; 1987 Eleanor Clarke Slagle Lecture. *American Journal of Occupational Therapy, 41,* 563–575.

Finger, S., & Stein, D.B. (1982). *Brain damage and recovery: Research and clinical perspectives.* New York: Academic Press.

Miller, R. (1981). *Meaning and purpose in the intact brain: A philosophical, psychological, and biological account of conscious processes.* New York: Clarendon Press.

Pope, A.M., & Tarlov, A.L. (Eds.). (1991). *Disability in America: Toward a national agenda for prevention.* Washington, DC: National Academy Press.

World Health Organization. (1991). *International Classification of Diseases,* 9th revision, 4th edition. Geneva, Switzerland: Author.

World Health Organization. (1980). *International Classification of Impairments, Disabilities, and Handicaps.* Geneva, Switzerland: Author.

# A